ECOLOGICAL MEDICINE

SM: 'To my lovely patients, who have been willing guinea pigs, faithful to the cause and most forgiving when my suggestions have not worked. However, in doing so, they have pushed forward the frontiers of ecological medicine.'

CR: 'To the Unknown ME Warrior. In the face of both untold abuse and neglect, the hurt of which is magnified by a cruel disbelief, you have shown in equal measure, a gentle grace and dignity, alongside a fortitude of unimaginable depth. I salute you.'

Small is beautiful – a study of medical science as if people matter – with apologies to EF Schumacher (19 August 1911 – 4 September 1977), German statistician and economist

Some people find the use of the word 'patient' as derogatory. They prefer 'clients', but as Dr Adam Kay points out in his entertaining book *This is Going to Hurt*, it is prostitutes that have clients. The word 'doctor' comes from the Greek for 'to teach'. Doctors should be teachers of health information. So that makes patients simply receivers of such. Not so derogatory after all!

To be a teacher in the right sense is to be a learner. Instruction begins when you, the teacher, learn from the learner, put yourself in his place so that you may understand what he understands and the way he understands it.
Kierkegaard 1813 –1855, Danish first existentialist philosopher

My education took off when I left medical school for the real world. Simply writing really makes me think further about my medical practice and how best to relay that information to my lovely patients. I so hope you enjoy reading this as much as I enjoyed writing it – these were happy days for me. (And me too! Craig)

My education was only interrupted by my schooling
Sir Winston Churchill, 1874 – 1965

ECOLOGICAL MEDICINE

The antidote to Big Pharma and Fast Food

Dr Sarah Myhill MB BS
and
Craig Robinson MA (OXON)

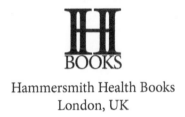

BOOKS

Hammersmith Health Books
London, UK

First published in 2020 by Hammersmith Health Books
– an imprint of Hammersmith Books Limited
4/4A Bloomsbury Square, London WC1A 2RP, UK
www.hammersmithbooks.co.uk

The information contained in this book is for educational purposes only. It is the result of the study and the experience of the authors. Whilst the information and advice offered are believed to be true and accurate at the time of going to press, neither the authors nor the publisher can accept any legal responsibility or liability for any errors or omissions that may have been made or for any adverse effects which may occur as a result of following the recommendations given herein. Always consult a qualified medical practitioner if you have any concerns regarding your health.

British Library Cataloguing in Publication Data: A CIP record of this book is available from the British Library.

Print ISBN 978-1-78161-170-8
Ebook ISBN 978-1-78161-171-5

Commissioning editor: Georgina Bentliff
Designed and typeset by: Julie Bennett, Bespoke Publishing Ltd
Cover design by: Madeline Meckiffe
Cover image by: Madeline Meckiffe
Index: Dr Laurence Errington
Production: Helen Whitehorn, PathProjects Ltd
Printed and bound by: Ashford Colour Press, Gosport, Hampshire, UK

Contents

PART IV. WHAT TO DO – THE BASICS

PART V. THE BOLT-ON EXTRAS

PART VI. HOW TO APPLY WHAT WE'VE LEARNT TO CURRENT BRANCHES OF MEDICINE

PART VII. CASE HISTORIES

PART VIII. APPENDICES

About the Authors

Dr Sarah Myhill MB BS qualified in medicine (with Honours) from Middlesex Hospital Medical School in 1981 and has since focused tirelessly on identifying and treating the underlying causes of health problems, especially the 'diseases of civilisation' with which we are beset in the West. She has worked in the NHS and private practice and for 17 years was the Hon. Secretary of the British Society for Ecological Medicine, which focuses on the causes of disease and treating through diet, supplements and avoiding toxic stress. She helps to run and lectures at the Society's training courses and also lectures regularly on organophosphate poisoning, the problems of silicone, and chronic fatigue syndrome. Visit her website at www.drmyhill.co.uk

Craig Robinson MA took a first in Mathematics at Oxford University in 1985. He then joined Price Waterhouse and qualified as a Chartered Accountant in 1988, after which he worked as a lecturer in the private sector, and also in The City of London, primarily in Financial Sector Regulation roles. Craig first met Sarah in 2001, as a patient for the treatment of his ME, and since then they have developed a professional working relationship, where he helps with the maintenance of www.drmyhill.co.uk, the moderating of Dr Myhill's Facebook groups and other ad hoc projects, as well as with the editing and writing of her books.

Stylistic note: Use of the first person singular in this book refers to me, Dr Sarah Myhill. One can assume that the medicine and biochemistry are mine, as edited by Craig Robinson, and that the classical and mathematical references are Craig's.

You never change things by fighting the existing reality. To change something, build a new model that makes the existing model obsolete

Buckminster Fuller

PART I
Introduction

Chapter 1
The inquisitive doctor

Mankind is fucked*. Humans are to the World what cancer is to humans: growing uncontrollably, invading parts where they should never be, and destroying the very Being that nourishes them. Life expectancy in Westerners is falling,[1] 19% of UK working-age adults have a disability,[2] infertility is rising with one in seven couples having difficulty conceiving,[3] average IQs of children are falling,[4] 54% of us have a chronic disease (including obesity)[5] and 10% of school children are now classified as SEND students (Special Educational Needs and Disability).[6] We are accelerating towards self-destruction and extinction. Stephen Hawking (English theoretical physicist, cosmologist and author, 8 January 1942 – 14 March 2018) predicted the extinction of *Homo sapiens* within a thousand years – a blink of evolutionary time.

James Lovelock (English scientist, born 26 July 1919), famed for his Gaia theory, also predicts a bleak future. He states that humans behave like a pathogenic micro-organism, or like the cells of a tumour, as far as the Earth is concerned. Lovelock is a remarkable man; entirely on his own, he invented the electron capture detector in his barn-turned-laboratory, which he calls his 'experimental station', and which is located in his back garden. In the late 1960s, he was the first to detect the widespread presence of CFCs in the atmosphere.

Doctors should be providing the intellectual imperative to stop this terrible decline. They are supposed to be the brainy elite, caring for us individually and as a population. Instead, doctors are responsible for over-seeing this degenerative process because they have been corrupted by Big Pharma. They are doing this with kindness, gentleness and great humanity. They even claim an evidence-based approach. They daily reassure people that all will be well with their five-a-day fruit and vegetables, that vaccinations can only do good, that cocktails of drugs will prevent heart disease and that the cure for cancer is on the horizon. Doctors fail to tackle the

---

*Linguistic note: The etymology of 'fuck' is not known with certainty, but it is probably cognate with the Germanic word *ficken*. It is an 'old' word but again the scholars are divided upon actual dates. What is certain is that it is a versatile word – it is both a transitive and intransitive verb, and an adjective, adverb and noun. This quality is admirably demonstrated by a story from Craig's past at a time during his 'Gap Year', when he was working as an odd-job porter at Stoke Mandeville Hospital, with his colleague, a Polish immigrant, 'Wodge'. Craig and Wodge were called in front of a hospital bigwig after dropping an expensive fridge. They were asked to explain themselves and here is how the conversation went:
Bigwig – So, Wodge, what happened?
Wodge – Some fucking fucker fucking fucked the fucking fucker.
Bigwig [head in hands] – And Robinson, what do you have to say?
Craig – I am impressed by Wodge's last sentence, Sir, it was 75% 'fuck'.

root causes of disease because that is difficult. It means changing our comfortable, addictive and convenient lifestyles. Unpleasant symptoms that are the essential, early harbingers of pathology are suppressed with toxic drugs. The underlying pathology grumbles on unrecognised until the heart attack manifests, the tumour becomes palpable or the dementia irreversible. 'What a shock! What a surprise! What bad luck,' I hear them cry. Doctors are being kind to be cruel.

During my work as an NHS GP I had to wear two hats. With all my patients I would launch into my enthusiastic diatribe to try to identify symptom and disease, causation and mechanism. That was fine until I got on to the difficult stuff that involved self-discipline – changing diet, taking exercise and tackling addiction. If the eyes glazed over I knew I was dealing with a 'Nah… don't do all that crap with me, just gimme the drugs' type. Out came the prescription pad, on went the NICE† Guidelines hat and off trotted the patient, apparently satisfied with his/her quick fix. Thankfully my medical life was blessed by patients who thought as I did. They immediately saw the logic, grasped the difficult straws and started to put in place the troublesome interventions.

Through a panoply of natural approaches, such as diet, nutritional supplements, sleep and exercise, detoxification regimes and other such, I watched intractable arthritis resolve; migraines, irritable bowels and bladders melt away; fatigue syndromes, psychoses, autisms and asthmas disappear. Suddenly I thought I could change the World of Medicine. What would you do in my shoes? Being naturally gobby, I shouted it out so all could hear. And that is when my real troubles began.

Up until 2000 it never even crossed my mind that doctors could be interested in anything other than doing their best to cure their patients.

It never occurred to me that doctors would not want to know about such safe, simple and effective medical interventions. It came as an intellectual tsunami to realise that not only did many doctors perceive me as a trouble-maker who undermined their authority, but so did the medical authorities themselves, from Health Boards right through to the General Medical Council (GMC), the UK regulator of doctors. They did not want their intellectually easy, drug-based, simple algorithms for management challenged. In their treatment of asthma, patients could be dismissed first with the blue inhaler, then with the brown inhaler and, for difficult cases, with both. Not only does this get patient out of the surgery in less than five minutes (a statistical triumph) but s/he also makes megabucks for Big Pharma. To my naïve amazement, the Establishment reacted furiously to the presumptuous, precocious, inquisitive doctor who was kicking the intellectual foundations of their ivory towers.

Between 2000 and 2012 I had to deal with 30 separate investigations from the GMC, making me the most investigated doctor in its history. No complaints came from patients; all came from jealous doctors, local Health Boards or the GMC itself. After the first few investigations I was unable to get medical indemnity for GMC hearings and so I conducted my own legal defence. In October 2010 I was suspended from the Medical Register because I 'lacked respect for my regulatory body, the General Medical Council'. In conducting my own defence, I demonstrated to the GMC that it was acting like a kangaroo court with the verdict having been decided upon before the hearing opened, with the GMC withholding evidence, with numerous GMC breaches of the Data Protection Act, and with the GMC denying me rights to call witnesses and refusing to tell me what allegations I faced. The last

---

†**Footnote:** NICE is the UK 'health' regulator, the National Institute for Health and Care Excellence, and provides national guidance and advice on health and social care.

person to whom this applied was Ann Boleyn, decapitated under the orders of Henry VIII in 1536. At least I had some reason to be grateful that I was being tried after the enactment of the Abolition of Death Penalty Act 1965!

I took the GMC decision to suspend me to judicial review in the High Court. But before that hearing could be held, the GMC ran an emergency hearing of its own at which my licence to practice was restored. By 2012, all GMC action against me had been cancelled, with no case to answer. This may have had something to do with GMC legal opinion, discovered through a Freedom of Information Act search, which advised that:

> '...the problem with the Myhill cases is that all the patients are improved and refuse to give witness statements.'

It is a lesson in how the collective Medical Establishment views the World that the fact my patients were 'improved' was considered to be a 'problem'.

Call me a slow learner. It has taken me 35 years to work out that I cannot change the World. But what I can do is to give those with the intelligence, discipline and determination, the Rules of the Game and the Tools of the Trade to diagnose, treat and cure themselves. In doing so they can slow the ageing process, prevent disease and live to their full potential.

But just as vital, when those who constitute the cancer of this world have succumbed to disease or degeneration, we shall be left with healthy human seeds who can repopulate the Earth with healthy stock. I want my family, my friends and my patients to survive the coming apocalypse. But to do so they must take control of their lives now. This too is part of Natural Selection. It means that those with minds that are sufficiently inquisitive to ask the right questions, intelligent brains to work out the answers

and diligent determination to apply those, will survive.

This may sound rather like a manifesto for eugenics, but that is not my intention in writing this – this is just the way Natural Selection works. Thomas Robert Malthus (English scholar, 14 February 1766 – 23 December 1834) had similar ideas. Malthusian theory argues that a population will outgrow its resources, and that disease and other catastrophes will inevitably lead to 'checks' on human population growth.[7]

What follows is the blue-print for survival. You just must do it.

References

1. Pasha-Robinson. Life expectancy plummets in parts of UK, data reveals. *The Independent* 17 January 2018. www.independent.co.uk/news/uk/home-news/life-expectancy-uk-plumments-ons-data-hartlepool-torridge-amber-valley-barnsley-a8164171.html (accessed 15 July 2019)
2. Panjwani A. How many people have a disability? *Full Fact* 3 May 2018. https://fullfact.org/health/how-many-people-have-disability/ (accessed 15 July 2019)
3. Infertility. NHS, 14 February 2017. www.nhs.uk/conditions/infertility/ (accessed 15 July 2019)
4. Dockrill P. IQ scores are falling in 'worrying' reversal of 20th Century intelligence boom. *Science Alert* 13 June 2018. www.sciencealert.com/iq-scores-falling-in-worrying-reversal-20th-century-intelligence-boom-flynn-effect-intelligence (accessed 15 July 2019)
5. 54% have chronic disease – CDC – 'Chronic Disease in America' - www.cdc.gov/chronicdisease/resources/infographic/chronic-diseases.htm
6. 10% of children now classified as SEND – 'afasic website' - https://www.afasic.org.uk/about-talking/what-are-speech-language-and-communication-needs-slcn/
7. Malthus. *Essay on the Principle of Population* - www.esp.org/books/malthus/population/malthus.pdf

Chapter 2

The roadmap from symptoms to mechanisms to diagnosis and treatment

Since we can no longer rely on the medical profession to guide us to a healthy lifestyle, we must do it ourselves. This can only be achieved by a true understanding of the underlying mechanisms by which Western diets and lifestyles negatively affect health and create disease.

The idea of this book is to empower people to heal themselves through addressing the root causes of their diseases. I hope that what follows is a logical progression from symptoms to identifying the underlying mechanisms, to the relevant interventions, tests and tools with which to tackle the root cause of those symptoms. This is how any garage mechanic would fix a car – first ask the driver why the car was not working (symptoms) and then have a look at the vehicle for tell-tale signs to obtain a working hypothesis of a diagnosis. Having established the mechanisms by which things are going wrong the mechanic is in a position to cure. Once the car is functioning normally the hypothesis becomes the diagnosis.

> *The expectations of life depend upon diligence; the mechanic that would perfect his work must first sharpen his tools.*
> Confucius, Chinese teacher and philosopher, 551 – 479 BC

So, first, this book discusses symptoms, not as something to be immediately squashed with powerful prescription drugs, but rather as signposts as to what might be going wrong. Symptoms are the early warning system of the body that all is not right. We must listen to them.

The next step along this logical path is an exposition of what mechanisms may be causing these symptoms and how one can identify which particular mechanisms are at play in this patient. The identification of these mechanisms is achieved through clinical symptoms, signs and tests.

At this point along the logical path, the reader will have identified their symptoms and also will have isolated the mechanisms causing those symptoms. The next step is to lay out the 'tools of the trade' – that is, the interventions that can be put in place to treat those mechanisms, as identified. These interventions are 'sustainable' in that they reverse, not escalate, disease processes. By contrast, symptom-supressing medication accelerates the underlying disease process.

The logical path is now complete:

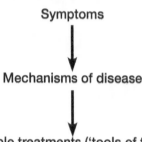

Symptoms

↓

Mechanisms of disease

↓

Sustainable treatments ('tools of the trade') to treat and reverse these mechanisms

Back to our broken-down car analogy, the responsible driver does not wait for something to go wrong. By feeding his car the best possible clean fuel and oil, ensuring it undergoes regular servicing and by driving with due care and attention, his car will motor on for hundreds of thousands of miles. This is disease prevention. My job as a doctor is to be the interface between the good science and the art of healing. My duty is to provide the necessary information to allow people to live to their full potential through identifying root causes of disease and treating them with logical interventions. In practice, there is a basic protocol that we should all be doing in order to be that 'responsible driver' and this I have called, 'Groundhog Basic'. In the film *Groundhog Day*, this refers to a time loop – this too is another sort of loop that bears constant repetition.

Groundhog Basic

Initially we have to identify and correct those aspects of contemporary Western lifestyles that are so damaging to health. The big issues are:

diet and nutrition
sleep
exercise
pollution and
infection avoidance.

Ideally, we should all put in place interventions now, before symptoms appear and before these problems trigger pathology. As mentioned, I call this set of interventions Groundhog Basic. It is the starting point to prevent and treat all disease. Do not be tempted to skip what is difficult. Done well, this may be all that is required.

These interventions are covered in the following chapters:

Chapter 20 – Groundhog Basic: what we should all be doing all the time to function at our full potential and prevent disease

Chapter 21 – The paleo-ketogenic (PK) diet plus essential micronutrients: multivitamins, minerals and essential fatty acids – what to eat, which supplements to take.

Chapter 22 – Sleep: common reasons for poor sleep and how to fix them

Chapter 23 Exercise– this must be the right sort to afford overall gains

Chapter 24 – Sunshine and light – why you should get as much of this as you can

Chapter 25 – Reduce the chemical burden: we are all poisoned – what you can do to minimise the effects

Chapter 26 – To love and be loved – sufficient physical and mental security to satisfy our universal need to love and care, and be loved and cared for

Chapter 27 – Avoid infections and treat them aggressively – be prepared so you can do this and get rid of them quickly

Chapter 28 – Diet, detox and die-off reactions – expect to get worse at first and see this as a good sign! Why this happens. What to do about it.

Without these difficult but vital foundations in place, other interventions will be to little avail. These interventions should be applied in all cases regardless of time, regardless of current state of health and regardless of current pathology. There is no excuse not to start now and, believe you me, I have heard all possible excuses under the sun. Groundhog Basic is non-negotiable.

None of us lives the perfect life. It is like the old Irish joke – when the traveller asked the way to Dublin, he was told by the local, 'If I were you, I would not be starting from here.' People do not seek medical help until they have a problem. For those that come to this book with established pathology, you may start with the specialty chapters, see what you have to do to recover and use the tools of the trade in addition to the Groundhog regimes to do so as quickly as possible. If you want to know the reason why, then plough your way through the early chapters.

In practice, with age and illness, we slowly have to move to the Groundhog Chronic strategies. Part VII of this book starts from a disease perspective, revises what has gone before and details the tricks of trade that have evolved proven and safe techniques.

This book is an introduction, a starting place, and, perhaps most importantly, a signpost for those patients who wish to take control of their own health. To do otherwise than this, and to try and write a book which covered every situation for every patient, would make for a dull old read. Furthermore, with experience, my ideas and advice will not stand still and so the fine detail of such a book would need constant updating. I make no apology for this state of affairs as, being old and female, I'm allowed to change my mind!

> *I'm not young enough to know it all.*
> Oscar Wilde, writer, 1854 – 1900

There is much more detail in our other books, namely:

- *Prevent and Cure Diabetes – delicious diets not dangerous drugs* supplies the WHY of the PK diet
- *The PK Cookbook – go paleo-ketogenic and get the best of both worlds* supplies the HOW of the PK diet
- *Diagnosis and Treatment of Chronic Fatigue Syndrome and Myalgic Encephalitis – it's mitochondria not hypochondria* takes a detailed look at energy delivery mechanisms and how they apply in practical reality
- *The Infection Game – life is an arms race* takes a detailed look at the role of infection as a driver of disease and what can be done to prevent and treat it.

Applying the principles of this book does take courage as well as determination. In the words of Earl Nightingale (12 March 1921 – 25 March 1989), American radio speaker and author, whose works focused on the issues of human character development, motivation and meaningful existence:

> *All you need is the plan, the road map and the courage to press on to your destination.*

Chapter 3
Stumbling and fumbling my way to the right questions

It's all about asking the question 'why?'

> *I keep six honest serving men*
> *(They taught me all I knew)*
> *Their names are What and Why and When*
> *And How and Where and Who*
>> Joseph Rudyard Kipling,
>> 30 December 1865 – 18 January 1936

> *Let's start with the bleeding obvious –*
> *when all else fails, use your brain.*
>> Dr Ada Marion Dansie, Medical
>> Consultant to George Bernard Shaw,
>> and my grandmother

Five years at medical school followed by one year in hospital jobs does little to prepare a doctor for the real world. I had no answers to the early questions thrown up by NHS General Practice:

'Why do I have high blood pressure?'
'Why do I get such awful headaches?'
'Why am I depressed?'

Correct conventional answers to these questions are deficiency of, respectively, anti-hypertensive drugs, painkillers and SSRIs (selective serotonin reuptake inhibitors – antidepressants such as Prozac). But this is not the 'why' of the matter. Indeed, it is hardly even the 'what' of the matter. Masking the symptoms does not explain them. The clues, which the symptoms represent, have been missed and the investigative detective work, which should have resulted from those clues, has been left undone.

> *The world is full of obvious things which*
> *nobody by any chance ever observes.*
>> Sherlock Holmes in
>> *The Hound of the Baskervilles*
>> by Sir Arthur Conan Doyle,
>> 22 May 1859 – 7 July 1930

One year on and I was breast-feeding my daughter, Ruth. She had terrible 'three-month' colic and all I could do to lessen the screams was to walk round the house, all night, with her in my arms. My husband Nick's reaction was 'You're the effing doctor – you sort it out.' He was right. It was not until I stumbled across advice for me to give up all dairy products that the problem was resolved. So too was my chronic sinusitis and rhinitis. At the time this was a momentous and life-changing discovery – but this information was nowhere to be found in the medical textbooks. Thirty-seven years later, this common cause and effect is still absent from conventional medical literature.

This made me worry about not knowing causation. I had been trained to elicit clinical symptoms and signs and recognise clinical pictures, but actually what patients wanted to know was, Why? What did they need to do to put things right? My standard line had been, 'Well, let's do a blood test and come back next week.' This gave me time to fumble anxiously through my lecture notes and textbooks, looking for answers. The answers my patients wanted were not there. It came as a great relief to me to find out that my patients really did not mind me telling them I did not know. Thankfully, they rated my ability to care higher than my ability to know. Thankfully, they were happy to help me with my researches and act as willing guinea pigs with the dietary and lifestyle experiments that actually addressed the root causes of their problems.

The investigation of a patient should be like a detective story – 90% of the clues come from the history and 10% from the examination and tests. Listen carefully and your patient will not only tell you the diagnosis but, most likely, also the causes. In my final practice medical exams in 1981 I had a darling patient with primary biliary cirrhosis. She told me exactly what was wrong with her and coached me through the questions that my examiners would ask!

> *Just listen to your patient, he is telling you the diagnosis.*
> Sir William Osler, 1st Baronet, FRS FRCP, Canadian physician, 12 July 1849 – 29 December 1919

Tests may confirm or refute the hypothesis, because every diagnosis is just a hypothesis. Then, once the diagnosis is further corroborated by test results, it has to be put to the ultimate test. The ultimate test is response to treatment. Is the patient better? If not, then the diagnosis is wrong.

> exitus acta probat – *the result validates the deeds.*
> Ovid 43 BC – AD 17/18

Doctors routinely confuse the making of diagnoses with merely the descriptions of symptoms and clinical pictures, neither of which constitutes a diagnosis. Examples include hypertension, asthma, irritable bowel syndrome and arthritis, all of which are descriptions of symptoms and none of which is an actual diagnosis. Clinical pictures include Parkinson's disease, heart failure and colitis. But these are convenient titles simply to slot patients into symptom-relieving categories which do little to reverse the disease process or afford a permanent cure. Symptom-relieving medication postpones the day when major organ failures result. Many patients are duped into believing that the drugs are addressing underlying pathology and will result in a cure. This is dishonest, wicked and unsustainable medicine.

My early days in NHS General Practice were exciting. I learned to expect miracles as the norm. I watched a child's 'congenital' deafness resolve on a dairy-free diet (see case history, Chapter 77); I saw patients with years of headaches find relief by cutting out gluten-containing grains; I saw women with chronic cystitis gain relief by cutting yeast and sugar out of their diets. A proper diagnosis establishing causation has obvious implications for management and the potential for cure. What was so astonishing to me was that when I tried to communicate my excitement and experiences to fellow doctors, they could not have been less interested and dismissed me as a 'flaky quack'.*

However, the greatest challenge came from seeing and treating patients with myalgic encephalitis (ME)/chronic fatigue syndrome (CFS).

***Historical note:** Why 'quack'? Quack is a shortening of the 'old' Dutch 'quacksalver' (spelled kwakzalver in the modern Dutch), which originally meant a person who cures with home remedies, and then came to mean one using false cures or knowledge.

This was the elephant in the room. There was absolutely no doubt that these patients were seriously physically unwell. I saw Olympic athletes, England footballers and cricketers, university lecturers, airline pilots, tough farmers, fire fighters and Gulf War veterans reduced to a life of dependency by debilitating pathological fatigue.

I concluded that I would never be able to write a book because it would be out of date as soon as it had been written. However, I now believe that, although I do not know, and will never know, all the answers, I do at least have sight of enough of the elephant to make a start. At least I am asking the right questions and so have a chance of recognising some of the answers when they present.

...dans les champs de l'observation, le hasard ne favorise que les esprits préparés (In the field of observation, chance favours only the prepared mind).
Louis Pasteur, French microbiologist, 27 December 1822 – 28 September 1895

In this book I hope to paint a recognisable picture that will deliver both the intellectual imperative and the reasoning behind my ideas and also inspire readers to make the difficult lifestyle changes that will result in long-term good health. But the devil is in the detail – read on.

What has been so unexpected is that the answers to treating ME/CFS have shed a whole new light on other common medical problems, such as cancer, heart disease, dementia and other such degenerative conditions. What follows is a blueprint for good health for all, for life.

This book is the end result of 37 years of trial and error, largely the latter. At first, I really did not know what I was doing but being a cocky little sod...

I couldn't wait for success, so I went ahead without it.
Jonathan Winters, American comedian, 11 November 1925 – 11 April 2013

I hope I am working towards the 'bleedin' obvious'.

PART II
Symptoms and clinical pictures

Chapter 4
Symptoms – our vital early warning system

Symptoms are our early warning systems, which protect us from foreigners and from ourselves. Do not suppress symptoms. They guide us back to health. And remember, the detective work starts with symptoms. The best clinical clues come from them – 90% of the diagnosis comes from the history, the patient's account of their illness.

Symptoms are desirable and therapeutic

The two commonest symptoms, pain and fatigue, are essential to protect us from ourselves. We all experience these symptoms on a daily basis – they tell us what we can and cannot do. Without these warning signs we would keep going until we dropped, either because the energy delivery ran out (so the heart and brain would stop) or wore out (healing and repair occur during sleep and rest). We ignore or suppress these symptoms at our peril.

Many other symptoms arise downstream of these two, the most common. This happens because we ignore the early warning signs that pain and fatigue represent, or interfere with them, or try to suppress them. Often pathology arises as a result of adopting this 'ignore, interfere and suppress' type of medicine. Therefore, symptoms

should always prompt us to ask the question 'Why?' Collections of symptoms may provide further clues as to causation.

> *We are too much accustomed to attribute to a single cause that which is the product of several, and the majority of our controversies come from that.*
> Baron Justus Von Liebig, German chemist, 12 May 1803 –18 April 1873
> Attrib.

'Evidence-based medicine'

Conventional medical treatments are based on 'randomised controlled trials' (RCTs). These are considered to be the 'gold standard' for evidence-based medicine, but there are many reasons why they are inadequate:

- Most, if not all, diseases have multiple causes and are not amenable to single interventions. However, the people participating in such trials are randomly allocated to either the group receiving the treatment under investigation or to a group receiving standard treatment (or placebo treatment) known as the 'control'. Already we can see that these trials effectively look at 'either/ or' choices and so exclude the possibility of multi-causal illness. For such multi-causal complex illnesses, the RCT fails at the first hurdle. This is part of what is called 'confounding' and is badly mitigated against. (Confounding is where the experimental controls do not allow the experimenter to eliminate plausible alternative explanations for the illness.)

- The RCT can be set up and the statistics manipulated in such a way as to get a positive outcome that promotes drug prescribing when in fact no such positive result has been achieved.
- Any drug trial that does not give a positive result is not published. This was the subject of a campaign run by Richard Smith, former Editor of the *British Medical Journal*, who advised that all drugs trials, regardless of outcome, should be published. He failed. Why? Follow the money – he who pays the piper calls the tune.

As Angus Deaton and Nancy Cartwright conclude in their article 'Understanding and misunderstanding randomized controlled trials':[1]

RCT results are…weak ground for inferring "what works".

The art of medicine should follow the long-established tradition of case studies. The best doctors are patient, patient watchers.

The good physician treats the disease; the great physician treats the patient who has the disease.
Sir William Osler, 1st Baronet, FRS FRCP, Canadian physician, 12 July 1849 – 29 December 1919

So, what follows in this book is not a list of RCTs giving quick-fix, symptom-suppressing, 'single' interventions, but rather a tool box of many interventions to address the many mechanisms at play that place the patient at the centre of the action. First, and in order to identify those mechanisms, we must investigate the symptoms… Read on!

Reference

1. Deaton A, Cartwright N. Understanding and misunderstanding randomized controlled trials. *Social Science & Medicine* 2018; 210: 2-21. www.sciencedirect.com/science/article/pii/S0277953617307359

Chapter 5
Fatigue: tired all the time

– how we know when we are running out of energy

Fatigue is the symptom that arises when energy demand exceeds energy delivery. If we think of energy as money, then so it is with energy:

> *Annual income twenty pounds, annual expenditure nineteen pounds nineteen and six, result happiness.*
> *Annual income twenty pounds, annual expenditure twenty pounds ought and six, result misery.*
> Mr Micawber from *David Copperfield* by Charles Dickens,
> 7 February 1812 – 9 June 1870

This means there is a two-pronged approach to treating fatigue – improve energy delivery systems and identify mechanisms by which energy is wasted. As I have said, I think of energy as money – it is hard work earning it and great fun spending it. In this chapter I look at energy delivery. How energy is wasted is discussed in Chapters 7 and 8.

Energy delivery

Energy delivery is all about the collective function of:
> the dietary fuel in the tank
> the mitochondrial engine and its controllers:
>>   the thyroid accelerator pedal and the adrenal gearbox.

Together these are responsible for producing the energy molecule adenosine triphosphate, or ATP. ATP is the currency of energy in the body and a molecule of ATP can buy any job, from muscle contraction to a nerve impulse, hormone synthesis to immune activity. Without ATP none of these things is possible. This explains the multiplicity of symptoms experienced when energy delivery mechanisms are impaired, because every cell and every organ of the body may be affected.

The symptoms may be described as 'mild' or 'severe', and the following checklists can be used as a rule of thumb* to decide whether energy delivery mechanisms are starting to fail.

Linguistic note: 'Rule of thumb' is often said to derive from a law that allowed a man to beat his wife with a stick so long as it is were no thicker than his thumb. The story goes that in 1782, Judge Sir Francis Buller made this legal ruling. In the following year, James Gillray published a satirical cartoon of Buller, caricaturing him as 'Judge Thumb'. Perhaps Buller has been mis-reported – the phrase was in use before 1782. He was known for being harsh in his punishments, but there is no evidence that he made this ruling. Edward Foss, author of *The Judges of England*, 1870, wrote that, despite investigation, 'no substantial evidence has been found that he ever expressed so ungallant an opinion'. (Craig's note: A little more than ungallant, I would say!)

Mild symptoms of poor energy delivery mechanism

When symptoms are mild, the patient will:

- become an owl – s/he won't be able to get up in the mornings, will sleep in at weekends (this may be a symptom peculiar to the underactive thyroid)
- start to use addictions to cope with fatigue – especially caffeine, sugar and refined carbohydrates
- have to consciously pace activity – and look forward to rest time and sleep
- dread Monday mornings, if in employment
- lose the ability (or it will become an effort) to enjoy him/herself
- treasure 'chill out' time in the evenings
- lose his/her usual stamina – s/he will not be able to achieve normal levels of fitness
- experience a decline in muscular strength
- become irritable, experience mild anxiety and low mood – these symptoms are imposed by the brain to prevent the person spending energy frivolously; having fun means spending energy
- feel mildly stressed – I think this symptom of stress arises when the brain knows it does not have the energy reserves to deal with physical, emotional and mental demands
- experience joint and muscle stiffness – for tissues to slide over each other with minimal friction requires them to be at just the right temperature; poor energy delivery means the body runs colder.

These symptoms are often seen as part of the ageing process. This is because mitochondria, which are the engines of cells that generate energy, are also responsible for the ageing process. Numbers of mitochondria fall with age. So, as we age, we have to pace our activities. This is because our body's ability to generate energy reduces hand in hand with the falling numbers of mitochondria. The obvious corollary is: 'Look after the mitochondria and slow down the ageing process.'

Severe symptoms of poor energy delivery and the molecular mechanism for such

At medical school one of the most dreaded subjects was biochemistry. The usual survival strategy was to mug up for the exam at the last minute, usually on caffeine and chocolate biscuits, sit the exam on an addictive high, adrenalin-fuelled by fear of failure, then forget those nasty biochemical formulae. This was permissible because biochemistry was given scant clinical application – energy delivery mechanisms, ATP and mitochondria were never mentioned on the wards. Now I find myself explaining much of Life in terms of energy and biochemistry. Like money, you don't know you've got it until you've lost it. Both bring fun and security. Energy is my most precious possession.

So, a little biochemistry must follow. The central player is one of Nature's most ancient molecules – namely, adenosine triphosphate, or ATP, as mentioned at the start of this chapter. The business of making energy focuses around the synthesis of its sister molecule, adenosine diphosphate (ADP). Spending energy involves ATP cycling back to ADP. ATP is a battery to deliver a bolt of energy and this powers nearly all tasks in the body, from conducting a nerve impulse to making a hormone. All living things need ATP and this molecule makes the difference between Life and Death.

As your ATP battery discharges and as energy reserves slip away, you will experience:

- **Poor stamina.** One molecule of ATP is converted to ADP and recycled back to ATP via mitochondria every 10 seconds. If this recycling is slow, then poor stamina (mental and physical) and muscle weakness will result very quickly.

- **Pain**. If you run out of ATP because mitochondria cannot keep up with demand, then there is a switch into anaerobic metabolism with the production of lactic acid. One molecule of glucose, burned aerobically in mitochondria, can produce 32-36 molecules of ATP (depending on efficiency). Anaerobic production generates just two molecules of ATP, together with one molecule of lactic acid. It is horribly inefficient. Furthermore, to clear the lactic acid requires six molecules of ATP. This is a particular problem for my severely fatigued patients who simply do not have the energy reserves to clear the lactic acid and therefore the lactic acid burn is prolonged. When this occurs in the heart, patients are told they have 'atypical chest pain', whereas what the patient is actually experiencing is angina.

- **Slow recovery from exertion and delayed fatigue**. As ATP is drained, the body can employ another metabolic trick. Two molecules of ADP (two phosphates) combine to form one molecule of ATP (three phosphates) and one of adenosine monophosphate, or AMP (one phosphate) – this is called the adenylate kinase reaction. The good news is that we have another molecule of ATP, but the bad news is that AMP is poorly recycled and drains out of the system. The body then has to make brand new ATP. This it can do from a sugar molecule, but this involves a complex and time-consuming piece of biochemistry – namely, the pentose phosphate shunt. Thus, there is delayed fatigue. This symptom is one that characterises the clinical picture of pathological fatigue because more severe tissue damage starts to occur at this point of very poor energy delivery.

- **Foggy brain**. The brain is greatly demanding of energy. At rest it consumes 20% of the total energy generated in the body. Poor energy delivery results in foggy brain, poor short-term memory and difficulty multi-tasking and problem-solving. These are the early symptoms of dementia and, indeed, much dementia is about poor energy delivery.

- **Dizzy spells** as if about to lose consciousness. These too are symptomatic of the brain running out of energy. This is commonly due to low blood pressure or blood sugar levels suddenly dropping (but the answer is NOT to eat more sugar – read on).

- **Very low mood and depression**, ATP multi-tasks. It is not just the energy molecule; it is also a neurotransmitter in its own right. To be precise, it is a co-transmitter – neurotransmitters such as dopamine, GABA, serotonin and acetylcholine do not work unless ATP is present. Disorders of mood, such as anxiety and depression, could be much better treated if energy delivery issues were tackled.

- **Anxiety and the feeling of severe stress**. This arises because sufferers know that they do not have the energy to deal with expected and unexpected demands. Anxiety creates another vicious cycle because it 'kicks' what I call an 'emotional hole' in the 'energy bucket' and interferes with sleep, thereby sending the energy balance further into deficit, and thereby increasing anxiety…

- **Procrastination**. This has the positive effect of postponing the moment when we have to spend energy.

> *I love deadlines. I love the whooshing sound as they go by.*
> Douglas Adams, English author,
> 11 March 1952 – 11 May 2001

- **Low cardiac output**. The heart is a pump which again demands energy. If ATP is not freely available, then it cannot pump powerfully. Weak beats result in poor circulation. The heart tries to compensate by beating faster, but this too is demanding of energy. Energy delivery cannot keep up and so blood pressure falls precipitously. Clinically this means my severe ME/CFS patients cannot stand for long, or sometimes even short, periods of time. These patients often have to lie down. Rest is much more restful if we lie down! And there is a further vicious cycle here. Low cardiac output compounds all the above problems of poor energy delivery because during periods of low cardiac output, suddenly fuel and oxygen delivery are additionally impaired. So, mitochondria go slow simply because they do not have the raw materials (fuel and oxygen) to function well. This is just one of the many vicious cycles I see in severe pathological fatigue. To expand on this a little: if mitochondria go slow, then the heart, being a muscle and so dependent on good mitochondrial function, will also go slow. The heart delivers fuel and oxygen to all cells in the body (and therefore to mitochondria in all those cells) and so, if delivery of fuel and oxygen is further impaired then this too further impairs mitochondrial function and so on, as shown in Figure 5.1.

- **Intolerance of cold**. Energy is needed to keep us warm and we need to be at just the right temperature. Too hot and energy is wasted. Too cold and we literally go torpid – indeed, this is part of energy-saving hibernation. My CFS patients are in a state of torpor.* Being cold results in another vicious cycle. Enzymes need heat – roughly speaking, a 10-degree rise in temperature doubles their rate of reaction. Being cold means that mitochondrial enzymes, thyroid enzymes and adrenal enzymes, all essential for function, will run slow. Indeed, measuring core temperature is a helpful way to measure energy delivery mecha-

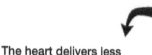

The heart is weak because of poor mitochondrial function affecting the cardiac muscle

The heart delivers less fuel and oxygen to all cells in the body (including those cells in the cardiac muscle), weakening all energy delivery systems

The heart delivers less fuel and oxygen to all cells in the body (including those cells in the cardiac muscle), weakening all energy delivery systems

The heart is further weakened by these lower levels of fuel and oxygen reaching the cardiac muscle

Figure 5.1: The vicious cycle of low energy

*Linguistic note: 'Torpid' means a state of being mentally or physically inactive or lethargic. 'Torpids' is the name given to a series of boat races at Oxford University – the name derives from the event's origins as a race for the second boats of the colleges, which were of course slower than the first boats.

nisms and monitor response to treatment (see Chapter 30).

- **Intolerance of heat**. We lose heat by pumping blood to the skin so it can cool. The skin is the largest organ of the body and pumping blood round the skin increases cardiac output by 20%. This explains why we all fatigue more quickly on hot days and this can be unsustainable for my severe pathologically fatigued patients.
- **Variable blurred vision**. The muscles of the eye demand energy and so, if energy delivery is poor, then the pathologically fatigued will be unable to contract their eye muscles to allow the lens to focus.
- **Light intolerance**. The retina, weight for weight, is the most energy demanding organ of the body. It consumes energy 100 times faster than the rest of the body. This is because the business of converting a light signal into an electrical signal requires massive amounts of ATP. Light intolerance is a feature of severe CFS/ME. It is also a feature of migraine which, I suspect, also has energy delivery as one possible cause. One cannot generate energy without the production of free radicals and these damage tissues. I suspect this explains the high incidence of eye pathology with ageing, such as cataracts, glaucoma and macular degeneration.
- **Noise intolerance**. Again, the business of converting vibrations of air and bone molecules into an electrical signal for the brain to interpret is greatly demanding of energy.
- **Shortness of breath**. If energy delivery at the cellular level is impaired, the brain may misinterpret this as poor oxygen delivery and stimulate the respiratory centre to breathe harder. This may result in hyperventilation, which actually makes the situation worse. Hyperventilation changes the acidity of the blood and so oxygen sticks more avidly to haemoglobin, so worsening oxygen

delivery. Shortness of breath may also result from heart failure, respiratory failure and anaemia.
- **Susceptibility to infection**. The immune system is greatly demanding of energy and raw materials.
- **Loss of libido**. This makes perfect biological sense – procreation and raising children require large amounts of energy.

Readers of George Orwell's *1984* will recognise many of these symptoms of fatigue in the protagonist, Winston Smith. This is not surprising as Winston's diet was appalling, often non-existent, and the demands of his work as a clerk in the Records Department of the Ministry of Truth, where he re-wrote the past, were emotionally, intellectually and physically exhausting. In short, Winston had very poor energy delivery and overwhelming energy demands. Orwell sums up the effect of this energy imbalance with characteristic succinctness and genius:

> *Winston was gelatinous with fatigue.*
> George Orwell (Eric Arthur Blair),
> 25 June 1903 – 21 January 1950

Signs of poor energy delivery

> Ut imago est animi voltus sic indices oculi.
> *The face is a picture of the mind as the eyes are its interpreter.*
> Cicero, 106 – 43 BC

The muscles of the face are largely unconsciously controlled and reflect not just thoughts but also energy. The brain that has a large energy bucket produces an 'attractive' mobile face that engages and smiles with shining eyes. No energy and even the most 'beautiful' face is rendered 'ugly', with flat unresponsive features and dull eyes that do not focus. Again, this makes perfect evolutionary sense – for obvious reasons we need to be able to assess the energy available to friends and foe.

'Attractive', 'beautiful' and 'ugly' may seem unusual words to find in a description of the signs of illness. But I use these terms because they are universally 'understood', not in any 'judgemental or 'discriminatory' way. The fact is that we 'look different' when we are ill, and evolution has 'taught' us to recognise these outward signs of illness as 'unattractive' – dark circles under the eyes, for example. Many of my most ill patients have become, as they have got better, the most attractive human beings.

Movement is another giveaway. When working, I always like to watch my patients coming into the surgery. So much can be learnt about energy and pain from gait, balance and poise.

Pathology that arises if poor energy balance symptoms are ignored or masked

Organ damage and organ failure arise as a result of ignoring or masking poor energy balance symptoms. The masking comes from suppressing symptoms with either prescription drugs or addictions, or both.

- **Heart failure**. Symptoms usually come before organ damage, but not always. The kidneys, for example, suffer in silence. However, if symptoms are ignored, then organ damage will result. As I have said, fatigue is the symptom that arises when energy demand exceeds energy delivery; when this occurs at the cellular level, levels of ATP, the energy molecule, within cells will fall. If levels of ATP fall below a critical amount, this triggers cell apoptosis – 'programmed cell death', or cell suicide in other words. Indeed, this is part of the ageing process – we literally lose cells and our organs slowly shrink. If the situation

becomes critical, either because total energy delivery fails, or the number of cells declines, we develop organ failure and ultimately die. Indeed, it is this process which prevents us from living for ever. A common organ failure that results in death is heart failure. We are currently seeing an epidemic of heart failure, which I believe partly stems from the prescription of statins. One of the side effects of statins is that they inhibit the body's own production of co-enzyme Q10, which is essential for mitochondrial function. (Interestingly, the benefits of statins seem to have little to do with their effect on cholesterol levels. Any benefit seems to arise because biochemically they look like vitamin D. Vitamin D is highly protective against heart disease, cancer and degenerative conditions. Statins are a particular hate of mine. See Chapter 58 for the statin story.)

- **Dementia**. This is brain organ failure – essentially it arises when the speed at which nerves process electrical signals slows down. That process is enormously demanding of energy. My CFS/ME patients exhibit early symptoms of dementia – happily reversible through improving energy delivery mechanisms (see Chapter 30). Another major cause of dementia is arteriosclerosis (arterial damage from metabolic syndrome), resulting in poor oxygen and fuel delivery to the brain. I suspect statins are also partly responsible for our epidemics of dementia. Another cause is the prion disorder of Alzheimer's associated with chronic infection and chemical poisoning.
- **Immune system failure**. The immune system is enormously demanding of energy and this probably explains why elderly people are much more likely to die from infection than younger people, simply because they do not have the energy to power their immune system to fight infections effectively. Infec-

tion has been, and continues to be, the single greatest killer of humans (see our book *The Infection Game – life is an arms race*).

- **Cancer**. The risk of this too increases as energy delivery mechanisms fail. It has always intrigued me that primary cancers of the heart are so rare. The heart is abundantly supplied with energy; it cannot stop beating for a second.
- **Pain**. This too may be a symptom of poor energy delivery because when aerobic metabolism cannot keep up with demand there is a switch into anaerobic metabolism with the production of lactic acid, as described earlier in this chapter – and this is painful. (In Chapter 6, we consider pain in detail.)

> *Of pain you could wish only one thing: that it should stop.*
> George Orwell in *1984*,
> 25 June 1903 – 21 January 1950

Here, we depart from Orwell's immediacy – one should not just wish to make pain stop, but rather one should wish to understand *why* one has pain, address the causes and make the pain stop that way.

The forgetting curve

Earlier in this chapter, I noted how my fellow medical students learnt biochemistry in order to pass the exam and then forgot it as quickly as they could. This book is large, and you may find yourself thinking that you cannot possibly remember it all. Thankfully, you don't have to recall all of it in detail – you can refer to it as often as you like, and in fact doing this will cement the contents in your memory.

The 'forgetting curve' hypothesises the decline of memory retention in time. It is an imperfect model but worth dwelling on. This curve shows how information is lost over time when there is no attempt to retain it. In 1885, Hermann Ebbinghaus collected data to plot a forgetting curve; it approximates an exponential curve as shown in Figure 5.2.

All is not lost. With regular sessions of 're-membering' – either by 'doing it' (here, following the advice daily) or 're-reading it', we can re-adjust the 'forgetting curve' to look more like Figure 5.3.

So, do not despair. Just do it – maybe re-read parts, and you will remember it, or at least pick out those essential to your health.

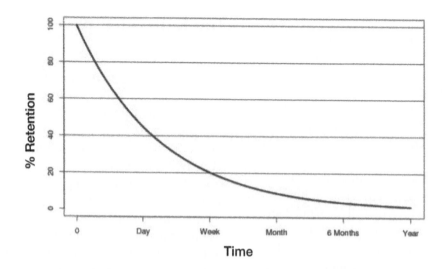

Figure 5.2: The 'forgetting curve' plotted by Hermann Ebbinghaus, German psychologist, 25 January 1850 – 26 February 1909

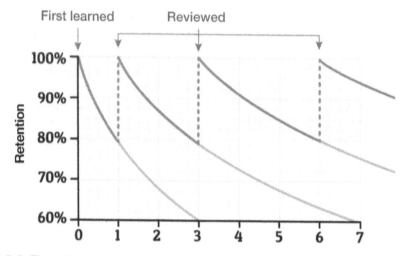

Figure 5.3: The effect on the 'forgetting curve' of regular 'remembering' sessions

Chapter 6
Pain

– pain is an early warning symptom of local damage
– there are different sorts of pain and this gives us clues as to the cause

*The art of life is the art of avoiding pain;
and he is the best pilot, who steers clearest of
the rocks and shoals with which it is beset.*
Thomas Jefferson, third president of the
United States, 1743 – 1826

As fatigue is the general symptom that protects the body from itself, then so pain is the local symptom that protects the body from damaging itself. Its function is to make us stop, so as to prevent further damage and rest the painful area to allow healing and repair. Pain is the red flag that warns us we are heading towards Thomas Jefferson's rocks. Allow pain to drive the motivation to steer another course. Leprosy causes digits and limbs to be lost simply because it destroys nerves – the body cannot protect a numb limb from damage. Pain is an essential part of life.

Modest amounts of pain are essential for good health. The body is very efficient – no energy resources are wasted. This has been an essential policy for evolutionary success – we have to be intrinsically lazy. However, in our modern world of plenty we become lazy because we can. Pushing the system (which in Nature occurs at least once a week during a predator-prey interaction) generates pain as a result of lactic acid burn together with mild wear and tear of muscles, connective tissue and joints. This modest pain is a powerful stimulus to lay down new tissue (muscle, tendons and bone) with its new complement of mitochondria, and this increases physical fitness. The difference between weak and strong, little and large muscles is the number of mitochondria.

Astronauts cannot remain long in space because there is no gravity and no mechanical stress on their bones – they quickly develop osteoporosis and muscle wasting. Putting a patient to bed is dangerous for the same reasons. Some of my more severe ME patients have no 'choice' but to spend long periods of time (sometimes years) in bed because of their extremely low energy levels, so low that organs begin to fail. The best example is POTs (postural orthostatic tachycardia syndrome) resulting from low cardiac output bordering on heart failure. Without proper ecological treatments they do not have the energy to recover.

Different types of pain give us clues to mechanisms

In taking a history from a patient I constantly think about mechanisms. The idea is to establish what these are because this has implications for treatment. The nature of the pain may provide useful clinical clues.

- **Mechanical.** In mechanical pain with tissue damage (which may arise additionally from subsequent inflammation), the sensitive coverings of organs are irritated. The pain from a broken bone comes from the periosteal membrane that covers the bone. The pain of an inflamed or ruptured gut (peritonitis) comes from the peritoneal membrane that wraps round the gut. The meninges covering the brain are highly sensitive and the pain of meningitis is severe. Pleural membranes when inflamed cause intense pain on breathing, called pleurisy. A feature of these pains is that the sufferer immobilises the area – any movement makes things much worse. Sufferers keep the affected area very still because movement is excruciatingly painful.

- **Muscle spasm from smooth muscle** ('unconscious' muscle, e.g. in the gut, womb, bladder). This produces some of the most severe pains. Examples include labour pains, renal colic (from kidney stones), gall stone colic (from gallstones), bowel colic from wind, constipation, adhesions or other such blockage. These spasms are mechanically caused as the muscles try to move an obstruction. A feature of this pain is that often movement is helpful, and the patient is restless. The pain is 'colicky', that is to say the severity waxes and wanes. Restlessness may

be part of treating the condition.*

- **Muscle spasm from skeletal muscle**. This is often extremely painful. I suspect it is often misdiagnosed as 'pinched nerve pain'. Often the pain occurs following a minor movement, not enough to cause any damage. It starts suddenly and is described as 'lancinating', knife-like, sharp or like an electric shock. The sufferer is completely floored. After a few minutes it settles, but any awkward movement may provoke it again. Cramp, stiff neck and 'stiff man syndrome' (fluctuating muscular rigidity and increased sensory sensitivity) are examples of acute muscle spasm which may be due to allergic muscles, mineral imbalances, dehydration or acidity. I suspect Jennifer Starzec of *Determination* is describing allergic muscles: 'People who don't see you every day have a hard time understanding how on some days – good days – you can run three miles but can barely walk across the parking lot on other days.'

- **Migraine** is such an interesting pain – however much it feels like it, we know the pain is not in the brain itself because the brain has no pain sensation. Neurosurgery is carried out with no anaesthetic. I suspect the pain of migraine has two facets – spasm of the scalp muscles (often due to allergy) together with poor energy delivery mechanisms. Perhaps this explains why the PK diet is so effective in abolishing migraine since it addresses both these issues.

- **Lactic acid burn from poor energy delivery**. In this event there is a switch into anaerobic metabolism with the production of lactic acid, which causes pain. It starts with a dull ache and, if not relieved, will continue up to the severe pain of a myocardial infarc-

---

*Footnote: The ignoble prize for medicine 2018 was won by Professor David Wartinger who described a cure for kidney stones. His patient reported that one of his kidney stones became dislodged after a ride on the Big Thunder Mountain ride of Walt Disney World. Wartinger demonstrated that rattling the patient around did indeed dislodge renal stones.

tion requiring morphine for relief. Athletes experience this daily and it allows and limits peak performance – no pain, no gain! Lactic acid burn in the heart is angina. The feature of this pain is that it comes with exercise and is relieved by rest, only to come again with exercise. However, in patients with very poor energy delivery (pathological fatigue) the lactic acid burn may be very persistent and not recognised as such. The best example comes from these pathologically fatigued patients who develop chest pain – actually this is angina, not due to poor blood supply, but due to poor mitochondrial function. Acute unremitting lactic acid burn as caused by an arterial obstruction causes severe pain such as that experienced in a myocardial infarction, pulmonary embolus or acute arterial obstruction. Pathologically fatigued patients also describe chronic headache which I suspect is lactic acid burn in the brain manifesting in the coverings of the brain with meningitis-like pain.

- **Muscle and joint stiffness**. This is a common but greatly overlooked cause of discomfort. The tissues do not slide smoothly over each other and the friction results in a sensation of stiffness as the body tries to protect itself from sudden movements. The sufferer has to 'warm up' slowly before attempting action. Recent work by the physicist Gerald Pollock on the fourth phase of water I believe explains much.[†] The idea here is that water molecules align themselves on surfaces in a graphite-like structure, which is slightly negatively charged. When two such surfaces come together the point of contact would be rendered almost frictionless. This may explain two recognised phenomena:

- why warmth relieves – the fourth phase of water requires background energy to power it
- why magnesium salts are so effective in treating such conditions since being markedly hygroscopic they 'hold' water and further reduce friction.

- **Inflammation** (see also Chapter 7) is nearly always painful, although mild inflammation may present with a lesser pain symptom of itch. Inflammation pains are often described as:
  - gnawing
  - burning in nature. My patients with inflammations from migrating silicone (from implants) often describe the pain as burning. I suspect much chronic low back pain is low-grade inflammation driven by allergy to microbes from the fermenting gut. Without effective treatment, or worse, with symptom suppression with drugs, degeneration follows, with a vicious downward spiral of pathology and pain.
  - throbbing, which is a feature of inflammation. Increased pressure makes the pain worse – the person with a severe toothache or sinusitis finds their symptoms worse lying down. The symptoms of inflammation may be reduced with cooling and worsened by heat.
  - worse with movement
  - (sometimes) worse at night – I suspect this is healing and repair pain.

- **Nerve pain** can be electric shock-like and markedly dependent on position or movement, implying a compression issue. Anyone who has banged their 'funny bone' (the ulnar nerve at the elbow) will recognise this. The pain follows the area that the nerve supplies,

---

†Note from Craig: I was fortunate enough to receive *The Fourth Phase of Water: Beyond Solid, Liquid & Vapor* by Gerald Pollock as a birthday gift from Sarah. It is a fascinating read and very 'accessible'.

so a careful mapping of the pain gives useful anatomical clues. Sciatica typically starts in the buttock and radiates down the back of the leg. One theory is that this arises from spasm of the piriformis muscle through which the sciatic nerve passes, and this may explain why some sufferers can be cured with the PK diet. Carpel tunnel syndrome involves the thumb, index, middle and part of the ring finger, sparing the little finger. It may arise because the nerve is pinched, which can be a mechanical problem or because of swelling of soft tissues from inflammation (often due to allergy) or the fluid retention of myxoedema (severely low thyroid hormones, which often becomes apparent with pregnancy as the need for these increases by 50%). Tic douloureux (or trigeminal neuralgia) is a severe, stabbing pain to one side of the face; I think of this as 'allergic nerves'. Perhaps the mechanism is similar to allergic muscle – sensitisation due to mechanical or infectious trauma and an inflammation maintained by allergy. This may be allergy to foods, microbes, chemicals and/or so on.

Pain is only perceived in the brain and modified by the brain

All pain is perceived more where there is fear, anxiety, depression and loss of hope – the mental and emotional state is critical. That is why it is so important to put the patient in control of the diagnostic process. A lovely example of this was given by Dr Henry Beecher, an American army anaesthetist. At the battle of Anzio, he received seriously wounded soldiers and asked if they needed pain relief; 75% did not. By contrast after the war, whilst working in a surgical unit he again asked – this time post-operative – patients who had suffered comparable tissue damage if they needed analgesics; 83% asked for such. State of mind determined the difference. Soldiers coming from a war zone thought of themselves as survivors – they were safe and on their way home. Yippee – what a relief! No morphine needed here.

> *The injuries that befall us unexpectedly are less severe than those which are deliberately anticipated.*
> Marcus Tulius Cicero, writer, politician and great Roman orator, 106 – 43 BC[‡]

Intuition is a wonderful thing. The untrained patient often makes a remarkably accurate diagnosis. Sometimes they dream and wake in the morning with an instinctive or 'gut feeling' for what is wrong. These are always worth considering. Even the vocabulary used to describe pain can be helpful in establishing causation.

Conclusion

The key to treating pain is not to mask it with painkillers but to ask the question 'Why?' before the clinical picture becomes blurred by inflammation and degeneration. Act immediately at the first symptom of pain. Use the pain to motivate to… well just do it.

Reference

1. Pollock G. *The Fourth Phase of Water: beyond solid, liquid and vapour.* 2013: Ebner & Sons, Seattle, Washington, US.

[‡]**Footnote:** I so admire Cicero. He was murdered on Mark Antony's order. He loved word plays. His last words are said to have been: 'There is nothing proper about what you are doing, soldier, but do try to kill me properly.'

Chapter 7
Inflammation symptoms

– pain, swelling, heat, redness and loss of function

Not all symptoms arise from inflammation,* but inflammation can cause almost any symptom. It is characterised by:

- pain
- swelling (with the potential for mechanical irritation)
- heat
- redness (due to increased blood flow)
- loss of function (as the body protects itself by shutting down that department).

Inflammation for healing and repair

Inflammation is an essential part of survival. We cannot live without damaging our bodies and inflammation is part of healing and repair. Surgical wounds heal with swelling, heat, redness, and pain (and consequent loss of function, i.e. we immobilise the wound). So does tissue damage due to physical damage, burns, over-use (repetitive strain injuries) or pathology. Feel the pain, rest the body and use the brain (and this book) to ask the question 'Why?'

Inflammation for dealing with 'foreigners'

Inflammation occurs when our 'standing army', the immune system, is activated. This should be for good reason against foreign microbes that want to invade our bodies. The living organism that we are represents a potential free lunch for such microbes. We fight a constant 'arms race' against invading microbes and parasites. There is much more detail in our book *The Infection Game – life is an arms race*.

Acute inflammation is the sudden reaction of part, or the whole, of the body, to an unrecognised, foreign incitant (an invader that 'incites' an immune reaction). This battle is characterised by symptoms (see below) evolved to physically

*Linguistic note: The word inflammation derives from the Latin verb *inflammare*, which combines *flammare* ('to catch fire') with the Latin prefix *in*, which means 'to cause to'. This is a good description of inflammation in the body. There is an interesting quirk in the English language here – the words 'inflammable' and 'flammable' mean the same thing in modern usage – 'capable of catching fire'. This is contrary to 'standard' English where the addition of 'in' as a prefix normally means 'not' as in, for example, 'inactive'. So, how did this arise? The story goes that in 1813, a scholar translated the Latin *flammere* to 'flammable' and after that 'flammable' came into common usage. The usage of 'inflammable' is decreasing, partly because many government regulations require 'flammable' to be used on products and official literature to avoid confusion, and 'non-flammable' is now the designated negative. Anyway, less of government regulations and back to the body...

expel, localise and 'kill' the incitant.

Chronic inflammation results when the battle of acute inflammation has failed, and the body is in a state of war against an incitant. This may be for good reason (if there is chronic infection) or bad (allergy and/or autoimmunity). Whichever, not only does this result in long-term pain and misery but it also drains precious energy reserves away from fun-loving life – we become physically fatigued, foggy and forlorn.

The key message, which is always of great disappointment to patients, is that one cannot know the cause of inflammation simply from the symptoms and signs. So, for example, looking at a hayfever sufferer, without clinical details, one may diagnose a cold. Looking at an inflamed patch on the skin, without clinical details, one's differential diagnosis would include allergic eczema, sunburn, chemical burn, infected cellulitis or viral or autoimmune rash. Any incitant may cause any symptom and good detective work is needed. The history is vital, tests may help, but it is the response to treatment that finally gives us the diagnosis. (See Chapter 16 for the mechanisms of inflammation.)

Table 7.1: Symptoms of acute inflammation resulting from one of the above incitants

Symptom	Mechanisms	Notes
Fatigue	A busy immune system kicks a hole in the energy bucket – most people are bedbound with acute influenza	Fatigue is an essential symptom to enforce rest so that the immune system has the energy available to fight
Malaise and 'illness behaviour'	Probably inflammatory mediators telling the brain…	…to rest up, keep warm and stay safe until the immune system has dealt with the invader
Depression	The inflamed body causes the inflamed brain	Stops us doing things and so conserves energy for the immune system to fight
Foggy brain, possibly an acute confusional state	The brain does not have the energy to function normally	Because all energy has been diverted to the immune army
Fever	Most microbes are killed by heat	All the more reason to run a fever
Swollen lymph nodes ('glands')	The lymph nodes are where white blood cells are being recruited and trained to fight this particular attack	Do not use symptom-supressing anti-inflammatory drugs, like aspirin and paracetamol, which handicap the immune army. Use antimicrobial weapons such as vitamin C, iodine, herbal remedies and supplements
General tendency to fluid retention e.g. puffy ankles	Inflammation is associated with oedema	Ditto
Mucus and catarrh	This physically washes out microbes	Ditto
Runny eyes	Ditto	Ditto

Cough and sneeze	Physically blasts out microbes from the airways	
Airway narrowing, wheeze, asthma	This results in the air we breathe becoming more turbulent, so microbes are thrown against, and stick to, the mucous lining of the airways to be coughed up, swallowed and killed in the acid stomach	Do not fill the stomach with fruit or sugar which will feed these microbes; leave it empty so microbes are coughed up and swallowed into a bath of concentrated acid
Vomiting	An essential defence against food poisoning and microbes that have been inhaled (then coughed up and swallowed)	Ditto
Diarrhoea and colic	Physically wash out the invaders	Ditto – again, do not feed the invaders in the gut
Cystitis	Empties the bladder of urine and therefore microbes	Ditto

With any acute infection, from childhood febrile illnesses to influenza (flu) and pneumonia, it is potentially dangerous to use symptom-suppressing medication which interferes with these natural defences. Any such medication hampers our defences and helps the invaders. I would caution against prescribing symptom-modifying medication which interfere with the body's natural processes of eliminating microbes. Indeed, I suspect this is why we are currently seeing epidemics of post-viral fatigue syndromes. At the first symptom of any infection, apply Groundhog Acute (Appendix 2, page A2).

Symptoms of chronic inflammation – infection, allergy, autoimmunity

Whilst any antigen can cause any symptoms (Dr John Mansfield described a case of osteoarthritis of the hip due to allergy to housedust mites), common things are common. Chronologically, infection and allergy symptoms often start in the nose and throat and extend to the lungs, gut, brain, and then any other organ. If a symptom has become chronic then I would consider the incitants listed in order of likelihood in Table 7.2.

Table 7.2: Incitants potentially causing chronic symptoms, in order of likelihood

Clinical picture	Common incitants	Notes
ENT symptoms such as catarrh, deafness, glue ear, post-nasal drip, polyps, snoring and obstructive sleep apnoea, voice changes, cough	Dairy products (cow, goat sheep) Yeast Mould infection	Chronic infection with yeast and mould is a greatly overlooked cause of symptoms – this is easily diagnosed through measuring urinary mycotoxins
Tinnitus, deafness, attacks of vertigo	Allergy to food or gut microbes Caffeine Perhaps chronic infection with bacteria and/or moulds Poisoning	I suspect this may also contribute to age-related deafness – Beethoven went deaf following salmonella infection
Asthma and chronic obstructive airways disease (COAD or COPD) – indeed, anyone using the blue and brown inhalers	Allergy to food, biological inhalants, and gut microbes Chronic infection with bacteria and/or moulds	Ditto – so often antibiotics are given 'blind' and the possibility of chronic fungal infection ignored. You will not see unless you look
Irritable bowel syndrome	Allergy to foods and upper fermenting gut problems	
Inflammatory bowel disease	Allergy to foods and upper fermenting gut problems	Microbes move under the mucous lining of the gut to drive inflammation
Headache	Aspartame, dairy Caffeine may cause a toxic headache	
Migraine has several causes	All the above...	...but there are other causes (see Chapter 49, Neurology)
All neurological and psychiatric/psychological symptoms	The inflamed brain driven by infection, allergy and autoimmunity	The brain, immune system, gut and body are inseparable and should be treated the same
Chronic pain syndromes (another terrible 'diagnosis' dished out to patients as a pretext to prescribe toxic drugs)	I suspect this is allergy to virus, especially all the herpes viruses which target the nervous and immune systems	Opioids, many of which had been prescribed, killed 70,000 Americans in 2017.[1]
Arthritis Allergic muscles, tendons, connective tissue	Allergy to foods and gut microbes	
Eczema and urticaria Venous leg ulcers	Allergy to foods and gut microbes Chronic staphylococcal infection of skin	

Acne and rosacea	Allergy to gut microbes and foods Chronic infection of skin	
Interstitial cystitis Chronic prostatitis/epididymitis Chronic vulvitis	Allergy to gut microbes, especially yeast	
The flitting arthritis of any microbial infection	Allergy to microbes – so-called 'palindromic rheumatism'	Rheumatic fever may damage the heart valves due to 'allergy' to streptococcus
Any pathology from cancer and coronaries to diabetes and dementia...	...may have an infectious incitant	There is much more detail on the diagnosis and treatment of chronic infection in our book *The Infection Game*

So, look for these symptoms, and you may suspect inflammation somewhere. As the Romans said:

ubi fumus, ibi ignis
...where there is smoke [the symptoms]
there is fire [inflammation]

Reference

1. Drug and Opioid-Involved Overdose Deaths — United States, 2013–2017 *CDC Weekly* January 4, 2019; 67(5152); 1419–1427 www.cdc.gov/mmwr/volumes/67/wr/ mm675152e1.htm?s_cid=mm675152e1_w

Chapter 8
Poisoning and deficiency clinical pictures

We love the simple paradigm of single poisonings (or toxicities) or deficiencies manifesting with simple clinical pictures which provide a diagnosis. Occasionally we see single gross deficiencies in calories, vitamins, minerals and essential fatty acids, and a clear clinical picture emerges. We all know the story of scurvy with gum disease, infection, neuropathy and death. Gross vitamin B3 deficiency results in the memorable dermatitis, diarrhoea, dementia and death of pellagra. Vitamin B12 deficiency may present with subacute combined degeneration of the spinal cord. I recall a case of a man who developed acute night blindness after some months of the prescription drug cholestyramine, designed to block absorption of fat from the gut. It also prevented absorption of fat-soluble vitamin A, hence his complete loss of vision in the dark. However, unlike the picture painted by the modern, medical, Sherlock Holmes, Dr Gregory House, it is unusual to see such singular pictures in clinical practice.

> *We are too much accustomed to attribute to a single cause that which is the product of several, and the majority of our controversies come from that.*
> Baron Justus Von Liebig, German chemist, 1803 – 1873 (Attrib)

The fact is that most deficiencies or toxicities present with:
Symptoms of poor energy delivery and/or
Symptoms of inflammation and/or
Growth promotion or inhibition
Organ failures and degeneration (dementia, osteoporosis, heart failure)

Common things are common and the clinical pictures that I see as a result of deficiency and/or toxicity are as listed in Table 8.1.

Table 8.1: Common clinical pictures associated with deficiencies and/or toxicities

Mechanism damaged or blocked or, perhaps, inappropriately switched on	Early symptoms	Late pathology
Energy delivery mechanisms	Fatigue, depression, anxiety, stress...	Premature ageing
	...chronic fatigue syndrome	Chronic infection, as the immune system does not have the energy to fight (Much more detail in *The Infection Game – life is an arms race*)
	Slowing of organ function	Organ failures such as heart, brain (dementia), kidneys etc
	Weakness, poor stamina	Loss of muscle (sarcopenia)
Hormone function e.g. insulin resistance	Hypoglycaemia as blood sugar level wobbles	Metabolic syndrome, diabetes, arterial disease, cancer, dementia (see our book *Prevent and Cure Diabetes – delicious diets, not dangerous drugs*)
Hypothyroidism	Fatigue	Premature ageing
Poor adrenal function	Ditto	Ditto
Low sex hormones	Sexual disorientation (for example, crocodiles may change sex in response to oestrogen mimics, such as xeno-oestrogens – a type of xeno-hormone that imitates oestrogen. These chemicals are found in some widely used industrial compounds such as PCBs (polychlorinated biphenyls) and phthalates)	Falling sperm counts Infertility (affects 14% of UK couples)
DNA and epigenetic changes	None – blissful unawareness until we are diagnosed with...	...cancer or teratogenicity (results in miscarriage, stillbirth or our babies born with birth defects). Birth defects include low IQ, learning disorders, slow development, cancers and much more

Direct damage to proteins	Prion formation (note these may also be part of chronic infection)	Alzheimer's, motor neurone disease, Parkinson's, multi-system atrophy, etc
Damage to the hardware and software of the immune system	Symptoms of inflammation which may be local or general	Allergy, autoimmunity
	Immune suppression	Increased risk of infection, cancer and degeneration
Growth control	Benign lumps, cysts, skin changes, poor quality connective tissue	Premature ageing, cancer
Nerves in the conscious brain	Mental slowing Lowering of intelligence Psychological disorders	Dementia Autism Psychosis (mania and schizophrenia)
Nerves in the subconscious	Poor balance and co-ordination Loss of senses (touch, vision, hearing, taste and smell)	Parkinson's disease
Nerves in the periphery	If dumbed down, then loss of sensation If dumbed up, then perhaps chronic pain syndromes	Peripheral neuropathy
Autonomic nerves	Inappropriate reactions e.g. fear, anxiety, sweating, fainting, diarrhoea, tachycardia and much more	
Electrical conduction in the heart	Palpitations Poor heart function with inability to get fit	Cardiac dysrhythmias
Healing and repair mechanisms	Degeneration	Premature ageing Osteoporosis

Indeed, I suspect it is chemical pollution of the external and internal environment that partly explains why the life expectancy of Americans has fallen for two years in succession.[1]

Many poisons and toxins are easily recognised, often by hazard warning signs. But so many are 'hidden in plain view' because we have become accustomed to having them 'around' us in normal life. Smokers are oblivious to the 'Smoking Kills' label. These 'hidden' or 'unrecognised' poisons are some of the most dangerous. In the UK, if a chemical in a food makes up less than 1% of the total, then it does not need to be declared – so pesticide residues can be eaten unannounced. As Shakespeare said:

> *Hide not thy poison with such sugar'd words*
> *[and sugar is very apposite here!]*
> The Second Part of *Henry VI*, Act 3 Scene II, by William Shakespeare, 26 April 1564 (baptised) – 23 April 1616

Food as a source of toxins

Food is potentially dangerous. If you look at life from the point of view of a plant, it does not want to be eaten, so it has evolved many poisons to protect it from such a fate. Examples include lectins,* alkaloids and alkylating agents (e.g. glycosides in cycad that cause motor neurone disease). Alternatively, it may become contaminated by mycotoxins (from moulds) and so on.

By contrast, meat and meat fat are non-toxic – animals have evolved other systems of defence; they can run away! I suspect the main ways in which meat and meat fat may be toxic arise from either cooking them at high temperatures, which results in toxic trans-fats being produced, or their fermentation (fermentation of protein) where there is an upper fermenting gut problem – both complications being recent evolutionary changes. When humans learned to cook and to farm, this introduced a new range of toxins as the carbohydrate-based foods involved may be fermented in the upper gut to a range of alcohols, D-lactate, hydrogen sulphide, ammonia and other such, as well as endotoxins being produced from fermenting microbes and mycotoxins from fermenting moulds.

Addictions as a source of toxins

These in particular are substances to be aware of and avoid:

Sugar and refined carbohydrates ('junk food') will result in a fermenting upper gut (which may produce hangover-like symptoms), sticky blood (sugar is sticky stuff) and hormonal swings (the 'blood-sugar roller-coaster'). See much more in our book *Prevent and Cure Diabetes – delicious diets not dangerous drugs*.

Alcohol – from drinking the stuff; we all feel poisoned with a hangover

Smoking

Caffeine – too much is toxic

Street drugs – cannabis, ecstacy, cocaine, morphine etc

Prescription medications – many psychotrophic drugs, such as SSRIs (selective serotonin re-uptake inhibitors), are addictive and simply replace one addiction with another, or add to one's addiction load, resulting in short-term gain with relief of symptoms but long-term pain with worsening of additional side effects.

The fermenting brain as a source of toxins

Professor Nishihara hypothesises that microbes, probably from the gut, get into the brain and ferment neurotransmitters into amphetamine- and LSD-like chemicals.[2] Clinically this would present with a huge range of psychiatric and psychological symptoms.

The vagus nerve is the major channel of communication between gut and brain. Vagotomy

---

Footnote: The Bulgarian dissident writer Georgi Markov was assassinated on Waterloo Bridge in 1978. He was stabbed with the point of an umbrella to embed a pellet of ricin in his calf muscle. He took four days to die. Ricin is a lectin.

(a surgical operation to sever the vagus nerve) is an operation performed to treat various gut symptoms, but it also protects against the development of Parkinson's disease. This suggests to me that microbes may get into the brain via nerve pathways. Interested readers should see reference 2 below together with Chapter 50: Psychiatry (page 50.1).

Mycotoxins as a cause of disease

Schoental hypothesised, with good reasons, that the plague of Athens in 430-426 BC resulted from poisoning by mouldy grains.[3] Thucydides described the clinical picture:

> *Violent heats in the head; redness and inflammation of the eyes; throat and tongue quickly suffused with blood; breath became unnatural and fetid; sneezing and hoarseness; violent cough, vomiting; retching; violent convulsions; the body externally not so hot to the touch, nor yet pale; a livid colour inkling to red; breaking out in pustules and ulcers. (2.49-2.50)*

Are you deficient or poisoned?

In people eating modern Western diets, micronutrient deficiencies are the norm – nowhere more so than in NHS hospitals. This is why Groundhog Basic is so important, because just by implementing this protocol, one narrows the diagnostic possibilities whilst improving the prognosis, whatever that may be. Indeed, instigating Groundhog Basic has become part of the diagnostic process with all my patients. I no longer bother to do basic nutritional tests on virgin patients because I know what the results will be – multiple minor deficiencies of vitamins, minerals and essential fatty acids. It is

much more important that patients spend their valuable resources on recovery so they can live life to its full potential.

Humans have evolved a fabulous detoxification system in the gut, liver and bloodstream to cope with these natural toxins, such as lectins, although the body can become overwhelmed if the exposure is chronic and/or large enough. However, we are all inevitably exposed to further unnatural toxins from the outside world (see Chapter 25). I have yet to do a fat biopsy or test for toxic metals and find a normal result! Possibly a more sensitive test is of function. The commonest manifestation of toxic stress is in the brain – think 'poisoning' with poor short-term memory, foggy brain and procrastination. Such toxic stress in the brain cannot always be diagnosed via the standard testing techniques – as ever, one should be aware of the clinical presentation. The signs and symptoms are our clues.

> *As an example, Richard Wetherill, an outstanding chess player, and retired university lecturer, began to notice that he could no longer think through the possible connotations of making a move in a game of chess. He used to pride himself on being able to look eight moves ahead. Just as a guide to this incredible feat of mental agility, at the start of a game of chess, after both players have made one move there are 400 possible positions for the pieces, after two moves by both players, there are 197,742 possible positions for the pieces, and after three moves there are about 121 million possible arrangements of the pieces! Back to Richard – he was concerned about what he saw as his mental decline and so, despite his wife telling him that there was nothing wrong, he went to see Nick Fox, a neurologist in London. The usual tests of memory and even a brain image revealed nothing amiss. Two years later, Wetherill*

died and a post mortem examination revealed a plethora of plaques and tangles in his brain, indicative of Alzheimer's disease. In fact such was the damage that most people would have been hardly able to function and yet Wetherill only noticed a reduction in his chess-playing prowess.[4] The lesson is not to ignore signs and symptoms and always to follow up on them and unearth the mechanisms that are causing them. It can even be more subtle than this – Craig's mum died from a brain tumour in 2004, a result of an undiagnosed lung cancer having metastasised. Craig and his mum used to have a reading club of two (!) and in late 2003, they decided to re-read Way Station by Clifford D Simack, having previously read it some 30 years before. Craig's mum kept on saying that the book appeared 'bland' and did not 'hit her emotions' as it had done before. This was put down to it being the second read-through but maybe it was an early indication of the tumour, which was diagnosed a few months later.

The key lesson here is that toxicity too can present with any symptom and must be considered as a part of any differential diagnosis. Again, it is unlikely to be the only cause – we live in a complex world so expect complex solutions.*

Read this book well and take this opportunity before opportunity takes you!

Healing is a matter of time, but it is sometimes also a matter of opportunity
Hippocrates, Greek physician, c. 460 BC – c. 377 BC, in *Precepts, 1*

References

1. Tinker B. US life expectancy drops for a second year in a row. CNN December 2017 https://edition.cnn.com/2017/12/21/health/us-life-expectancy-study/index.html
2. Nishihara K. Disclosure of the major causes of mental illness – mitochondrial deterioration in brain neurons via opportunistic infection. *Journal of Physics and Biochemistry* 2012; 12: 11-18. www.drmyhill.co.uk/drmyhill/images/d/dc/NISHIHARA.pdf
3. Schoental R. Mycotoxins in food and the plague of Athens. *Journal of Nutritional Medicine* 1994; 4: 83-85. www.tandfonline.com/doi/abs/10.3109/13590849409034541
4. Melton R. How brainpower can help you cheat old age. *New Scientist* 14 December 2005. www.newscientist.com/article/mg18825301-300-how-brainpower-can-help-you-cheat-old-age/ "

---

†**Personal note from Craig:** I think this is why I disliked biology and chemistry at school and why I chose to drop them in favour of Latin and Greek as soon as I could. (I dropped biology aged 12). They were too complex. Mathematicians look for simplicity – they are lazy. Newton, my mathematical hero, said:

Truth is ever to be found in the simplicity, and not in the multiplicity and confusion of things.
Sir Isaac Newton, British mathematician, 4 January 1643 – 31 March 1727

Well, Newton was right, if discussing things mathematical, and the briefer a mathematical proof, the more elegant and satisfying. However, my ongoing battle with ME, and working with Sarah, have taught me that interwoven complex (biological) systems have multiple feedback systems, all of which have to be considered when looking for answers.

Chapter 9
Hormonal clinical pictures

Symptoms are so often ascribed to 'hormones' when it must be remembered that hormones are simply the messengers. The word 'hormone' derives from the Ancient Greek *hormon*, the present participle of *horman*, to set in motion. So yes, we must be able to make hormones to communicate, but also, we must be ready to ask the question, 'Why are hormones present in too great or too small an amount?' if that situation arises. We have hormones to control energy delivery mechanisms, to control growth (including healing and repair) and to allow reproduction. The summary below is a huge simplification – there are many subtle overlaps and interplays – but this gives the key principles.

Hormones to control energy delivery mechanisms

As described in Chapter 5, these are the thyroid and adrenal hormones. Problems here manifest as poor energy delivery symptoms.

Growth hormones and sex hormones

These include the male sex hormone testosterone, the female sex hormones oestrogen and progesterone, and others.

The only evolutionary reason we live at all is to procreate our 'selfish genes', to quote Richard Dawkin. What is a good survival strategy for our genes is not necessarily a good survival ploy for our brains and bodies. You and I will die, but by contrast our genes will live on in subsequent generations until the species becomes extinct. The strategies for a good life (what I personally and selfishly desire) are different from, and maybe in conflict with, those for gene procreation. The point here is that sex hormones are essential for the survival of the genes, but procreation is a high-risk activity for the survival of individual brains and bodies. Indeed, sex hormones drive us to participate in outrageously risky and antisocial behaviour from downright dangerous, competitive actions (to impress and attract the opposite sex) to treachery and promiscuity (when an opportunity permits).

Infidelity and promiscuity have been with us always, as Shakespeare's Balthasar states in *Much Ado About Nothing* Act 2, scene 3, 62–69:

> *Sigh no more, ladies, sigh no more,*
> *Men were deceivers ever,*
> *One foot in sea, and one on shore,*
> *To one thing constant never.*
> William Shakespeare, 26 April 1564
> (baptised) – 23 April 1616

Sex hormones are intrinsically dangerous. Sexual activity (yes, I know it is great fun!)

brings exposure to very nasty diseases, some of which remain with us for life and drive cancer and/or organ failures. Furthermore, pregnancy and childbirth kill many women – not that evolution 'cares' two hoots about that provided the genes have a chance of survival. Thankfully we have great brains and have evolved wonderful systems that allow relatively safe pregnancy and childbirth. I would take full advantage of such. As obstetrician Dr Adam Kaye said in his wonderful book *This is going to hurt*, 'Home delivery is for pizzas, not babies'.*

Having produced a baby, Nature ensures its survival with the love hormone oxytocin. This is further produced in response to the nipple stimulation of breast-feeding. This reflex is another way by which men induce women to love them and do mad things as a result.†

Oxytocin was what Puck must have used to persuade Titania to fall in love with Bottom. This hormone also turned me from a logical, intelligent, goal-driven woman into a burbling, cooing, emotional wreck who could only think about a hungry baby and nappies. I even do this with other babies! Oxytocin also reprogrammed my memory cells. Whilst in labour with my firstborn I promised myself never, ever again. Within nine months I was again pregnant.

Further mechanisms by which why oestrogens and progesterones (and so the Pill and HRT) are so dangerous are given in Table 9.1.

Table 9.1: The dangers of oestrogens and progesterones

Mechanism	Increase risk of:
They are growth promoting – it is hormones that drive breast, ovary and uterine development at menarche (onset of periods)	Breast, cervical, uterine and probably ovarian cancer Also bowel cancer and melanoma Should such develop during pregnancy, then termination is essential if the mother is to survive
They make us do mad things – as anyone falling in love can testify to	Risky behaviour, depression and suicide
They are immunosuppressive – this is essential to prevent the pregnant mother rejecting the foetus as a 'foreigner' since half its DNA is non-self	All infections acute and chronic become potentially more serious
They induce metabolic syndrome, so women can get fat in anticipation of pregnancy and breast-feeding	All the complications of metabolic syndrome – namely, obesity, hypertension, diabetes and so heart disease Increased clotting tendency so risk of thrombosis, pulmonary embolism and stroke

*Aside from Craig: Not that we are advocating the eating of pizza! The word *pizza* is Italian for 'pie'. The previous derivation of the word is uncertain. It may have come from the Greek *pitta*, meaning bread. It is even possible that the word originated in a Langobardic word, *bizzo* meaning 'bite'. Langobardic is an extinct West Germanic language that was spoken by the Lombards (Langobardi), a Germanic people who settled in Italy in the 6th century AD.

†Note from Craig: The best course of action for me here is to remain utterly silent. As my mother once said to my father, 'Men! They should be seen and not heard!'

Menopausal symptoms

We know these result from falling levels of oestrogens and progesterone and this causes problems for two reasons. Sex hormones impact on energy delivery mechanisms and this explains the fatigue, mood swings and depression some suffer. It is often at this time that an underlying hypothyroidism is unmasked. We then have the horrible hot flushes – see Chapter 54 for the why and how to treat these.

Testosterone

I suspect testosterone levels, after puberty, are directly related to energy delivery mechanisms. They are at their highest at puberty then decline with age, paralleling energy delivery mechanisms. This permits more mitochondria and bigger muscles. Too little testosterone is associated with fatigue. By contrast, athletes are tempted to use them for performance enhancement – we know that in the past the East Germans and Russians greatly improved their Olympic medal tally using male sex hormones. Testosterones (and they come in several forms) are not as intrinsically dangerous as the female sex hormones simply because men have a completely different set of physiological requirements to procreate and these are not intrinsically dangerous when testosterone is present in physiological doses. Many people, men and women, as they age, feel much better for using physiological doses of testosterone – to improve muscular strength. Whilst some believe that testosterone is a risk factor for cancer, this does not make sense. Risk of cancer increases with age as testosterone levels fall. Prostate cancer cells are present in 16% of post-mortem samples in the male population over the age of 80, and are associated with low serum testosterone. I suspect testosterone in physiological doses is cancer protective. The key is *physiological doses*, which amount to 1-2 grams daily of testicular glandulars.[‡]

[‡]**Historical note:** The Ancients may not have had a good understanding of hormones, but they did make various attempts at 'controlling' their effects. For example, during Thesmophoria (a festival in honour of the Goddess Demeter, whose domain included the fertility of the Earth), Athenian women placed Agnus leaves under their bed in order to remain agnes (pure). The same cannot be said to be true of Athenian men.

PART III
Mechanisms

The mechanisms by which symptoms and diseases are produced, how to identify these mechanisms through tests and why the basic 'tools of the trade' are effective

Chapter 10
Diagnosis starts with detective work

– looking for mechanisms
– how to organise and manage your recovery plan
– please see Chapter 79 for real-life examples of these management frames in action

We humans love a mystery, we love crime detective TV series, we love 'working something out', we are inquisitive, and this inquisitiveness has led to great things. Alongside Shakespeare, Agatha Christie tops the league of best all-time bestsellers, with an estimated 2-4 billion books sold (cripes Craig – we have a bit of catching up to do...). The Ancient Greeks loved a mystery too. Sophocles' play *Oedipus Rex* has Oedipus trying to solve the mystery of a plague that is decimating Thebes; the play is a dramatisation of how he ultimately 'detects' the culprit responsible for the plague, a culprit who shall remain nameless in this book! But when this detective work concerns our own health, it takes on a more important, and less recreational, aspect. Just as Oedipus did, we must look for clues as to the culprit(s), and only once identified, can we begin to deal with these murderers.

How do we look for those clues? We have touched on this earlier, but let's pull it together so you can create your own diagnostic process to guide you down the correct paths of management. We have to use the combined acumen of doctor, patient and laboratory to deliver a result and make it work for the individual patient – and every patient is unique. And if you are working 'alone' on this, not having a doctor to guide you, then you must be both the doctor and the patient. This is completely possible and the books I have written with Craig are our best attempt to empower patients to be their own 'health detectives', or their own doctors. A helpful tool, and one that I use all the time, is the management frame below. There are lots of examples in the case history section to help you to build your own, and in particular Chapter 79.

The patient history 'frame'

Start with the past. Confucius knew this:

> *Study the past if you would define the future.*
>
> Confucius, Chinese teacher and philosopher, 551 – 479 BC

Symptoms, their chronology and the circumstances which trigger or relieve them, provide important clues as to the underlying biochemical, immunological and hormonal lesions. Always start with the past – put in all you can remember, in date order. Establishing the chronology of symptoms is essential to work out mechanism. Start with the frame shown in Table 10.1 – fill it in as things come to mind – the joy of these frames is that they can be filled in piecemeal and the logic follows effortlessly. Simply organising my thoughts like this has revolutionised my practice of medicine.*

Table 10.1: The patient history frame to be completed – add as many lines as needed, and keep adding

Date	Symptom	Mechanism

Past problems
Past problems give clues – think of:
- Baby and toddler problems
- Vaccinations
- Diet
- Reactions to medications, foods, biological pollens, animals, dusts, moulds, chemicals (perfume, cleaning agents, cosmetics, etc), metals (nickel and jewellery); electrical sensitivity (wifi, cordless phones, mobiles)
- Infectious triggers of symptoms, food poisoning
- Abuse or bullying as a child – includes situations where a child is constantly stressed, by, for example, an abusive family situation. This can lead to 'hypervigilance', which has implications for understanding the mechanisms of disease in some patients
- Housing (chemicals and moulds)
- Travel and insect bites
- Workplace: pesticides, toxic metals, sick building syndrome (see Chapter 15: Poisonings)
- Hobbies
- Local pollution: industry, waste-sites
- Unexplained oddities.

---

*Note from Craig: These frames have also revolutionised my understanding of Sarah's thought processes and, in consequence, I now ask better questions. Indeed, I think we should call these boxes, 'Myhill Frames' – used well, they simplify and explain so much that previously was confused and mysterious. One sees patterns.

Family history

Problems run in families and, indeed, so do answers to problems:

- Mitochondria come down the female line, and so I often see mother–daughter or mother–son combinations, both with CFS/ME, where mitochondrial failure is the central cause. Mitochondria also determine longevity, so look to your mother and her mother for this.
- The gut microbiome comes down the female line – we acquire our mother's gut-friendly, immune-tagged, 'safe' microbes at the point of birth, possibly in utero.
- Problems of the immune system run strongly in families i.e. allergy, autoimmunity and cancer. Indeed, I don't think I have ever seen a case of cow's milk allergy and failed to find a close relative with this as a likely diagnosis.
- Don't forget thyroid disease - if your mother had it, so will you.

Noted responses

Include patterns. Are symptoms better or worse with:

- the seasons
- alcohol
- medication
- exercise
- temperature changes
- warm climate
- house move
- dietary change
- antimicrobials (symptom-supressing medication and addictions do not count!)
- divorce, bereavement… and so on…

Remember, just because an intervention has not been effective does not mean it can be dropped. For example, energy delivery mechanisms involve several players, all of which have to be working well to see a clinical result. We live in a complex world and that demands complex solutions.

Detail the tests that you have already had done

So often these are poorly interpreted because high normal and low normal results are ignored. Use Appendix 4 to assist here. Again, you can see some examples in the 'management frames' in the case histories, and especially in Chapter 79.

Table 10.2: The 'test results management frame'

Test	Significant result	What it means	Action

Move on to the present

Use Chapters 4 to 9 to try to fit your symptoms into the mechanisms in Table 10.3. You may need to put one symptom into more than one category. Enjoy the 'eureka' moments that jump out of the pages as you start to make the links between symptoms and mechanisms. It is even more fun when the actions result in cures.

Table 10.3: The mechanisms and actions 'frame'

Symptoms	Mechanism	Action
	Poor energy delivery	
Clinical score		
		Basic package of supplements
	Mitochondria going slow	
		Diet
	Sleep problems	
	Thyroid problems	
	Adrenal problems	
	Allergy	
	Fermenting gut	
	Infection with bacteria	
	Infection with virus	
	Infection with yeast/mould	
	Dental problems	
	Poisoning	Detox
Connective tissue/bone problems		
	Other/unknown	

Diet

In recording what you are eating and drinking, be completely honest – there is no point cheating yourself! It is all too easy to overlook the addictions. Put in *everything* you eat or drink.

Also record dietary supplements – put these into the category that addresses the reason that you are taking them.

Using these management frames greatly helps pattern recognition. With this tool, we can all become expert in our own bodies and minds and, given the right clues, can work out these mechanisms. This is the point of this book. Indeed, the word 'doctor' comes from the Greek 'to teach'. I must teach my patients the methods of this book, so they can take control – and in turn teach me! As William Osler said:

> *To study the phenomenon of disease without books is to sail an uncharted sea, while to study books without patients is not to go to sea at all.*
> Sir William Osler, 1st Baronet, FRS FRCP, Canadian physician, 12 July 1849 – 29 December 1919*

Having analysed the symptoms to come to possible mechanisms of disease, this gives us a hypothesis of why that patient is ill. We then need to put that hypothesis to the test by appropriate investigations and treatments, choosing the relevant tools to treat and, most importantly, assessing the response to treatment. If the response to treatment is that there is no improvement, then we must think again.

> *It is not a case we are treating; it is a living, palpating, alas, too often suffering fellow creature.*
> John Brown, physician, 1810 – 1882[1]

So, a proper diagnosis is always retrospective.

> *Life can only be understood backwards; but it must be lived forwards.*
> Søren Aabye Kierkegaard, Danish philosopher, theologian and poet, 5 May 1813 – 11 November 1855

> *A reckoning up of the cause often solves the malady.*
> Celsus, Roman scholar and author of the encyclopaedic *De Medicina*, *Prooemium*, 25 BC – 50 AD[†]

All diagnosis starts with a hypothesis which has to be put to the clinical test of response to treatment. The huge variation between individuals, what they can do and how they respond, means that every case is unique. You will make mistakes. Heaven knows, I have made my share of mistakes too. You will have to fly in the face of perceived wisdoms. I too have been and still am there. It will be a bumpy ride. But therein lies the reason why medicine will always be so interesting and life so engaging.

You may receive some ridicule or even incredulity, but soldier on, safe in the knowledge that a brain no lesser than Voltaire knew this:

---

*William Osler used to holiday at Gull cottage, Landermere, on the Essex coast, where all my childhood holidays were taken. The local gossip there was that he was Jack the Ripper. However, I subscribe to Patricia Cornwall's brilliant analysis which names Walter Sickert – another wonderful detective story.

†Historical note: Not much at all is known about the life of Aulus Cornelius Celsus. In fact, it is not known for sure whether his first name was Aulus. Of the many volumes of his encyclopaedia, only one remains intact – *On Medicine (De Medicina)*. He follows the division of medicine, established by Hippocrates, into diet, pharmacology and surgery. In his treatments, Celsus's preferred method is to observe the 'operations' of Nature, and to regulate these operations, rather than to oppose or, as we might say, 'squash' or 'suppress' them. So, for example, he believed that a fever was an effort by the body to 'throw off some morbid cause'. How right he was. Celsus was not a symptom-squasher.

Our wretched species is so made that those who walk on the well-trodden path always throw stones at those who are showing a new road.

François-Marie Arouet, known by his *nom de plume*, Voltaire, 21 November 1694 – 30 May 1778

...and know also that your life will be lived to its full potential.

Reference

1. Brown J. *Lancet* 1904; 1: 464. Interested readers should see: McDonald P. *The Oxford Dictionary of Medical Quotations*. OUP 2003, p 16.

Chapter 11
Fatigue mechanisms: the fuel in the tank

– diet, micronutrients and gut function
– tests

I spend more time discussing diet, micronutrients and gut function than all others put together. Craig and I have written two other books which supply much more detail – namely, *Prevent and Cure Diabetes – delicious diets, not dangerous drugs*, which answers the question *why* to do the PK diet and *The PK Cookbook – go paleo-ketogenic and get the best of both worlds*, which answers the question of *how* to do the PK diet. The details that follow are a distillation of the *why*.

The paleo-ketogenic (PK) diet

Let food be thy medicine and medicine be thy food!
Hippocrates, father of western Medicine, c 460 – 370 BC

Humans, and indeed all mammals, evolved over millions of years eating a PK diet based on protein, fat and vegetable fibre. Even vegetarian mammals rely on vegetable fibre that is fermented to short-chain fatty acids – they too power themselves with fat.

The human brain was able to grow in size and complexity quickly because primitive man hunted meat, fish and gathered shell fish. Meat and fat provide the perfect raw materials for brain structure and function together with the necessary stimuli for growth through social co-operation for successful hunting. There may have been the occasional carbohydrate bonanza. In the autumn we ate carbohydrates in an addictive way (a useful survival tool) and this allowed us to lay down fat, with helpful survival value for the winter. But when autumn finished, we returned to hunting because we had no choice. Fossilised human turds look like dog turds! Primitive man was primarily a carnivore. Cave paintings show hunters.

Fat is a wonderful fuel. It is energy dense, not fermented in the gut and easily utilised. So, the human gut shrank. This made man a much more successful hunter because he was not carrying a huge fermenting belly. It is only in the last few thousand years, negligible in evolutionary time, that carbohydrates have crept into the diet as man has learned to farm and to cook. It is only in the past few decades that sugar and refined carbohydrates have replaced fat as our fuel, with disastrous metabolic consequences. Since the Neolithic, or Agricultural, revolution human brain sizes have decreased by 8%. Even now through their lives, vegetarians suffer much more brain shrinkage than meat eaters, vegans even more. For example, a study in the journal *Neurology* in September 2008 found that brain volume loss was associated with the low levels of vitamin B12, often found in vegans and vegetarians.[1] This study also found associations with Alzheimer's disease and other cognitive failures. Also, a study in the *BMJ* in August 2019 concluded that choline (an 'essential' nutrient that cannot be produced by the body in amounts needed for human requirements and so therefore needs to be consumed) is essential for brain function and that 'accelerated food trends towards plant-based diets/veganism could have further ramifications on choline intake/status'.[2] Finally, although direct causality has yet to be conclusively proven, Michalak et al concluded that: 'In Western cultures vegetarian diet is associated with an elevated risk of mental disorders.'[3]

> *Fat is the most valuable food known to man.*
>
> Professor John Yudkin, British physiologist and nutritionist, 1910 – 1995

I recommend all my patients read Barry Grove's excellent presentation on this topic[4] and the book that summarises his thinking, *Trick and Treat – how 'healthy eating' is making us ill*,[5] though this is now a relatively old book. For many, a good understanding of the evolutionary imperatives is enough to make them change their diet.

Some vegetable fibre is still essential to nourish the lining of the large bowel. This is dependent for its fuel source on the fermentation of vegetable fibre by friendly anaerobic microbes, mainly bacteroides species. Complete lack of bacteroides may result in major pathology, such as ulcerative colitis.

Fruit would only have been consumed once a year, when the fruit tree ripened. Modern fruits are also different, carefully bred to appeal to modern man's addictive sweet tooth. Primitive humans' idea of an apple would have been a crab apple.*

There may have been, as noted, the occasional carbohydrate bonanza and so metabolic syndrome evolved as a mechanism to store these carbohydrates in the short term, as muscle and liver glycogen; in the long term, as fat. Female sex hormones encourage metabolic syndrome so as to lay down fat in preparation for the energy-sapping business of pregnancy and breastfeeding. However, with the advent of winter, primitive man had to revert to his primitive, low-carb, high-fat hunter diet. By contrast, modern Westerners live in a permanent state of 'autumn' because they can. Constant carbohydrate consumption leads to metabolic syndrome and is defined by the contents of the supermarket trolley. My daughter lives in Paris and is a people watcher. I am a supermarket trolley watcher and am fascinated by what goes in; I look with a combination of horror and disgust at the piles of junk which masquerades as food. Serious disease results. This starts in the classrooms and nurseries, with fat, unfit and fatigued kids and falling intelligence, and progresses to premature death with diabetes and dementia, cancer and coronaries.

So, if meat and fish are such perfect foods, then why did humans move on to other foods? Increasing population, hunger and intelligence to improve the propagation of our genes. As detailed earlier, Nature is only interested

---

*Footnote:** Craig used to scrump crab apples from his neighbour's garden, but these trees are no longer there; the humble crab apple is out of fashion. (Craig's note to Her Majesty's law enforcement agencies – this offence is, in my opinion, now time limited.)

in procreation of selfish genes (see Richard Dwarkins *The Selfish Gene*[6]). I am on the evolutionary scrapheap – no matter if I cark it[†]... I have passed my genetic Olympic torch on to my daughters and it is too late for me to do any more such. Bringing carbohydrates into the diet allows more of us to get to breeding age. The fact that the cost of this is reduced longevity is of little evolutionary interest.

I doubt that anyone has fully adapted to cope with the recent addition of unrefined carbohydrates. What I do know is that this ability to cope declines with age. I know that my CFS/ME patients are carnivorous evolutionary relics. I do not have CFS/ME myself, but I too function much better eating a PK diet. There are many interventions I can suggest which are clinically helpful, but in the treatment of almost any patient a good PK diet is almost invariably the single most important and most difficult intervention required.

In particular then, it is important to look in detail at metabolic syndrome – what happens when we fuel our bodies with carbohydrates.

Metabolic syndrome: carbohydrate intolerance and hypoglycaemia, *the* major cause of ill health in Westerners

The fuel for our mitochondrial engines is ultimately acetate groups. Evolution intended that these come from, in order of importance, three possible sources:
* beta oxidation of fat
* short-chain fatty acids from the fermentation of vegetable fibre in the large bowel
* glycogen stores in the liver and muscle.

The problem with eating sugar, fruit sugar and refined carbohydrate is that the primary fuels of fat and fibre are bypassed. This is dangerous metabolism because it exposes us to that inflammable (or flammable – see page 7.1) petrol of a fuel – namely, sugar. Sugar is NOT an essential fuel. It is highly toxic. The problem is that, if the body has got used to running on sugar and carbs (and this is called metabolic syndrome), then wobbly blood sugar levels result and this in turn results in serious symptoms. If the blood sugar level falls too low, energy supply to all tissues, particularly to the brain, is impaired. However, if blood sugar levels rise too high, then this is very damaging to arteries, and the long-term result of arterial disease is heart disease and stroke. This is caused by sugar sticking to proteins and fats to make AGEs (advanced glycation end-products), which accelerate the ageing process. Glycosylated haemoglobin, or HbA1c, is just one such AGE. Poorly controlled diabetics have high levels of AGEs and are at high risk of disease and death (from arterial disease, sticky blood, dementia and cancer).

Excess sugar flooding into the system after a high-carbohydrate meal should be mopped up by the muscle and liver glycogen sponge, but only so long as there is space there for both to act as a metabolic sponge. The sponge empties when we exercise. Exercise depletes glycogen in the muscles, so squeezing the sponge dry. This system of control works perfectly well until it is overwhelmed, by either eating excessive

---

[†]**Linguistic note:** The verb 'to cark it' is Australian slang for 'to die'. As to its derivation, there are a few possibilities put forward. Some say that it is onomatopoeic, sounding like a dying person. Others say it is a shortening of the word 'carcass'. There is even a suggestion that it derives from the Hindi *Khak* (meaning dust), and therefore relates to the phrase 'dust to dust, ashes to ashes' used at funerals, and that it arose during the British Raj and was then 'exported' as a phrase to Australia. The reader can make up her own mind as to the most likely. There are over 1000 words meaning 'to die' in the English language![7]

carbohydrate and/or not exercising. On a PK diet there are no blood sugar control problems at all. Modern-day keto-adapted humans can run a blood sugar of 1.0 mmol/l (reference range 4-7 mmol/l) and experience no poor energy delivery symptoms. The US National record for running the furthest distance in 24 hours is held by Mike Morton, a keto-adapted athlete, who covered 172 miles.

Nowadays the situation is different: we eat large amounts of sugar and refined carbohydrate and do not exercise enough in order to squeeze dry the glycogen sponge. The body therefore has to cope with this excessive sugar load by other mechanisms. The key player here is insulin, a hormone secreted by the pancreas. This is effective at bringing blood sugar levels down and does so by shunting the sugar into fat. The amount of insulin released is proportional to the rate at which blood sugar levels rise – this is what makes dietary sugar so pernicious; it is rapidly absorbed, and blood levels rise rapidly. Indeed, this rapid rise gives an addictive hit – the faster the better! A video of blood sugar levels on a high-carb diet would look like the Rocky Mountains. Beer is particularly high in sugar and alcohol, and drunk quickly gives the best addictive hit of all carbohydrates. Many foods achieve the same hit and we call this 'comfort eating' – we use it to deal with stress because, in the short term, it masks the symptoms of such. Sugar, fruit sugar and refined carbohydrates (white flours, white rice, cooked potato and other root vegetables) are addictive – especially sugar. I know because I am an addict. I have kicked that addiction but once an addict always an addict!

In the short term, the brain loves this addictive carbohydrate hit, but it is highly damaging to the body. Insulin is poured out to deal with this high. Remember the rate at which the blood sugar rises determines the amount of insulin released. Blood sugars come crashing down as insulin

shunts sugar into fat cells via triglycerides. The body is saved from sugar damage (hurrah!), but as blood sugar levels fall quickly, the brain goes into panic mode – it cannot afford to run out of energy, which means going unconscious and becoming easy prey for the local sabre-toothed tiger. The main panic hormone is adrenalin (there are others) and this is poured out in response to the falling blood sugar levels. We associate the falling blood sugars with adrenalin, and indeed it is adrenalin and other stress hormones which are responsible for the symptoms we call hypoglycaemia.

The clinical picture that arises from using sugar and carbohydrates as a primary fuel for our mitochondria (the power stations of our cells) is called metabolic syndrome. Doctors often wait until a patient is obese and has high blood pressure before diagnosing such – but that is too late. Metabolic syndrome further progresses to diabetes, cardiovascular disease, mental disorders, degenerative conditions (including arthritis and osteoporosis) and cancer. Alzheimer's disease has been dubbed 'type 3 diabetes'.

The symptoms of hypoglycaemia are varied (and worsened by the upper fermenting gut because of the alcohols produced – see page 11.7) and derive from the various mechanisms that give rise to the stress response and result from it.

Symptoms of hypoglycaemia

The symptoms of hypoglycaemia arise from:
- Adrenalin release: disturbed sleep, shakiness, anxiety, nervousness, palpitations, tachycardia, sweating, feeling of warmth, pallor, coldness, clamminess, dilated pupils, numb feelings, 'pins and needles'
- Glucagon and other gut hormone release: hunger, rumbling gut, nausea, vomiting, abdominal discomfort, headache
- Poor energy delivery to the body and brain (see Chapter 5).

Tests for hypoglycaemia

One can test for hypoglycaemia, but in practice the clinical picture is so characteristic that I rarely request any tests. A one-off blood sugar test tells us very little because timing is all – we do not know at which point of the blood sugar roller-coaster of metabolic syndrome we are looking. Ideally, we need a 'video' of blood sugar levels taken over several days. Purchase your own blood sugar monitor and measure several times through the day. A blood glucose reading taken when the adrenalin hypoglycaemia symptoms occur may be misleading because it is the rate at which blood sugar falls (not the absolute level) that determines the amount of adrenalin released.

The most practical diagnostic tools are:
- One's total bill at the supermarket checkout for carbohydrate-based foods
- Being apple shaped – fat is dumped where the immune system is busy so being apple shaped points to having an upper fermenting gut. And yes, sigh, my young daughters delighted in loudly exclaiming this diagnosis during supermarket trips
- High body mass index (BMI) – but a normal BMI does not exclude the diagnosis!
- Raised glycosylated haemoglobin – a measure of sugar stuck to haemoglobin as described above; this is a very useful measure of average blood sugar levels (see Appendix 4)
- High LDL cholesterol and low HDL cholesterol relative to total cholesterol (see Chapter 42 for the 'why')
- A 12-hour fasting blood sugar – this should be below 5.6 mmol/l but ideally below 5.0
- Variable blood pressure initially (as a result of the adrenalin released with falling blood sugar levels), then continuous high blood pressure as arteries become stiffened through scarring. Again, one can easily purchase home blood pressure monitors

- High normal erythrocyte sedimentation rate (ESR) and high normal plasma viscosity. (Be aware, the 'normal range' for ESR has changed over time. It used to be 1-10 mm per hour. That has been increased to 1-20 mm/hour, rising with age. This reflects the fact that metabolic syndrome is now considered 'normal', but it isn't normal, and it is actually driving inflammation.)

Micronutrients

Westerners all need micronutrient supplements in addition to a PK diet because:
- Modern agriculture results in micronutrient-deficient crops
- Food storage and processing further depletes micronutrient levels
- We are physically inactive, we need less food and therefore consume fewer micronutrients
- We are all inevitably exposed to more toxins in the environment which require additional micronutrients to help detoxify them; these may be persistent organic pollutants (POPs – pesticides, volatile organic compounds, heavy metals), noxious gases, food additives, social addictions or prescribed medications. Many of these require micronutrients for their elimination from the body.

Tests of micronutrient status can be done through blood, sweat or urine testing. It is important to consult with the lab because some tests can be misleading. For example, a serum magnesium is unhelpful since serum magnesium is maintained by the body at the expense of magnesium levels inside cells. Most doctors do not understand the difference between a serum magnesium and a red cell magnesium. The point is, serum levels must be kept within a tight range, or the heart stops. Therefore, serum levels are maintained at the expense of levels inside cells. Most labs just do serum levels and patients are told their magnesium is normal. Hair tests also can be misleading. In practice I rarely do these tests on a 'virgin' patient because I know they will be deficient. We should all be taking a basic package of multivitamins, minerals and essential fatty acids (see Groundhog Basic, page A1).

In addition to the above, there are some interesting evolutionary wrinkles which have implications for modern diets and supplements:

- **Vitamin C** – During our evolution humans, together with fruit bats, guinea pigs and dry-nosed primates, lost their ability to manufacture their own vitamin C. This explains why your dog does not get scurvy from eating a pure meat diet. Humans invariably have levels of vitamin C that are too low for optimum health. I recommend taking vitamin C daily, at least 5 grams (5000 mg) for Groundhog Basic, and to bowel tolerance for Groundhog Acute and Chronic. Vitamin C multitasks – it is highly protective against both the upper fermenting gut and chronic infection. I see vitamin C and sugar as two sides of the same coin and any condition associated with metabolic syndrome is reversed by vitamin C (see Chapter 31, and, for even more detail, our book *The Infection Game – life is an arms race*).

- **Vitamin D** – Humans evolved in Africa, running naked under the African sunshine, and developing a dark skin to protect against burning ultraviolet light was a huge evolutionary advantage. We evolved the ability to make vitamin D from the effect of UV light on cholesterol in the skin – vitamin D is markedly anti-inflammatory and further protected the skin from damaging inflammation in response to this UV. Vitamin D diffuses through the rest of the body, where it acts

as a general anti-inflammatory. What this means clinically is that the further away from the Equator one lives, the greater the tendency to pro-inflammatory conditions. Sunshine is by far and away the most important source of vitamin D. One hour of Mediterranean sun produces about 10,000 iu (international units) of vitamin D. As primitive man migrated away from the Equator, he started to run into problems with vitamin D deficiency and so a lighter skin became an evolutionary advantage – so modern Mediterraneans are olivaceous, and Northerners, white. Indeed, Northerners followed sea routes with high fish diets so much of their vitamin D was derived from eating fish. Most modern Caucasians are vitamin D deficient. There is an inverse relation between sunshine exposure, vitamin D levels and incidence of disease as one moves away from the Equator. Vitamin D protects against osteoarthritis, osteoporosis, fractures (vitamin D improves muscle strength, thereby improving balance, movement and preventing falls), cancer, hypertension, high cholesterol, diabetes, heart disease, multiple sclerosis and susceptibility to infections. In the absence of sunshine, I recommend at least 5000 – and up to 10,000 – iu of D3 daily. No toxicity has ever been seen at these doses.

- **Vitamin B3** – This is not, strictly speaking, a vitamin. The body can synthesise vitamin B3 (niacin, niacinamide) from the amino acid tryptophan. However, it needs large amounts of protein to do so. Paleo diets were high in protein, modern diets are lacking, and so now for most people niacin has become a vitamin. I recommend 1500 mg slow-release daily.

- **Glutathione** – This is almost invariably deficient because it is in such demand to detoxify a variety of modern pollutants. I recommend at least 250 mg daily.

- **Minerals** – A good diet with good micronutrient content is only of use if it can be assimilated into the body. Colonel Danny Goodwin Jones of Trace Element Services (see page A33) uses minerals to treat, with great results, a wide range of problems in farm animals, from failure to thrive to prevention of TB in cattle. I was puzzled why I was not seeing the same dramatic benefits in humans taking mineral supplements until the penny dropped. Farm animals are fed their evolutionary correct diet of grass. They have normal gut function. By contrast, humans eating high-carbohydrate, high-allergen diets all have upper fermenting gut with inflammation and high levels of microbes in the upper gut. The supplements were simply feeding these abnormal microbes. The upper fermenting gut occurs when the amount of carbohydrate eaten overwhelms our ability to digest it. When fermented, the immune system has to act to prevent the fermentation products invading, and we know that where the immune system is busy, there is dumped fat. Upper gut fermenters are apple shaped, as I have said.

The upper fermenting gut

Gastroenterologists like to call this condition 'small bowel bacterial overgrowth' (SIBO) but I do not like that name because it excludes the possibility of fermentation in the stomach, and fermentation by yeast and other microbes. Infection with *Helicobacter pylori* (the major cause of stomach and duodenal ulcer) is one example of a fermenting microbe.

We can all develop a fermenting upper gut if we eat sufficient carbohydrate to overwhelm our body's ability to digest and absorb it. I do that when I eat too much at Christmas. However, lack of stomach acid and pancreatic enzymes and bile salts, all of which kill microbes, further predispose us to upper fermenting gut. So does poor energy delivery since the business of digesting, absorbing and dealing with the results of such in the liver is greatly demanding of energy. I now know that virtually all people eating Western carbohydrate-based diets eventually develop upper fermenting gut and this drives many pathologies.

The consequences of upper fermenting gut are many, as shown in Table 11.1.

Hypochlorhydria in more detail

We need an acid stomach for protein digestion, absorption of micronutrients (especially minerals and vitamin B12) and protection against infection. Altogether, 90% of infection comes in through the mouth by eating or inhalation. Those inhaled microbes should get stuck on sticky mucus which is eventually swallowed, and which should then meet their Maker in the acid bath of the stomach. Insufficient stomach acid, hypochlorhydria, results in poor protein digestion, malabsorption of minerals, upper fermenting gut and susceptibility to infections. Symptoms of acidity and acid reflux (GORD – gastro-oesophageal reflux disease) may be due to what I call a 'half acid' stomach.

The normal oesophagus is neutral at pH 7. Normal stomach contents are extremely acid at pH 2-4. The normal duodenum is alkaline at pH 8. As foods are eaten and enter the stomach, the effect of the food arriving dilutes stomach contents and the pH rises (acidity goes down). The stomach pours in more acid to allow proper digestion and sterilisation of food and the pH falls back to its normal value of 2-4. The key to understanding GORD is the pyloric sphincter, which is the muscle which controls emptying of the stomach into the duodenum. This muscle is acid sensitive, and it only relaxes when the acidity of the stomach is correct – that is, 2-4.

Table 11.1: The consequences of upper fermenting gut

What	Why
Hypochlorhydria – i.e. low levels of stomach acid	See below for the detail, but in a nutshell this leads to leaky gut, which means acid cannot be concentrated in the upper gut
Hypochlorhydria results in reflux (often diagnosed as hiatus hernia) and oesophagitis	The stomach cannot empty downstream, so it bubbles upstream
Hypochlorhydria results in belching, bloating and possibly colicky pain	Foods ferment to gases which distend the gut
Hypochlorhydria results in susceptibility to infections	Ingested and inhaled microbes (which are coughed up and swallowed) are not killed in a bath of stomach acid
Hypochlorhydria results in osteoporosis	One needs an acid environment to absorb minerals
Fatigue – products of fermentation include various alcohols, hydrogen sulphide, D-lactate and other such…	…which have the potential to inhibit mitochondria as well as kick a 'detox' hole in the energy bucket – at rest the liver (the body's 'detoxer') consumes more energy than the brain and heart combined
Foggy brain – the fermenting gut is also known as the auto-brewery syndrome	It makes us 'drunk' – indeed, this may contribute to drink-driving cases (perhaps another reason for calling it the auto-brewery syndrome – boom boom!)
Hypoglycaemia – alcohol stimulates insulin release, which directly causes blood sugar levels to drop	This is why alcohol is so dangerous in the diabetic on blood sugar-reducing medication
Allergies – one can sensitise to gut microbes which, contrary to conventional medical opinion, translocate into the bloodstream and get stuck at distal sites[8]	I suspect this explains many allergic symptoms which do not respond to allergy elimination diets, such as arthritis, polymyalgia rheumatica, interstitial cystitis, vulvitis, prostatitis, connective tissue disease, temporal arteritis, urticaria and, possibly, asthma, varicose eczema, acne and rosacea, tinnitus, age-related deafness and many others
Psychological and psychiatric disorders – work by the Japanese researcher Professor Nishihara suggests that gut microbes appear in the brain with the potential to ferment brain neurotransmitters to neuro-active and psycho-active substances like LSD and amphetamine.[9]	This may explain a loss of touch with reality, such as severe mood swings, paranoia, hallucinations, obsessive compulsive disorders, eating disorders and behaviour disorders.

At this point stomach contents can empty into the duodenum (where they are neutralised by bicarbonate released from the liver via the bile ducts).

If the stomach does not produce enough acid and the pH is only, say, 5, then the muscle which allows the stomach to empty (the pyloric sphincter) will not open. The stomach contracts in order to move food into the duodenum, but the progress of the food is blocked by this contracted pyloric sphincter. So, the pressure of food in the stomach increases and gets squirted back up into the oesophagus. Although this food is not very acidic (not acid enough to relax the pyloric sphincter), it is sufficiently acid to burn the oesophagus and so one gets the symptoms of gastro-oesophageal reflux. The paradox is that this symptom is caused by insufficient stomach acid – in other words, the reverse of what is generally believed.

Acid blockers, such as proton pump inhibitors (e.g. omeprazole) and H2 blockers (e.g. zantac) may afford short-term relief of hyper-acidity symptoms but spell disaster for gut function. Minerals are malabsorbed (resulting in osteoporosis), proteins are not broken down (resulting in allergies as large, antigenically interesting molecules appear downstream) and the gut is not sterilised, resulting in fermenting gut, susceptibility to infection, increased risk of cancer, osteoporosis and dementia. I often ask my patients if their prescribing doctor has advised them of these long-term side effects; the result is a resounding never.

Tests for hypochlorhydria
The following are easy to do yourself:
- 'The burp test': Swallowing bicarbonate, say ½ teaspoon in ½ pint water, on a fasting, empty stomach should result in belching within two minutes as carbon dioxide is released by the action of acid on bicarbonate. If it does not, then suspect hypochlorhydria.
- Finding meat fibres present in a stool analysis (but this may also be due to poor pancreatic function).

Tests for fermenting gut
In order of clinical usefulness, these are:
- Comprehensive digestive stool analysis, which screens out major pathology, gives a good handle on the ability to digest and indicates which microbes are fermenting (not that this matters terribly since the starting point to treat is the same – PK diet and vitamin C to bowel tolerance)
- Breath tests for *H pylori* and other upper gut fermenters (hydrogen, lactose and lactulose breath tests). Remember, a negative test does not mean there is no gut fermentation.

Pancreatic function
In the duodenum and small intestine, pancreatic enzymes and bile salts are essential to emulsify, digest and absorb proteins, carbohydrates, fats, essential fatty acids and fat-soluble vitamins. They further help reduce numbers of microbes in the upper gut. If one's ability to digest is overwhelmed, then proteins are fermented downstream to produce foul-smelling wind. This happens to me at Christmas when I am greedy. Thankfully I expect to be out on my horse on Boxing day, so others do not suffer the consequences!

Fat in the stools may produce greasy floating stools, another indication of digestive function being overwhelmed.

Tests of pancreatic function
Useful tests include:
- Faecal elastase
- Comprehensive digestive stool analysis – to measure levels of enzymes and bile sales in the stool, together with the presence of meat fibres and fats

- Blood amylase is a test of damage to the pancreas and is only abnormal where there is severe pathology.

However, the best test for fermenting gut is response to treatment – starve the little wretches out with a paleo-ketogenic diet and kill them with vitamin C to bowel tolerance (see Chapter 31; Tools of the trade plus much more in *The Infection Game – life is an arms race*)

Over time, you may feel that you are sliding down the forgetting curve illustrated in Chapter 5, but fear not. Remember, 'doing it' and occasionally dipping into the text will do the trick. In any case, the forgetting curve hypothesis is imperfect. Among its imperfections are that memory is enhanced by, for example, a good night's sleep, and you will have enhanced sleep if you follow Groundhog Basic. Another serious limitation in the forgetting curve hypothesis is its lack of taking account of the 'flashbulb memory' phenomenon. This is where people have vivid 'imprinted' memories of important moments, such as your wedding day, or the day you got your decree nisi through. These imprinted memories often happen because they are reinforced by emotions felt at the time – so when you no longer feel 'that fatigue', or when you 'have a good night's sleep' or when you 'don't feel that familiar pain in your shoulder', this may well 'imprint' the contents of this book in your memory!

References

1. Vogiatzoglou A, Refsum H, Johnston C, Smith SM, et al. Vitamin B12 status and rate of brain volume loss in community-dwelling elderly. *Neurology* 2008; 71(11): 826-832. DOI: 10.1212/01.wnl.0000325581.26991.f2
2. Derbyshire E. Could we be overlooking a potential choline crisis in the UK? *BMJ Nutrition, Prevention and Health* 2019; 0: 1-4. doi:10.1136/bmjnph-2019-000037
3. Michalak J, Zhang XC, Jacobi F. Vegetarian diet and mental disorders: results from a representative community survey. *Int J Behav Nutr Phys Act* 2012; 9: 67. doi: 10.1186/1479-5868-9-67
4. Groves B. http://files.meetup.com/1463924/Homo%20Carnivorous-WAPF2.pdf
5. Groves B. *Trick and Treat – how 'healthy eating' is making us ill* 2009: Hammersmith Books Limited.
6. Dwarkin R. *The Selfish Gene* OUP, 1978 (4th revised edition 2018).
7. Crystal D. A thousand words of death. *The Guardian* 13 September 2014. www.theguardian.com/books/2014/sep/13/a-thousand-words-for-death-lexicon-dying-david-crystal (accessed 18 November 2019)
8. Berg RD. Bacterial translocation from the gastrointestinal tract. *Adv Exp Med Biol* 1999; 473: 11-30. www.ncbi.nlm.nih.gov/pubmed/10659341
9. Nishihara K. Disclosure of the major causes of mental illness – mitochondrial deterioration in brain neurons via opportunistic infection. *Journal of Biological Physics and Chemistry* 2012; 12: 11-18.

Chapter 12
Fatigue mechanisms: the engine and fuel delivery

**– the engine of our car – mitochondria
– fuel and oxygen delivery – the heart, circulation and lungs
– tests**

An analogy we often use in our other books, and on my website, is that of the body as a car. In brief, here is how this analogy works:

Engine...	mitochondria
Fuel...	diet and gut function
Oxygen...	lungs
Fuel and oxygen delivery...	heart and circulation
Accelerator pedal...	thyroid gland
Gear box...	adrenal glands
Service and repair...	sleep
Tool kit...	methylation cycle
Cleaning – oil...	antioxidants
Catalytic converter...	detoxification
A driver...	the brain in a fit state!

In this chapter we look primarily at the body's engine(s) – the mitochondria.

All mammals are made up of about 300 different cell types – muscle cells, nerve cells, skin cells and so on – all of which have a different job of work to do. Whatever that job happens to be, it will require energy. The way that energy is supplied to cells is the same for all cells and, indeed, all living creatures. Energy is delivered by tiny engines within cells that take fuel from the bloodstream and burn it in the presence of oxygen to make energy in the form of ATP. These engines are called mitochondria. The mitochondria in X Files-fan Craig's pet frog Gillian, are the same as those in me. A heart cell may contain 2000 to 3000 mitochondria, and a heart by weight is 25% mitochondria.

ATP is the currency of energy in the body. With ATP we can buy any job, from contracting a muscle to making a hormone. ATP is present in every living cell and makes the difference between a living cell and a dead one. Indeed, if ATP levels fall low this triggers apoptosis – that is, cell suicide. If energy delivery is impaired, then the cell will go slow; if the cell goes slow, then the organ goes slow. Poor ATP delivery – in other words, poor energy delivery – can therefore result in many different symptoms.

For good energy delivery, not only must the mitochondria be working well, but there must be enough of them. The business of getting physically and mentally fit and staying fit is all about putting in place interventions to allow mitochondria to work to their full potential, and then getting more of them. There is much more detail in our book *Diagnosis and Treatment of Chronic Fatigue Syndrome and Myalgic Encephalitis – it's mitochondria not hypochondria*; these people are mitochondriacs, not hypochondriacs!

Since 2005 we have done over 900 mitochondrial function tests and published three papers on the subject[1, 2, 3] (thank you again John, Norman and Craig*). What we know is that our mitochondrial engines can go slow for four possible reasons:

- They do not have the raw materials to function efficiently (raw materials for the molecular machinery)
- They do not have the raw materials to function efficiently because they are being starved of fuel and oxygen; this depends on good function of the heart, lungs and bloodstream
- They are blocked by a toxin from the outside world (pesticide, volatile organic compound, toxic metal) or the inside world (products of the fermenting gut, or of chronic inflammation)
- The control mechanisms of the thyroid accelerator pedal or the adrenal gear box are faulty.

To explain in more detail why mitochondria might not function properly:

- **Not enough raw materials for mitochondria to work** – The common rate-limiting steps are deficiencies of magnesium, vitamin B3, acetyl L-carnitine, co-enzyme Q10 and D-ribose. However, there will be others.
- **Mitochondrial membranes are not in good nick** – It is the membranes of the mitochondria that hold the bundles of enzymes (cristae) in just the right 3D configuration to allow all the biochemical steps to proceed efficiently. These membranes contain cardiolipin which is unique to mitochondria. They need the right combination of fats to achieve this.
- **The mitochondria are blocked by a toxin** – These toxins can come from the body (e.g. aldehydes from poor antioxidant status, products of the upper fermenting gut, mycotoxins) or from outside the body (e.g. pesticides, heavy metals, volatile organic substances and, again, mycotoxins). Mitochondria can also be blocked by lactic

---

*Note from Craig: My involvement was limited as follows – after obtaining 'mito scores' for a number of patients and listing all these out with their ability levels, Sarah sent a spreadsheet of these results to me in 2005. About three hours later I emailed Sarah, saying, 'The correlation coefficient is 0.8, or thereabouts. You've got something here.' This was a genuine 'Wow!' moment.† Then the really hard work of writing a formal scientific paper fell to Sarah, Professor Norman E Booth and Dr John McLaren-Howard. Sadly, Norman Booth passed away in August 2018. He was a tireless advocate for CFS/ME, and was often seen at Oxfordshire ME Group for Action (OMEGA) meetings, but in addition, we should not forget that he was an accomplished academic, with 158 research items listed on his research gate page: www.researchgate.net/profile/Norman_Booth

†Footnote from Craig: The Wow signal is a famous signal picked up by the SETI project – 'Search for Extraterrestial Intelligence' – on one of its radio telescopes in 1977. The signal was repetitive and ticked all the boxes for having been transmitted by an extraterrestial intelligence. The scientist who first noticed this signal, Jerry R Ehman, wrote 'Wow' on the printout next to it, thereby naming it for all time. When I (Craig) left Oxford in 1985, I made only two job applications – one to Price Waterhouse, Chartered Accountants, and one to SETI. I was shortlisted down to the final two for the SETI job but then Ronald Reagan introduced an 'Americans only' policy to some US departments and SETI was included. I went off to be a beancounter.

acid. This represents just one of the many vicious cycles we see in pathologically fatigued patients – the more one slips into anaerobic metabolism, the harder it is to get out of it. This is a 'cycle' because when mitochondria function poorly, the body switches into anaerobic respiration more quickly than it would for a 'fit' person, and a product of anaerobic respiration is lactic acid, which can block the mitochondria, thereby making their function even worse, and so more lactic acid is produced via further anaerobic respiration, and so on we go. This is an obvious mechanism by which the body protects us from ourselves – it stops us spending energy before we run out of it completely (which results in death).

- **The control mechanisms of the thyroid accelerator pedal or the adrenal gear box are faulty** – See Chapter 13.

Relevant tests to correct mitochondrial function

- Tests to identify deficiencies – blood tests for co-enzyme Q10, vitamin B3 levels (red cell NAD), acetyl L-carnitine, red cell (not serum) magnesium
- Tests to identify blockages – Genova core test for pesticides and VOCs; Toxic metals in urine following a chelating agent
- Tests for membrane integrity – Biolab essential fatty acids
- Tests for antioxidant status – Biolab blood antioxidant profile and/or urine.

How to increase the number of mitochondria – we need a big engine

For good energy delivery not only must mito-chondria be working efficiently but we need lots of them. To increase the numbers (and so the 'size' of our engine) we need exercise and thyroid and adrenal hormones (see Chapter 23: Exercise, and Chapter 13: Fatigue mechanisms II, for the thyroid accelerator pedal and the adrenal gear box.)

What we also know from our third scientific paper[3] is that by using the tools of the trade (Chapter 30), then correction of mitochondrial function occurs reliably well. If this is not paralleled by clinical improvement, then there must be other causes of the fatigue.

Energy delivery to the brain – relies on fats

There is a further interesting peculiarity with respect to the energy supply to the brain which is different from that used by the rest of the body. Although the brain weighs just 2% of total body weight, it uses 20% of total energy generated in the body. There are not enough mitochondria in the brain to explain this, which means there must be another energy-generating source. Brain cells are also very different from normal cells. They have a cell body, and very long tails – or dendrites – which communicate with other cells. Indeed, if a nerve-cell body from the spinal cord that supplied one's toes was sitting on my desk and was the size of a football, the tail would be in New York assuming one was in London. These tails (dendrites) are too narrow to contain mitochondria, but it has been suggested that the energy supply comes directly from the myelin sheaths which wrap around nerve fibres. Myelin has adopted mitochondrial biochemistry to produce ATP and it is this that supplies the energy for neuro-transmission. Myelin sheaths are made up almost entirely of fats, so we need to look to oils and fats for improved energy supply to brain cells.

Humans evolved on the East Coast of Africa eating a diet rich in sea food. It is suggested that the high levels of oils, particularly fish oils, allowed the brain to develop fast. Primitive humans came to have bigger brains, so allowing intelligence to develop. Essential fatty acids are vital for normal brain function. We need two types of fat for good brain function – firstly, medium-chain fats as fuels, such as meat fat (lard and dripping), butter, coconut oil, palm oil and chocolate fat; secondly, fats for building membranes for energy delivery in the myelin sheaths – these are long-chain fats from vegetable, fish, nut and seed oils. Our modern so-cial phobia of cholesterol and fat is producing an epidemic of depression and dementia.

There is much more on the importance of these fats in Appendix 3 of our book *Prevent and Cure Diabetes - delicious diets not danger-ous drugs* and in Appendix 1 of our book *The PK Cookbook – go paleo-ketogenic and get the best of both worlds.*

Oxygen supply and fuel delivery – heart, lungs, blood and blood vessels

Oxygen – even I know what happens when my cylinder runs out!
Coal miner from Annesley Woodhouse, Nottinghamshire, with pneumoconiosis, c. 1985
(Craig's beloved Scully, of *The X Files*, made a similar comment in season 1 episode 8.)

Oxygen and fuel delivery require a healthy pair of lungs for oxygen exchange to take place, good oxygen-carrying capacity (that is, good levels of haemoglobin in the blood), open arter-ies and a strongly pumping heart. Symptoms of failures of the above would include all the symp-toms of poor energy delivery. In addition, one may see shortness of breath, pallor and/or cold extremities, and – in extreme cases – blueness, or 'cyanosis', of extremities and lips.

The heart

Cardiac output may be reduced for several possible reasons, all of which come under the umbrella of 'heart disease'. The mechanisms are as follows:

- **Poor energy delivery mechanisms to the heart:** This may be due to poor blood supply (arteriosclerosis) or poor mitochondrial function. This is one area where there is an obvious vicious cycle for my pathologically fatigued CFS/ME patients – poor energy delivery to the heart means that it does not beat strongly as a pump and therefore this will further impair fuel and oxygen delivery and therefore worsen mitochondrial function. This explains the symptoms of postural orthostatic tachycardia syndrome,[‡] often seen in severe CFS/ME. The heart cannot increase output by beating more strongly because it does not have the energy delivery to do so. It tries to increase output by beating more quickly, but this is only sustainable for a few minutes or seconds. Blood pressure then drops precipitously, and the patient has to lie down or will black out.
- **Cardiac dysrhythmias:** The heart is beating too slowly, too quickly or irregularly. Any of these renders the heart less efficient.
- **Valve problems**: These could be either the narrowing of a heart valve or a leaky heart valve (which may be heard as a heart murmur).
- **Loss of heart muscle** due to infarction (a heart attack) or muscle disease (cardiomyopathy – which is also a mitochondrial disorder).
- **Inflammation of the heart coverings,** such as pericarditis. (This is usually painful and may produce an audible 'rub'.)

The lungs

The lungs are designed for peak athletic performance. In Nature we would achieve this around once a week, where there is a predator/prey interaction – you have to literally run for your life, either to save it or to secure your next meal. What this means is that, at rest, the lungs only have to achieve a fraction of what is needed during fight or flight.

Unfortunately, this means that a great deal of lung damage can be sustained before a person realises what is going on (especially if they do not exercise to test the system). So, for example, chronic obstructive airways disease (COAD or COPD) and emphysema in a smoker often present after years of smoking damage to the lungs. Poor lung function is usually an obvious cause of poor energy delivery.

Blood vessels

The main cause of impaired blood supply to organs in Westerners is hardening and narrowing of the arteries, or 'atherosclerosis'. Arteries have a delicate lining which can be easily damaged by turbulent blood flow. Of course, this is going to happen when the blood pressure increases and typically occurs where one blood vessel divides into two and therefore there is more turbulence at this junction. High blood pressure occurs as a result of stress because the stress hormone adrenaline is released. The commonest cause of adrenaline release is metabolic syndrome, as we saw in Chapter 11.

There's another double whammy here – if blood sugar levels spike then this will damage the artery directly. Sugar is sticky stuff and forms AGEs (advanced glycation end-products). So, with high-carbohydrate diets the arteries are damaged by the sugar and then again by the turbulent flow created by adrenaline-driven blood pressure. (Remember that high blood sugars are brought down by insulin, but if brought down too low, the body 'panics' and pours out adrenaline.)

Pathology arises when the immune system moves in to heal these areas of damage – the healing and repair process involves laying down fibrous tissue (to prevent the artery rupturing) and this will narrow the blood vessel further, leading to more turbulence and more damage. This is why controlling blood pressure and blood sugar are such an important part of preventing arterial damage. This combination of high blood pressure, loss of control of blood sugars and obesity is called 'metabolic syndrome' by the medical profession and results in a host of other problems downstream. Remember, metabolic syndrome can be defined by the contents of the supermarket trolley – this makes for much earlier and easier diagnosis. Contrary to popular opinion, obesity does not drive any pathology – it is a symptom. This is a further illustration of how doctors routinely confuse a causal effect with a casual association.

Anaemia

Insufficient haemoglobin (the oxygen-carrying molecule) may arise because of insufficient raw material (usually iron, zinc or vitamin B12), low numbers of red blood cells (poor bone marrow function) or abnormal haemoglobin (sickle cell anaemia, thalassaemia) or haemolytic anaemia (several possible causes).

---

‡Footnote: Postural orthostatic tachycardia syndrome (POTS) is a condition in which a change from lying to standing causes an abnormally large increase in heart rate. This can cause very distressing symptoms such as light-headedness, trouble with thinking, blurry vision, fainting or weakness. Many sufferers are effectively 'reduced' to having lie down all the time.

Hyperventilation

If one over-breathes, carbon dioxide is washed out of the bloodstream. This makes the blood more alkaline, making oxygen stick more avidly to haemoglobin and therefore be less available to cells. Hyperventilation is a stress response which, in Nature, would be most often in preparation for fight or flight. The lactic acid produced by such would mitigate the alkalosis of hyperventilation.

Tests for problems with oxygen and fuel supply

Tests for the above problems include:

- For anaemia/haematology – full blood count. Anaemia is a symptom that must always be taken seriously – unrecognised blood loss may be the first symptom of serious pathology. This always needs investigating as a matter of urgency.
- For nutritional causes of anaemia – measure ferritin, white cell zinc and active vitamin B12.
- Consider poor energy delivery mechanisms as applies to the bone marrow – this is greatly demanding of energy to make new blood, and of course raw materials. I suspect this explains the 'anaemia of chronic disease' since there is a great increase in demand for new blood cells and the bone marrow simply cannot keep up with demand. In patients with chronic infections I often see low white cell counts.

- For arterial function – Doppler scans[§] for blood flow, angiograms.
- For cardiac output – the best test is exercise. Inability to get fit or inability to walk briskly up a hill without serious shortness of breath, or pain, could point to heart disease and/or poor energy delivery mechanisms.
- For lung function – the best test, again, is exercise tolerance. 'Pink puffers' represent the smokers' disease of emphysema; they do not have the surface area of lung for oxygen to be absorbed (but the heart is okay) or 'blue bloaters' who have poor cardiac output (but their lungs are okay). Lung function tests available through a respiratory physiologist are very helpful.

References

1. Myhill S, Booth N, McLaren-Howard J. Chronic fatigue syndrome and mitochondrial dysfunction. *International Journal of Clinical and Experimental Medicine* 2009; 2: 1-16.
2. Booth N, Myhill S, McLaren-Howard J. Mitochondrial dysfunction and pathophysiology of myalgic encephalomyelitis/chronic fatigue syndrome (ME/CFA). *International Journal of Clinical and Experimental Medicine* 2012; 5(3): 208-220.
3. Myhill S, Booth N, McLaren-Howard J. Targeting mitochondrial dysfunction in the treatment of myalgic encephalomyelitis/chronic fatigue syndrome (ME/CFS) – a clinical audit. *International Journal of Clinical and Experimental Medicine* 2013; 6(1): 1-15.

[§]**Historical and literary note:** Doppler scans employ the 'Doppler effect' to generate imaging of the movement of tissues and body fluids (often blood) and their relative velocity to the probe. By calculating the frequency shift of the tissue/body fluid under observation, its speed and direction can be determined and 'visualised'. The Doppler effect (or the Doppler shift) is the change in frequency or wavelength of a wave in relation to an observer who is moving relative to the wave source – it accounts for the change in pitch of an approaching and then receding train, or to determine which galaxies are approaching us or moving away from us. This effect is named after Christian Andreas Doppler (29 November 1803 – 17 March 1853), an Austrian mathematician and physicist. Author Alan Garner used the title *Red Shift* for his novel concerning three intertwined 'time-shift' love stories, one set in the present, another during the English Civil War of the seventeenth century, and the third in the second century AD – it comes highly recommended.

Chapter 13
Fatigue mechanisms II

– the thyroid accelerator
– the adrenal gearbox
– tests

Engines work most efficiently when energy requirements are closely matched to energy delivery. An excellent example of this is the 'centrifugal governor'. This is a governor with a feedback system that controls the speed of an engine by regulating the amount of fuel admitted. This maintains a near-constant speed, irrespective of the load or fuel-supply conditions. Centrifugal governors were invented by Christiaan Huygens in the 17th century and these governors regulated the distance and pressure between millstones in windmills. In 1788, James Watt adapted one to control his steam engine where it regulates the admission of steam into the cylinder. For interested readers, there are many great YouTubes that show centrifugal governors in action.*

In the body, one can think of the collective function of the thyroid and adrenal glands as being the centrifugal governor that achieves this matching of energy demand with energy supply. This careful gearing of energy delivery to energy demand is vital to evolutionary success. By doing so, vital reserves are conserved for lean times.

It is the thyroid gland which 'base loads' to allow sleep and cope with the seasons. We must save energy when we can and spend it when we must. We warm up by day and cool down at night and this is part of the mechanism which determines the circadian rhythm. In winter, we save energy by hibernating – so it is normal to experience energy-conserving mild fatigue (and, indeed, depression) in winter to help us survive. We then have a boost of energy in the spring and summer to allow us to secure food supplies.

*Footnote: This idea resonated with Alfred Russel Wallace (8 January 1823 – 7 November 1913), who used governors as a metaphor for the evolutionary principle: 'The action of this principle is exactly like that of the centrifugal governor of the steam engine, which checks and corrects any irregularities almost before they become evident; and in like manner no unbalanced deficiency in the animal kingdom can ever reach any conspicuous magnitude, because it would make itself felt at the very first step, by rendering existence difficult and extinction almost sure soon to follow.'

The thyroid accelerator pedal

Both an underactive and an overactive thyroid are major risk factors for disease. Both conditions impact hugely on energy delivery. The problems of underactive thyroid are much more common than overactive (see Chapter 41: Endocrinology). Diagnosing a thyroid problem is not straightforward. The biggest mistake that doctors make is to rely exclusively on tests. The clinical picture is just as important and for some patients one can only know by prescribing a trial of thyroid hormones. Remember, all diagnosis is hypothesis – which must then be put to the test.

We are currently seeing an epidemic of thyroid disease. We know 8% of the UK population is hypothyroid but, like diabetes, it is hugely underdiagnosed. Consultant endocrinologist Dr Kenneth Blanchard reckons that possibly up to 40% of Westerners are hypothyroid – it is especially common in my CFS/ME sufferers.

Causes of hypothyroidism

For normal thyroid function we need the cooperative action of the pituitary gland in the brain, the thyroid gland in the neck, liver, heart and muscle, and responsive hormone receptors, all working together, as explained in Table 13.1.

Table 13.1: The factors needed for normal thyroid function

What	Why	How damaged or blocked	Action
Pituitary gland in the brain	To make TSH to kick the thyroid into life	Head injury Major haemorrhage (e.g. Sheehan's syndrome) Poisoning Tumour	I doubt the pituitary can recover from a permanent injury Detox may help Treat the hormone deficiency that arises downstream, especially thyroid and adrenals
Thyroid gland in the neck	To make thyroxine (T4)	Micronutrient deficiency, especially iodine, zinc, iron and/or selenium	Basic package of supplements Tests not essential but could do: iodine in urine, white cell zinc, ferritin, red cell selenium
		Poisoning – see list below Goitrogens – see list below	Avoid and detox See Chapters 15, 25
		Autoimmune destruction	Blood tests for auto-antibodies; if positive this increases the risk of other autoimmune conditions (see Chapter 51); especially avoid vaccination
		Viral destruction, especially herpes viruses	I know of nothing that can heal a destroyed thyroid gland. Sufferers will have to take thyroid hormone supplementation for life

Liver, heart and muscle	Converts inactive T4 to active T3	Blocked from making the conversion by stress hormones and toxins as below Micronutrient deficiencies	Avoid stress as much as you can and toxins as listed below Take a thyroid supplement that contains T3
Receptors that respond	Without such hormones are ineffective	Blocked by toxins as listed below	Avoid toxins as listed below There is no test for thyroid hormone receptor resistance; it is diagnosed from the clinical picture, and the dose of T3 determined by clinical response. Indeed, blood tests are misleading
			All the above will need thyroid hormone replacement therapy – for details see Chapter 41

Poisoning and toxic stress

Sources of toxic stress include halides (other than iodine), such as fluoride (drinking water, toothpaste and dental treatments), bromide (PBBs), radioactive iodine (medical treatments, Chernobyl, Fukoshima).

Other chemical thyroid insults include perchlorates (in washing powder and rocket fuel), phthalates and bisphenol A (in plastic wrappings), pyridines (in cigarette smoke), PCBs and PBBs (fire retardants in soft furnishing), UV screens (sun blocks), cosmetics, pesticides and probably many more.

Autoimmune hypothyroidism

Autoimmune hypothyroidism is also becoming increasingly common, with 20% of Westerners having an autoimmune conditions.

Natural goitrogens

The key fact to remember here is that goitrogens (substances that interfere with uptake of iodine by the thyroid gland) manifest through iodine deficiency. So long as you have adequate iodine in your diet (and I reckon 1 mg daily is the minimum for optimum health) you need not worry about the goitrogenic potential of foods such as brassicas, peanuts and soya.

The signs and symptoms of an underactive thyroid

These signs and symptoms result from poor energy delivery (physical and mental fatigue, muscle weakness, cold intolerance etc... see Chapter 5). In addition, there are symptoms which are typical and particular to an underactive thyroid, vis:

- Fluid retention which causes swelling, so swollen tissues: the tongue may swell so the imprints of teeth show on the tongue; if the patient sticks her/his tongue out, it will fill the mouth and touch the lip corners), vocal chords may swell causing voice changes, face and ankles swell causing puffiness, deafness owing to swelling of the middle ear structures
- Nerve pinching, resulting in carpel tunnel syndrome, sciatica, peripheral neuropathy, slow Achilles tendon reflex
- Poor quality dry skin, hair and flaky nails
- Slow heart rate (often less than 60 beats per minute - but note, the heart of a fit

athlete may be slow because the heart beats so powerfully). A normal heart rate at rest should be 70 beats per minute

- Goitre – a swelling of the thyroid gland that causes a lump to form in the front of the neck
- Muscle stiffness
- Sleep disturbances – the thyroid is centrally involved in our circadian rhythm; hypothyroidism (low thyroid levels) may present with being an owl, poor quality sleep and the constant need for more sleep
- Ketogenic hypoglycaemia (see Chapter 28: Diet, detox and die-off reactions).

Tests of thyroid function

A blood test to measure thyroid hormones – namely, free T4, free T3 and TSH – is an essential start. However, for the purposes of treatment the clinical detail is as important as the blood tests. Indeed, I see the blood test as the coarse tuning, with the clinical input being the fine tuning. Often the diagnosis is only made following a trial of thyroid hormones. This is done in conjunction with diet and mitochondrial function using core temperature (see Chapters 30 and 41 for the clinical nitty gritty of how to treat).

The adrenal gear box

Whilst the thyroid gland does the coarse tuning, the adrenal gland does the fine tuning to match energy demand to energy delivery on a more immediate basis. Adrenaline (or 'epinephrine'), noradrenaline (or 'norepinephrine') and dopamine from the adrenal medulla can massively increase energy delivery on a second by second basis. Adrenaline stimulates glucose release from glycogen stores in the liver and muscles to provide an abundance of fuel and increases mitochondrial output. This is an essential survival strategy to allow us to achieve peak performance and deal with an acute stress, such as being chased by a

sabre-toothed tiger. If the hunt continues, there is an outpouring of the adrenal cortex medium-term stress hormone, hydrocortisone. This maintains energy output again by increasing blood sugar levels (and stimulating appetite) and stimulating mitochondria. Indeed, such an outpouring of adrenal hormones allows mitochondria to increase their output by 200%. This explains why it is only at world events that world records are broken. It may be that for peak athletic performance, when fast-twitch muscle fibres are employed such as for sprinting or weight lifting, a dual fuel of ketones and glucose produces the best result.

However, this is not sustainable in the long term. Unremitting high blood sugar is very damaging. Unremitting stress results in adrenal exhaustion – this protects mitochondria because if mitochondria fatigue then ATP levels fall too low, in which case cells will die.

A normally functioning adrenal gland is essential for life – absence of function kills (Addison's disease), too much maims (Cushing's syndrome or steroid hormones). What I see most commonly is adrenal exhaustion – that is, partial failure resulting from chronic unremitting stress (see Chapters 30 and 41 for the details of treatment).

A certain amount of stress is essential for a healthy and productive life. Getting the balance right is the tricky bit. Stress can come in many guises. I think the symptom of stress arises when the brain realises that it does not have the energy resources to deal with demands. The main stressors which result in adrenal fatigue in order of clinical frequency are I suspect:

- Fluctuating blood sugar levels because of sugar and carbohydrate addiction, resulting in…
- Lack of sleep – either poor quality or insufficient hours of sleep or both
- Other addictions – alcohol, nicotine, drugs, prescription medications. We use these to suppress the symptoms of stress because

they allow our brains to ignore those distressing symptoms. This is dangerous medicine and creates further obvious vicious cycles

- Emotional/psychological stress
- Financial and time stress
- Infectious stress – often it is the viral infection which is the last straw that breaks the camel's back and tips an under-functioning person into a full blown CFS; rarely is the virus the sole cause
- Micronutrient deficiencies
- Undiagnosed allergies
- Toxic stress and poisoning – from environmental exposures (polluting industry), occupational exposures (pesticides), social exposures (cosmetics, hair dyes), prescription medications.

There are many other possibilities, but the starting point to address all of the above is Groundhog Basic.

Symptoms of adrenal fatigue

All the symptoms of poor energy delivery (physical fatigue, mental fatigue, muscle weakness, depression etc, as detailed in Chapter 5), plus:

- inability to rise to the challenge and deal with any of the above stressors
- lack of enthusiasm, which may manifest as poor libido (dare I say it – inability to rise to the occasion‡)
- poor temperature control (so core temperature fluctuates), possibly with a tendency to excessive sweating. Menopausal hot flushes are more severe where there is adrenal fatigue.

Poor adrenal function – tests and treatment

Conventional testing for adrenal function relies on a short synacthen test in which the patient is injected with ACTH, a hormone that gives the adrenal gland a powerful kick. This will pick up complete adrenal failure as occurs in Addison's disease, but will not pick up partial failure or adrenal fatigue. The adrenal stress profile is a very useful test that can be easily done on salivary samples (see Chapter 30) and is often done in parallel with thyroid function tests. Chapter 30 details how to balance the thyroid with the adrenals for optimal energy delivery.

Treatment is two pronged. First, try to identify and deal with the cause of the stress. Secondly, use adrenal glandulars to provide physiological replacement therapy whilst the glands recover.

The blood tests for thyroid function and the salivary tests for adrenal function allow the 'coarse tuning' of your car engine. We then have to look at the fine tuning. Allowing the body to heal from any condition is like conducting an orchestra. Not only do we need to know who all the players are, but these players also need to be playing the right tune at the right time. Then you get a melody (see Chapters 30 and 41 for the clinical nitty gritty). Remember, all diagnosis starts with hypothesis and depends on response to treatment to confirm such.

Coping with stress

We use addictions to cope with stress. They work by illusion and masking:

- **Illusion:** Some addictions mimic stress hormones and give us the illusion that we have an abundance of energy. Cocaine, amphetamines, ecstasy and, to a lesser extent, caffeine, all have, amongst others, noradrenaline-like actions, which increase

---

‡**Footnote from Craig:** I think you just did, Sarah!

energy output. They give us false energy which dupes us into feeling that we can change the world singlehandedly. Once the drug wears off, the brain realises that it is sailing very close to the wind because it has used up vital energy reserves. The brain gives us a feeling of acute fatigue to allow recovery time to regain energy stores. We call this, withdrawal. 'Train spotting' results from prolonged addictive use and prolonged withdrawal. Remember, unlike the banks with money, we cannot 'borrow' energy. If we run out of energy, then mitochondria stop, and we die. Indeed, I suspect this is one of the mechanisms by which these drugs kill. When one hears of an ecstasy user dropping dead, I suspect this is because the body runs out of energy for life.

- **Masking:** Other addictions work by masking the unpleasant symptoms of stress by stopping us from caring. The socially acceptable ones are sugar and alcohol, vaping and smoking, tranquillisers and (shockingly) prescription opiates. There is now a fad for prescription cannabis. Indeed, many prescription drugs are addictive and simply replace one addiction with another.

These addictions bring us immediate relief – a smoker will tell you that the comfortable sensation starts within milliseconds of inhalation and, indeed, even in anticipation of relief. Addictions mask the very symptoms which tell us something is going wrong and lead us into further disease. However, the relief does not last, and a further dose of addiction is necessary to feel 'normal'.

We all know this, but it does not prevent addiction. The power of short-term emotional gain is much stronger than cold-blooded intellectual knowledge. It takes an iron will and much self-discipline to start to deal with addictions.

I see the Western progression through life as an addictive ladder which starts with sugar and refined carbohydrates and moves up through nicotine, alcohol, cannabis, ecstasy and heroin. The addict either dies prematurely or realises his errors and climbs back down the addiction ladder, but often is left on the first rung of sugar and refined carbohydrate. In terms of scale, this is the most serious addiction because it is not recognised as such – indeed, it is socially acceptable.

The good news is that adrenaline is also an addiction. One strategy is to swap unhealthy for healthy addictions, like walking, gardening, the Arts and Culture. These healthy addictions provide more adrenaline where there is a competitive edge. I ride my horse risking falls and fractures. Bridge players risk being shot by their partners for playing the wrong card!‡

‡**Footnote:** The bridge murder case, also known as the 'bridge table murder case' was the trial of Myrtle Adkins Bennett, a Kansas City housewife, for the murder of her husband, John G Bennett, over a game of contract bridge in September 1929. She died in 1992 and her estate was valued at more than $1 million. She left most of the money to family members of John Bennett, the husband she had killed more than six decades before.

Chapter 14
Mechanisms: sleep

– the why and how for the regular servicing of our bodies

Sleep is the golden chain that ties health and our bodies together.
Thomas Dekker, English dramatist and pamphleteer, c.1572 – 1632

Why to sleep

During sleep the glymphatics, the rubbish disposal systems of the brain, open up to allow cleaning, healing and repair. An example of such rubbish is amyloid, the pathological protein of Alzheimer's disease. This is cleared from the brain during sleep. If sleep is lacking, then amyloid builds up in the brain. Lack of sleep is a, possibly *the*, major risk factor for dementia. Indeed, there is no disease process that is not worsened by lack of sleep. It really is a risk factor for all disease. Quantity and quality of sleep are non-negotiable.

All living creatures have times in their cycle when they shut down their metabolic activity for healing and repair to take place. In higher animals we call this sleep. During the flu epidemic after the First World War, a few sufferers developed neurological damage in which they lost the ability to sleep. All were dead within two weeks; this was the first solid evidence that sleep is an absolute essential for life. Happily, the body has a symptom which tells us how much sleep we need. It is called tiredness; ignore this at your peril!

During sleep we heal and repair; during our waking hours we cause cell damage. If there is insufficient sleep, then the cell damage exceeds healing and repair and our health gradually ratchets downhill. Lack of sleep is a major risk factor for all degenerative conditions, from heart disease to cancer and neurological disorders.

Without a good night's sleep on a regular basis, all other interventions are to no avail. There are at least three aspects to pay attention to: the quantity of sleep, when to sleep (circadian rhythm) and the quality of sleep.

The quantity of sleep

Modern Westerners are chronically sleep deprived. We average 7.5 hours sleep when the biological average requirement is nearer 9 hours, perhaps a bit more in winter, less in summer. To show how critical this balance is, imagine dividing the day into 12 hours of activity and 12 hours of rest. One extra hour of damaging activity (13 hours awake) means the loss of one hour of rest and healing sleep (11 hours). The difference is two hours. It is vital to observe a regular bedtime and to be able to wake naturally, without an alarm clock, feeling refreshed.

When to sleep (circadian* rhythm)

Humans evolved to sleep when it is dark and wake when it is light. Sleep is a form of hibernation when the body shuts down in order to repair damage done through use, to conserve energy and to hide from predators. The normal sleep pattern that evolved in hot climates is to sleep, keep warm and conserve energy during the cold nights and then sleep again in the afternoons when it is too hot to work and to hide away from the midday sun. As humans migrated away from the Equator, the sleep pattern had to change with the seasons and as the lengths of the days changed. In winter we need to shut down to conserve energy – this means more sleep. Mild fatigue and depression in winter prevent us from spending energy unnecessarily. Conversely, in the summer we need to expend large amounts of energy to harvest the summer bounties and accumulate reserves to carry us through the winter – we naturally need less sleep, can work longer hours and have more energy. But the need for a rest (if not a sleep) in the middle of the day is still there. Therefore, it is no surprise that young children, the elderly and people who become ill often have an extra sleep in the afternoon, and for these people that is totally desirable. Others have learned to 'power nap', as it is called, during the day, and this allows them to feel more energetic later. If you can do it, then this is an excellent habit to get into; it can be learned.

The average daily sleep requirement is 9 hours, ideally taken between 9.30 pm and 6.30 am – that is, during the hours of darkness – but allow for more in the winter and less in the summer. An hour of sleep before midnight is worth two after; this is because human growth hormone is produced during the hours of sleep before midnight.

The symptom of jet lag is a powerful illustration of the existence of a circadian rhythm. Circadian rhythms start with light which impacts on the skin (interestingly not necessarily through the eyes) and switches off melatonin production. As darkness ensues, melatonin is produced to create the hormonal environment for sleep. Melatonin stimulates the pituitary gland to produce thyroid-stimulating hormones, and this peaks at midnight. The thyroid is stimulated to produce T4 (thyroxin) which spikes at 4:00 am. This is converted to the active thyroid hormone T3, which spikes at 5 am. T3 kicks the adrenals into life and the rising levels of adrenaline, cortisol and DHEA wake us up at 6:00-7:00 am. My guess is that it is the varying levels of all these hormones through the night that determine the proportion of non-REM to REM sleep (see opposite) and this too is critical for good health. Good thyroid and adrenal function are essential for good quality sleep. A further likely mechanism for sleep is the effect on core temperature. Indeed, there is a very clear relationship between onset of sleep and falling core temperature, and this is achieved by increasing blood flow to the skin, so heat is lost.

> *An hour of sleep before midnight is worth two after*
> Well known saying... and Mother was right again!
>
> *Early to bed and early to rise, makes a man healthy, wealthy and wise.*
> Benjamin Franklin,[†] 17 January 1706 – 17 April 1790

---

*Footnote: Franz Halberg (5 July 1919 – 9 June 2013) coined the word 'circadian' in 1959 by combining two Latin words – circa (about) and diem, accusative singular of dies (day). Halberg was a maverick, working seven days a week, right up to his death, who spoke of the 'quicksand of clinical trials on groups' and that 'These [clinical trials] ignore individual differences and hence the individual's needs'.[1]

The quality of sleep

There are two recognisable types of sleep, called rapid eye movement (REM) sleep and non-REM sleep. We see a cycle of such every 90 minutes. Non-REM sleep comes first and during this time we sort through the experiences of the day and store the important ones, essential to survival, as memory. We then slip into REM sleep during which we dream, and problem solve. All sorts of odd connections are made. We start the night with a high proportion of non-REM to REM sleep and finish it with more REM sleep. I suspect the proportions of such are determined by the changing hormone levels of melatonin, thyroid and adrenal hormones which occur through the sleep cycle. It is easy to see how both sorts of sleep confer survival advantage. We do not want to clog up the brain with useless memories and we need to make lots of bizarre connections for problem solving. This has been known for a long time.

For non-REM sleep:

I consider that a man's brain originally is like a little empty attic, and you have to stock it with such furniture as you choose. A fool takes in all the lumber of every sort that he comes across, so that the knowledge which might be useful to him gets crowded out, or at best is jumbled up with a lot of other things, so that he has a difficulty in laying his hands upon it. Now the skilful workman is very careful indeed as to what he takes into his brain-attic. He will have nothing but the tools which may help him in doing his work, but of these he has a large assortment, and all in the most perfect order. It is a mistake to think that that little room has elastic walls and can distend to any extent. Depend upon it there comes a time when for every addition of knowledge, you forget something that you knew before. It is of the highest importance, therefore, not to have useless facts elbowing out the useful ones.

Sherlock Holmes from *A Study in Scarlet*
by Sir Arthur Conan Doyle
22 May 1859 – 7 July 1930[†]

For REM sleep we have:

The key to having good ideas is to get lots of ideas and throw out the bad ones.

Linus Pauling, American chemist, biochemist and peace activist, 28 February 1901 – 19 August 1994

We end with more from Thomas Dekker, this time his lullaby which Craig's wife, Penny, used to sing to their children every night:

[†]**Historical note:** We do have Franklin to thank for bringing this well-known phrase into common usage (my mother said this to me an awful lot during my teenage years, always with a strong emphasis on the 'wise' – Craig) but there are earlier versions, showing that indeed this wisdom has been known for hundreds of years. In *The Book of St Albans*, printed in 1486, we have:

As the olde englysshe prouerbe sayth in this wyse. Who soo woll ryse erly shall be holy helthy & zely.

The Middle English word *zely* had numerous meanings in 1486 but foremost were 'auspicious' or 'fortunate'. So 'holy helthy & zely' meant 'wise, healthy and fortunate'. *The Book of St Albans* contains advice on hawking, hunting and heraldry, with a chapter on fishing added in 1496.[2]

Golden slumbers kiss your eyes,
Smiles awake you when you rise;
Sleep, pretty wantons, do not cry,
And I will sing a lullaby,
Rock them, rock them, lullaby.
Care is heavy, therefore sleep you,
You are care, and care must keep you;
Sleep, pretty wantons, do not cry,
And I will sing a lullaby,
Rock them, rock them, lullaby.

The Cradle Song, by Thomas Dekker,
English dramatist and pamphleteer, c.
1572 – 25 August 1632

References

1. Halberg F, Cornelissen G, Katinas G, Syutkina EV, et al. Transdisciplinary unifying implications of circadian findings in the 1950s. *Journal of Circadian Rhythms* 2003; 1(2). DOI: http://doi.org/10.1186/1740-3391-1-2 (www.jcircadian-rhythms.com/articles/10.1186/1740-3391-1-2/)
2. Full text of the 'Boke of Saint Albans'. https://archive.org/stream/bokeofsaintalban00bern/bokeofsaintalban00bern_djvu.txt

‡**Footnote:** Conan Doyle was buried in 1930 and again in 1955. He was not a Christian, considering himself a Spiritualist, and so he was first buried on 11 July 1930 in Windlesham rose garden. His body was later reinterred together with his wife's in Minstead churchyard in the New Forest, Hampshire.

Chapter 15
Poisonings

– where they come from and how we detoxify

Shakespeare thought gold worse than poison to one's soul:

> *There is thy gold, worse poison to men's souls,*
> *Doing more murder in this loathsome world,*
> *Than these poor compounds that thou*
> *mayst not sell.*
> Romeo and Juliet, Act 5 Scene II, by
> William Shakespeare, 26 April 1564
> (baptised) – 23 April 1616

Well, far be it from me to disagree with the Bard himself, but as far as bodies are concerned, poisons (toxins) wreak havoc and we must have systems in place to deal with unavoidable exposures. These come naturally from:
- the gut: food and microbes
- mitochondria: the business of energy generation
- inflammation: which includes healing and repair
- recycling of raw materials from normal metabolism.

However, this toxic burden is further increased by toxins from the polluted environment in which we all exist. In order of importance (which changes according to the dose) these include:
- unnatural foods, such as sugar, refined carbohydrates and artificial additives, such as sweeteners, colourings and preservatives
- products of the upper fermenting gut (if you are eating any amount of carbohydrates, expect such)
- toxic metals from vaccinations, dental work, surgical implants (including silicones), cooking pans
- pesticide residues in food
- smoking – carcinogenic tars (cadmium, nitrosamines, radioactive and benzene compounds), carbon monoxide, nitrogen oxides and cyanides; altogether, 3800 different compounds have been identified. Remember, even passive smoking is a risk factor for cancer. Nicotine is one of the safer components
- social drugs: alcohol, nicotine (vaping), caffeine, 'legal highs'
- prescription and over-the-counter drugs, with paracetamol a major toxin
- household chemicals and cleaners
- cosmetics, especially hair dyes* and

*Footnote:** In the words of PG Wodehouse, English author and humourist (15 October 1881 – 14 February 1975): 'There is only one cure for grey hair. It was invented by a Frenchman. It is called the guillotine.'

aluminium-based deodorants
- mycotoxins from water-damaged buildings and from fungal infection of the airways and gut
- occupational hazards: pesticides in agriculture, chemicals used indoors and out and many others
- air pollution: ozone, particulate matter, sulphur dioxide, nitrogen dioxide, carbon monoxide and lead.

Endogenous sources of toxic stress

Endogenous sources are those inside us or that we are producing ourselves.

The gut: food and microbes

I have come to suspect that this is the single largest source of toxic stress. Blood draining from the gut passes in the portal vein directly to the liver, the job of which includes dealing with toxins. If this blood passed directly into the systemic circulation, we would soon die – indeed, the mechanisms of death in liver failure could be explained by such a poisoning. At rest, the liver consumes a massive amount of energy: 27% of total energy consumption, to deal with this toxic load.

As I have said in earlier chapters, if you look at life from the point of view of a plant, it does not want to be eaten and renders itself as poisonous as possible. Indeed, the vast majority of plant matter in the world is too toxic to eat. Even foods that we do eat regularly have toxins, such as lectins, alkaloids and possible carcinogens. The cycad seed consumed on the Island of Guam causes motor neurone disease which killed 10% of its inhabitants.

More toxic stress also arises from the upper fermenting gut. We normally ferment vegetable fibre in the lower gut to produce fuel in the form of short-chain fatty acids – one such, n-butyrate,

is essential for nourishing the lining of the large bowel. However, where there is abnormal fermentation of carbohydrates and proteins in the upper gut, there is production of many toxins, such as ethyl, propyl and butyl alcohols, hydrogen sulphide, D-lactate, oxalates, ammonia and many others.

Mitochondria: the business of energy generation

No machine is 100% efficient and the business of burning sugar in mitochondria in the presence of oxygen will produce toxins in the form of free radicals. These are mopped up by antioxidant systems within cells, extracellular fluid and the bloodstream. The antioxidant system is a way of safely dealing with free radicals, passing them from front-line antioxidants such as co-enzyme Q10, superoxide dismutase and glutathione peroxidase, to second-line antioxidants such as vitamins B12, A, D and E, and thereon to the ultimate repository, vitamin C.

Inflammation: which includes healing and repair

Normal metabolism of protein and carbohydrates, immune activity, hormones, neurotransmitters, enzymes, haemoglobin, muscle fibres, and all other aspects of the body's functioning, result in many breakdown products, all of which have to be detoxified, recycled and/or excreted. These include urea, creatinine, uric acid, oxalates, purines and porphyrins together with alcohols, esters and many others.

Recycling of raw materials

When cells are damaged or replaced through wear and tear, injury or inflammation, large molecules are released which are too big to get into the bloodstream. These are mopped up by the lymphatic system – a system of drains which course throughout the body and the brain (where they are called glymphatics). The contents are broken down for recycling in lymph nodes to produce chyle and finally empty into the inferior vena cava vein in the neck via the thoracic duct. It is the glymphatics in the brain which open up during sleep to allow drainage of toxins, including prion proteins (the pathological particle of many degenerating brain conditions). Sleep is a vital part of detoxing the brain as explained in Chapter 14.

Exogenous toxins from the polluted environment

Because we live in an increasingly polluted world, we are putting more stress on our detox systems. Our detox systems did not evolve to deal with such. However hard we try, we are all contaminated with pesticides, volatile organic compounds and heavy metals, which bioaccumulate in tissues. I have yet to find a single person with a normal fat biopsy or absence of toxic metals in urine following the taking of a chelating agent. In addition, there are noxious gases and background ionising radiation (see Chapter 8 for the clinical pictures).

The problem of detoxifying a combination of toxins

It may be that in isolation toxins can be dealt with, but in combination problems arise because of:

- The biochemical bottleneck effect – All toxins have to be cleared by the body by the same mechanisms. It takes longer for the total load to reduce if there are multiple toxins, so they hang around longer with greater potential for harm.
- Cocktail effect – Pollutants may interact, perhaps to form new and more toxic compounds

- Electromagnetic pollution, with electro-toxicity and electro-sensitivity, is compounding the above problems.

We are all poisoned

We are inevitably and unavoidably exposed, so it is impossible to completely avoid every 'nasty' chemical. As I said, I have yet to do a fat biopsy or measure toxic metals in urine following chelation (DMSA challenge – see below) and find a normal result. We live in equilibrium with our environment and the best we can do is keep the total toxic load as low as reasonably possible. Anything which can be done to reduce the toxic chemical load will be helpful in allowing our bodies to recover.

Dr Paula Baillie Hamilton, in her book *The Detox Diet*, explains how chemicals in foods and the air interfere with internal metabolism to make us fat and lethargic. Indeed, she points out that farm animals are deliberately fed hormones, antibiotics and pesticides to make them fat and lethargic, and therefore they do not have to eat so much in order to put on weight (which gives us cheap meat). Effectively, we are feeding our farm animals to produce a metabolic syndrome. Many chemicals are persistent and concentrate through the food chain; it is very likely that if Westernised humans were a farm animal, they would be declared too toxic to eat.

What this means is that modern 21st-century *homo sapiens* must put in place all possible interventions to reduce the toxic load and help the body to rid itself of these potential nasties. Again, there is a two-pronged approach – do one's best to:

1. reduce the toxic load (by avoidance) and
2. help the body's own detox mechanisms.

How do we know we are carrying a clinically relevant toxic load?

FIRST, record a good history. Consider the clinical pictures and toxic possibilities detailed in Chapter 8. This gives an idea of what exposures have taken place, with implications for avoidance and /or detox regimes.

THEN do tests. These may be direct measurements of toxicity or indirect measurements of toxic effects. Remember, toxicity and immuno-toxicity go together.

Some toxins get into the body, do severe damage but evaporate or are detoxed before testing is possible. Such examples include formaldehyde, noxious gases like carbon monoxide, sulphur dioxide, nitrous oxide and radiation damage. Drugs of addiction, such as heroin, cannabis and ecstasy, have the potential to cause permanent damage (including death). However, these are likely to be undetectable by the time of testing.

Tests for toxic metals

Measuring toxic metals in urine, blood and hair is unreliable because heavy metals are very poorly excreted and bio-concentrate in organs such as the heart, brain, bone marrow and kidneys, so are not available to measure. A normal test does not mean all is well. The answer is to use a chelating agent, such as DMSA (captomer) which is well absorbed from the gut, grabs toxic and friendly minerals alike, and pulls them out through the urine. It is excellent for diagnosing toxicity of heavy metals such as mercury, lead, arsenic, aluminium, cadmium, nickel and probably others. Anyone can do this test at home by ordering the kit from Biolab or Genova. On the day of testing, first empty the bladder, then take DMSA at a rate of 15 mg per kg of body weight, collect all pee for six hours, measure the total, then send a small sample to the lab. DMSA is a good chelator of friendly minerals so expect to see high levels of some, especially copper, manganese, zinc and probably others. This is a very useful test that I often request.

Indeed, I am constantly surprised by this test which often shows a problem despite no obvious clinical symptoms. The first symptom may be the onset of cancer or a prion disorder. Doing this test may be a useful screening test in anyone looking to live to 100!

Tests for pesticides and volatile organic compounds (VOCs)

There are two good options here:

1. I am so fortunate to work with Acumen laboratories whose tests include DNA adducts, translocator protein studies, fat biopsies and other such. Fat biopsies are so interesting; pesticides and VOCs may be found in our fat in mg/kg. This would be similar to the sorts of levels in blood of a drug we would expect to see if we were taking it therapeutically. This partly explains why people get sick when they lose weight – these pesticides are mobilised to cause an acute poisoning. OR

2. Blood and urine tests from Genova's toxic effects CORE tests look at urine and blood samples to give a measure of pesticides and VOCs such as alkylphenols, organochlorines, organo-phosphates, plasticisers, preservatives and polychlorinated biphenyls (PCBs). This test is available through Natural Health Worldwide – naturalhealthworldwide.com.

Tests for mycotoxins

Increasingly I am using this simple urine test, MycoTox Profile – Mold Exposure by the Great Plains Laboratory Inc, which is easily available. Positive results are very common. It measures the toxic products of fungi, many of which are seriously dangerous, causing organ damage,

damage to mitochondria, immunotoxicity and much more.

Test for toxic metals causing immuno-toxicity

An excellent test for toxic metals is the MELISA test developed by Dr Vera Stejskal (see www.melisa.org/melisa-clinics/) and available in UK through Biolab. This should be done in the case of almost any inflammatory process of unknown origin, including all cases of autoimmunity, arthritis, chronic pain and degeneration that are not responding to Groundhog Chronic interventions.

Tests for other toxins causing immuno-toxicity

Again, I am lucky to be able to do immunotoxicity (lymphocyte sensitivity) tests for pesticides and VOCs at Acumen laboratories, but currently these are not otherwise available. However, toxicity and immunotoxicity (sensitivity) go hand in hand, so where is a toxic load then it is very likely the immune system will be activated. The bottom line is that the detox heating regimes work reliably well and if there is any clinical hint of a problem then these should be put in place (see Chapter 34).

How do we know how well we are dealing with toxins?

Tests of ability to detox

Standard blood tests of biochemistry (urea and electrolytes, liver function tests, kidney function tests etc) give some handle on ability to detox. These are crude tests and if normal do not mean all is well. They include liver function tests (bilirubin, enzyme levels), kidney function (urinalysis, urea, creatinine, eGFR) and uric acid.

- **Urea and creatinine** are measures of kidney function. Using an algorithm, glomerular filtration rate can be calculated from the creatinine, age and sex. Ideally it should be above 90 ml/minute; do something if

it falls below 60. The creatinine level in the blood is partly determined by muscle mass and protein intake – high protein turnover increases creatinine in the blood so excessive amounts may give a false impression of a renal problem which can be simply resolved by reducing protein intake (see Chapter 21: The PK diet, for details of how much protein is desirable).

- **Bilirubin** – In the absence of liver pathology, a high bilirubin indicates Gilbert's syndrome (see below).
- **Gamma glutamyl transferase** – This enzyme is induced in response to a load; typically it is raised in response to excessive alcohol consumption. Some prescription medication has the same effect, but it may be raised in response to alcohols generated by the fermenting gut.
- **Lactate dehydrogenase** – This is the enzyme necessary to clear lactate which results when there is a switch into anaerobic metabolism with production of lactic acid. I suspect high levels of this enzyme are symptomatic of such a tendency and point to poor energy delivery mechanisms. It may also be an indication of tissue damage and for this reason has been used as a cancer marker.

The above are crude tests and just because they are normal does not mean that all is well. More sensitive tests include:
- **Homocysteine** – This is a marker of the efficiency of the methylation cycle, an essential detox process.
- **Glutathione** – This has to be in abundant supply as part of methylation and also the final repository for many exogenous toxins, such as toxic metals. It is commonly deficient. Indeed, my view is that we live in such a toxic world we should all be taking glutathione 250 mg daily.

- **Liver detoxification profile** – This measures the ability of the body to excrete substances such as aspirin, caffeine and paracetamol, so one can infer which enzyme pathways are deficient.

Test of antioxidant status

An easy screening test is the Genova oxidative stress urine profile. Whilst this does not tell us why there is a problem, it does tell us if there is an issue. If you find there is, visit Chapter 36 and quench the inflammatory fire with antioxidants. Retest to make sure these interventions have been effective.

A common detox disease is Gilbert's syndrome[†]

Gilbert's syndrome may affect up to 10% of the population. Although this is said to be a benign biochemical abnormality, actually it is symptomatic of inability to detox through glucuronidation. Sufferers are less able to clear a toxic load and so more susceptible to poisoning from endogenous and/or exogenous toxins. Many suffer from fatigue and Gilbert's is common in my CFS/ME patients, many of whom have high or high normal levels of bilirubin. Although Gilbert's is diagnosed when the bilirubin runs above 19 micromols per litre (mcmol/l), in clinical practice I like to see levels running below 10. The treatment of Gilbert's is to help another detox pathway which deals with similar toxins – namely, the glutathione pathway. This is achieved by supplementing with glutathione, 250 mg per day for life.

[†]**Historical note:** Gilbert's disease is named after Augustin Nicolas Gilbert (15 February 1858 – 4 March 1927), a French physician, born in the Ardennes to a family of farmers. As a young boy, his brilliance as a scholar was clear to all and so he broke with family tradition. 'Gilbert's sign' is also named after him; this is where patients with liver cirrhosis pass more urine when fasting than after a meal, contrary to expectations.

Chapter 16
Inflammation mechanisms

**– why and how the immune system is switched on
– tests of inflammation**

Inflammation occurs where and when the immune system, our standing army,* is active. This is good for fighting infection and for healing and repair, but bad when switched on as in allergy and autoimmunity. This is civil war or military *coup d'etat*.

The immune system is switched on when it perceives a foreigner that has the potential to do harm. There is an inertia in the system, so it takes time to switch on. In the case of an acute infection, say measles, this inertia allows the measles virus to get ahead of the game so measles illness results. Then this virus is killed and cleared away by inflammation. The immune system learns, so at a subsequent exposure to the measles virus, the inertia has gone, and the virus is immediately killed. We call this immunity and it is highly desirable.

Precisely the same principles apply to invaders that may be metals, chemicals, silicones or other such foreign material. In small amounts the immune system perceives no danger and ignores them. In larger amounts, inflammation is switched on to kill and clear the foreigner. But metals, silicones and many chemicals are tough molecules that cannot be broken down and cleared away – so the immune system goes on fighting with chronic inflammation. We call this allergy and it is highly undesirable.

It may be that through sheer chance, the combined effects of microbial material, toxic metals and other such switch on a completely inappropriate reaction to the body's own tissues. We call this autoimmunity and it is highly undesirable. This explains why vaccination is so good at switching on autoimmuinity (see Chapter 51: Immunology).

So the immune system may be switched on, for good reasons or for bad.

---

*__Historical note:__ The British are suspicious of having a standing army. Many may not know that the UK Parliament must approve the continued existence of the British Army by passing an Armed Forces Act at least once every five years. This requirement goes back to the Bill of Rights, 1689. The Royal Navy, Royal Air Force and Royal Marines along with all other forces do not require this Act. The point is that there is a recognition that, although there are clear advantages to having a standing army, there are dangers too; here the dangers are perceived as the army gaining too much political power and ultimately being a threat to the 'people'. The same is true of the body's standing army, our immune system. We need it to fight off invaders, but there are dangers too, as we shall see.

Table 16.1: Possible causes of an immune response

Incitant	Good or bad? – is having an immune response 'generally' a good or bad thing?	Comments
Acute infection	Good – but so important to fight this early and hard[†]	Life is an arms race – you and I are a free lunch. Let's kick the bugs out before they enter and drive chronic disease. (See *The Infection Game* for much more detail)
Toxic metals	Bad – pro-inflammatory to switch on autoimmunity and allergy	From vaccinations, dental work (amalgam, braces, bridges, root fillings), piercings, surgical plates, screws, implants, cosmetics, tattoos… AVOID! Test with MELISA available through Biolab (see page A6.1)
Poisonous plants	Good	We learn not to eat them again
Food that is not directly poisonous	Bad. This is called allergy. Immediate IgE allergy to food such as peanuts can and does kill	We need food to nourish us
	I suspect, but do not know, that many delayed allergy reactions are not food allergies but…	…allergies to the microbes in the gut which ferments that particular food. This explains the delay factor and why vitamin C to bowel tolerance is often so helpful. The vitamin C kills the microbes and so there is nothing (or very little) left to be allergic to
		…or to toxins in foods, such as lectins. This may explain why many people are intolerant of wheat although 'allergy tests' are normal
Tree, grass and weed pollen, animal hair, house dust and house dust mites	Bad. This is a damned nuisance. These antigens are not dangerous	The immune system has its wires crossed. It is possible this is linked to lack of gut parasites, such as worms, in Western guts. The idea here is the IgE immune system goes 'looking for parasites', does not find them but instead 'sees', and tries to kick out, the innocuous. We know pollen allergy is switched on by diesel exhaust fumes

[†]**Footnote**: Acute infection is a common trigger for chronic inflammation – so always be prepared to treat this aggressively.

Moulds	Mostly good but they can cause chronic infection	Moulds have the potential to cause chronic infection, especially in the airways. This is a greatly over-looked driver of disease – e.g. chronic sinusitis and chronic obstructive airway disease (COAD or COPD)
	...and/or allergy	Again, allergic asthma and chronic obstructive pulmonary disease (COPD) such as 'farmer's lung'. I suspect horse COPD is also mould infection/allergy from damp hay
	Moulds produce mycotoxins	Mycotoxins, such as ochratoxin, fumonisins, and aflatoxin produced by aspergillus, penicillium strains, fusarium etc may drive cancers, switch on allergy and autoimmunity, damage organs and cause chronic fatigue syndromes
Chemicals	Mostly good because...	...many chemicals are toxic and we need to learn to avoid them and take action to eliminate them from the body, perhaps with heating regimes
	...however, some people become exquisitely sensitive to chemicals in doses too low to cause toxicity	This is called multiple chemical sensitivity, is a damned nuisance and difficult to treat
Microbes from the upper fermenting gut	Mostly bad. Some will always get into the bloodstream	Friendly microbes with which the immune system is familiar will be ignored and excreted in the kidneys and urine
	Unfriendly microbes which are unfamiliar...	...may get into the gut wall and drive inflammatory bowel disease
	...may get into the bloodstream and then get stuck in distal sites to drive inflammation...	...in the joints, connective tissues and bones: arthritis, rheumatics, fibromyalgia, bursitis, tendonitis, fasciitis and other such
		...in the genitourinary tract: nephritis, interstitial cystitis, prostatitis and other such
		...in the skin: chronic urticaria and venous ulcers
		...in the brain: psychological and psychiatric conditions such as OCD, autism, dementia, psychosis

Incitant	Good or bad? – is having an immune response 'generally' a good or bad thing?	Comments
		…in the immune system: autoimmunity (possibly by molecular mimicry)[§]
Electromagnetic pollution, especially from cordless phones, mobile phones and wifi	Bad	This disrupts voltage-gated calcium channels across all cell membranes and makes cells more 'twitchy' so they react at much lower thresholds to other incitants

Apply Groundhog Acute at once (see Appendix 2). If you do not have *The Infection Game*, then take it from Craig and me, prevention and early aggressive treatment are all. Do not wait for a doctor's diagnosis but get stuck in straight away. It is much easier to sweep the invaders off the beach from a position of strength than wait for them to occupy the castles of your body. If you wait for chronic[‡] inflammation to become established before doing something about it, you risk life-long disease and premature death. Listen to your symptoms, do not suppress them but ask about the mechanism driving them at once and put in place the necessary interventions to prevent the inevitable progression from health and happiness to disability and death. The sooner you can do this the better; it is never too late to start. Remember, pathology is accelerated by conventional symptom-suppressing medicine with short-term gain and long-term pain. Time is of the essence, so be prepared. Many of my post-viral ME sufferers have their life-long illness triggered by glandular fever (Epstein-Barr virus), often at a time of exam stress at university, with symptom-suppressing medication prescribed and a complete absence of Groundhog Acute. For the intellectual imperative that under-pins this approach, see *The Infection Game*. One of my favourite quotes is:

> *The patient should get large doses of vitamin C in all pathological conditions while the physician ponders the diagnosis.*
> Dr Frederick Robert Klenner, BS MS, MD, FCCP, FAAFP, 1907 – 1984

[‡]**Linguistic note:** Just for clarity of language, when talking of disease processes, 'acute' means of rapid onset and 'chronic' means persistent or otherwise long-lasting in its effects. It is interesting how usage of the word 'chronic' has changed over time. In 'UK informal English', chronic can mean 'very bad' as in the sentence 'The acting was chronic'. It is thought that this transition has occurred because of a misunderstanding of such phrases as 'The teacher shortage was chronic', which means that there has been a shortage of teachers for a long time, but which has been interpreted as a very bad shortage of teachers.

[§]**Footnote:** The idea here is that the immune system reacts to an antigen, such as a food or microbe, in the gut. Through pure chance this antigen is the same shape as a cell type in the body. Autoimmunity is switched on because the body 'sees' the cell type as an antigen. Perhaps the best example is ankylosing spondylitis. In this condition, there is molecular mimicry between klebsiella bacteria in the gut and the spinal ligaments of people who are HLA B27 positive. So, in essence the body makes antibodies against klebsiella bacteria in the gut and then these antibodies cross-react with spinal ligaments and cause the condition of ankylosing spondylitis.

Tests which indicate inflammation in the body

- **Body core temperature** is a very useful cheap test. Running a fever is symptomatic of generalised inflammation. Remember, with age one's ability to do such declines as energy delivery mechanisms decline. However, a temperature spike over and above a low average may well signify chronic inflammation.
- **Local heat**. Thermography is a very useful and sensitive tool for identifying local areas of inflammation in the body. Essentially it takes a 'heat' photograph and of course inflammation is characterised by heat. I love this technique because it involves no radiation, and so scans can be regularly repeated to check clinical progress. Heat photographs are as individual as light photographs so changes are easy to see. I look forward to a DIY phone app that anyone can use (hurry up you boffins!). I need one to help me diagnose and locate 'gravel' in my lame horse.
- These tests tell us the immune system is busy but not why:
  - Erythrocyte sedimentation rate (ESR)
  - Plasma viscosity
  - C reactive protein.
- **Cell-free DNA**. This is a measure of DNA which is not packaged up within a cell – any lying outside must derive from a severely damaged cell. This test is very helpful in my CFS and ME patients who nearly always show raised levels. This test alone puts CFS and ME into a category of significant pathology.
- **Faecal calprotectin**. This is typically raised in inflammatory bowel disease. It may also turn out to be a better screening test for bowel cancers than looking for blood in the stool.
- **Tests for chronic infections**. These are listed in Appendix 5, which is taken from *The Infection Game* section 'Principles of diagnosis of chronic 'stealth' infections – which tests?'

Be mindful that for low grade inflammation there may be no positive test. This is a particular problem for PWME ('People with ME') whose illness is often infection driven but conventional tests lack the sensitivity and specificity to diagnose it. Shamefully they are told by doctors, who should know better, that there is nothing wrong because all the tests are normal. In addition, and because inflammation problems are so common in Westerners eating high-carb diets, living on addictions, with severe micronutrient deficiencies and toxicities, the 'normal ranges' for inflammatory markers have been changed. When I qualified as a medical student, an ESR was considered normal up to 10 mm/hour. Now normal is up to 20 mm/hour and some labs 30. I like to see it running below 5. (For treatment of inflammation, see Chapter 36.)

Chapter 17
Mechanical damage

– structure
– friction
– degenerative disease

Structure

Humans are probably at greater risk of mechanical damage than any other mammal because, relatively recently in evolutionary terms, they (we!) chose to walk around on two legs. This brought great evolutionary advantages: humans are not the fastest predator, but they could run great distances without fatigue and hunt down their prey; in addition, their arms and shoulders were freed up, so they could throw spears and rocks. This made them excellent hunters. In a mammal-Olympics, humans would have won the marathon and the javelin competitions. Cheetahs would have won the 100 metre sprint.

However, a vertebral column that evolved to work from the horizontal now had to function in the vertical position. This it continues to achieve marvellously well so long as all else is well. The vertebral column is inherently unstable and what keeps it functioning well and free from pain is a powerful system of muscles and connective tissue which holds the skeleton in place. There are many wonderful mechanical interventions to help us achieve this most efficiently, and discussion of these is outside the scope of this book. Being a physician, I tend to view

the body from the point of view of essential organs like the brain, gut and heart, but the osteopaths take the opposite view – the body is a physical machine with brain, gut and heart as merely the support staff. Get the physical aspects right and the support structure falls into line. A great deal of athletic training has to do with correct posture/poise, and there are very few people who would not benefit from such training.

Most people stand incorrectly. Furthermore, if we injure ourselves to cause pain, we will adjust the way we stand to deal with that in the short term. This may well leave us with even worse posture. Within the brain we have a three-dimensional map of how the body should be and this is maintained by the fabulous cerebellum, which is responsible for balance and posture. Each muscle has to be set at just the right degree of tension to hold us in place. I suspect that many of the subtle manipulative techniques, such as Bowen therapy and Reiki healing, which cannot be explained by simple mechanical means, could be explained by a re-mapping of the brain. It could be that there are learned muscle spasms which may in the short term be a response to pain but in the long term cause pain in their own right, and that these could be re-mapped by appropriate techniques to afford relief. Whatever the explanation, there has to be one because I see so many people benefit from these techniques for which modern medicine appears to have no good explanation. It may be hard work, but remember (or learn from!) Ovid: *'exitus acta probat'* (the end justifies the deed, or the 'means' as we tend to say). I often see people whose health has been restored simply through attention to posture and exercise.

Friction

I have thought much about the mechanism by which pain is perceived. Remember there is no 'pain' in the body – it is all in the brain. Pain is simply the ploy the brain uses to make us protect ourselves... and very effective it is too! What to my mind is biologically plausible is that some pain is a symptom of friction. The obvious example is a displaced bone fracture where the misplaced bone shard causes massive friction and of course massive pain.

Friction between biological surfaces is damaging. It results in wear and tear and is energy sapping. All moving machines use tricks to minimise friction, such as finely engineered weight-bearing surfaces, ball-bearings and lubricating oils. The body is no different and employs similar techniques to minimise friction. These include the ultra-smooth surfaces of joints, synovial lubricating fluid within joints, special pockets of such fluid to minimise the friction of moving tendons (bursae) together with a softer matrix of fibrous/elastic material we call collagen. This is further steeped in a semi-solid colloidal, mucus matrix. Finally, we have the fourth phase of water – this mechanism means water molecules are aligned on all biological membranes in a graphite-like structure on surfaces to create an almost friction-free interface. (Interested readers

are directed to Gerald Pollack's wonderful book, *The Fourth Phase of Water*.)

Collectively we call this connective tissue.* This is a terribly boring name for a divine conglomeration that allows our soft tissues to look gorgeous and function beautifully despite being suspended from an unforgiving skeleton.

Indeed, there is a seamless transition from rock-hard bone into soft pliable muscles and internal organs via these tough tendons and elastic tissues. These tissues are bathed in a mass of electrical charges which give just the right degree of stickiness – not so much that tissues sag but sufficient to allow tissues to glide smoothly over each other, and not so much that a limb seizes up completely. Furthermore, this stickiness must be absolutely uniform through the tissues, otherwise areas of relative stiffness will concentrate the lines of force, and concentrations of such are painful. We call these painful concentrations by many names, including fibrositis, rheumatics, spondylitis, lumbago, screws, bursitis, tendonitis, fasciitis, repetitive strain injury, stiff neck and other such.

The physical properties of all the above further rely on good hydration and this comes not just from drinking water but also from being able to hold that water in the correct cell space. This needs a diet rich in fat, salt and minerals, together with heat (energy is needed in the form of far infrared radiation for the slippery graphite-like properties of the fourth phase of water). Meat and bone broth provide the raw materials to make new connective tissue. (See our book *The PK Cookbook* for these practical details.) There is little doubt that modern diets high in carbs and low in fat and salt have been a disaster for our physical structure and function. I seem to be seeing epidemics of Ehlers Danlos syndrome (EDS),† characterised by poor quality

---

*Linguistic note: I suggest that we rename connective tissue *mollic corporal splendidis*, translated (roughly), idiomatically, as 'gorgeous soft body'. Craig

connective tissue. It is common in my CFS and ME patients and I suspect results in leaky membranes, leaky gut, leaky blood vessels and leaky brain – so there is much potential for other pathology to ensue. I am wondering if EDS results from a poisoning. We know the antibiotic ciprofloxacin damages tendons. It is routinely fed to factory-farmed chickens and pigs and inevitably gets into the food chain. All the more reason to eat organic food.

An understanding of the magnificent properties of connective tissue explains why so many different therapies are effective. This includes TENS, acupuncture, massage therapy, magnets and manipulative treatments such as osteopathy, shiatsu, McTimoney chiropractic and many others. We know these treatments are effective because they are so widely used by patients who get relief. Again, remember Ovid.

Healing and repairing

There is a general view that as we age our joints wear out and arthritis is inevitable. Nonsense. The joints and bone of our body are not like stones in a river that gradually erode with time. They are very good at healing and repairing – we know this from bone fractures which knit together well. However, to heal and repair we need raw materials, the energy to repair, freedom from toxins and infection, the right stimulus, time and good sleep. Groundhog Basic (page A1) gets us a long way.

---

†**Historical note**: EDS was perhaps first noted by Hippocrates in 400 BC in his writing, 'Airs Water and Places'. He recorded that some Scythians were 'unable to draw their bow because their shoulder joints were too lax'. Scythians lived in areas to the north of the Black Sea and were the first peoples to master mounted warfare, especially with the use of Scythian bows and arrows. They were great mounted archers, and this is probably why Hippocrates especially noted those examples of an inability to draw a bow because this would have been a source of enormous disgrace to Scythian men.

Chapter 18
Mechanisms of growth promotion*

– benign, malignant and prion disorders

Benign and malignant (cancerous) growths

Growths too are an inevitable result of modern Western diets and lifestyles. They are virtually absent in people living paleo lifestyles. Interested readers should read Challa et al for a useful overview.[1] They state that: 'Whalen KA, et al have done studies on the Paleolithic diet, comparing it to the Mediterranean diet. In one study of over 2000 people, participants in each group consumed the list of foods that would fit into each diet pattern. The results were similar in both the groups, although the consumers of a Paleolithic diet decreased their all-cause mortality, decreased oxidative stress, and also decreased mortality from cancers, specifically colon cancers.'

In addition, there is a detailed list of studies supporting the health benefits of a PK (paleoketogenic) diet in our book *Prevent and Cure Diabetes – delicious diets not dangerous drugs*.

We are seeing epidemics of benign breast lumps, polycystic ovarian disease, skin lumps and nodules, neuromas, fibromas, thyroid lumps, prostate hypertrophy and so on. Some benign lumps increase the risk of malignant lumps, so any such should be seen as an imperative to put in place Groundhog Basic (page A.1). Benign lumps arise because of growth-promoting factors in modern Western diets and lifestyles. For a cancer to result, there are two clear mechanisms involved – namely, genetic damage followed by growth promotion.

1. Genetic damage

DNA is constantly being damaged by free radicals which may come from within the body (as a result of energy delivery mechanisms or inflammation) or from outside the body as a result of factors such as background radiation. This produces about 10,000 DNA mutations every second. (Interested readers are directed to Forster et al, 2002 for more detail on this.[2])

Happily, we have enzymes such as the

---

*Editorial note: This is an area where one could reference many hundreds of studies to support the premises of this chapter. Instead, the decision has been taken to direct the interested reader to a few articles that demonstrate the range of evidence. This book is not a reference book or textbook, but rather a book to empower and enable readers to take charge of their own health.

zinc-dependent DNA ligase, which spend their lives trotting up and down DNA cutting out the damaged sections and repairing them. But if the rate of damage exceeds the rate of repair, then DNA will be permanently damaged with the potential for gene blocks or gene activation. This is genetic damage. If a gene involved with cell replication is affected, then uncontrolled cell division may occur – in other words, an early cancer.

Damage to DNA may occur as a result of:

- free radicals from energy delivery mechanisms (worse when these are inefficient)
- free radicals from inflammation (infection, allergic or autoimmune)
- direct damage from toxic stress caused by pesticides, toxic metals, persistent organic pollutants (see Chapter 25) and mycotoxins among others
- all the above effects being worsened where there is poor antioxidant status (antioxidants mop up the free radicals created by toxic and inflammatory stress) and/or micronutrient deficiencies resulting in poor ability to heal and repair DNA.

2. Growth promotion

For cancers and other growths, the second step is that these uncontrolled cells have to grow and multiply, and this will be enhanced by growth promoters. In order of importance these promoters include:

- sugar[†] (and carbohydrates) because cancer cells can only run on sugar
- insulin (which is produced in response to a sugar load)

- sex hormones in the Pill and HRT (not testosterone in physiological doses)
- inflammation driven by chronic low-grade infection
- dairy products (which contain natural growth promotors – yes, even the organic, unpasteurised and fermented versions – I can offer no excuses for the dairy addicts)
- hormone mimics – these include organochlorines (pesticides), polychlorinated biphenyls (fire retardants), and phthalates (plasticisers)
- other toxins which stick onto genes, interfering with cell division and growth controllers.

Prion disorders

Prion disorders include Alzheimer's disease, Parkinson's disease, Creutzfeld-Jacob disease (CJD), probably motor neurone disease, multi-system atrophy (MSA) and others. Cancers, it is well known, are immortal cells which replicate themselves and build up to cause problems. Viruses are strips of DNA which replicate themselves and build up in the body to cause problems. I think of prion disorders as protein cancers. They are proteins which are normally present in the body and perform essential functions. However, if they come into contact with a particular toxin or heavy metal, or another twisted prion (rotten-apple effect), then they too twist and distort. They twist in such a way that they cannot be broken down by the body's enzyme systems and effectively become immortal. Difficulties arise because they obstruct normal biochemistry and so cells

---

[†]**Historical note**: An article by Kearns et al published in November 2017 in the journal *PLOS Biology* cites internal documents by the Sugar Research Foundation (SRF), suggesting that knowledge of a possible link between sugar and cancer goes back as far as the 1960s and yet these results were not published.[3] Kearns et al state: 'The sugar industry did not disclose evidence of harm from animal studies that would have (1) strengthened the case that the CHD risk of sucrose is greater than starch and (2) caused sucrose to be scrutinized as a potential carcinogen.'

malfunction. Pathologically the substance that arises is known as amyloid.

Although amyloid can occur anywhere in the body, the biggest problem is in the brain, perhaps partly because it is a closed box and therefore there is no room for all this excess protein to be dumped and partly because each part of the brain is so vital that any loss of function is quickly noticed. Amyloid is cleared from the brain during sleep by the glymphatic system. We know that lack of sleep is a major risk factor for all diseases of the brain, including dementia. Do not wait for disease – go sleep! Interested readers are directed to the article by Shokri-Kojori et al which states that: '...losing just one night of sleep led to an increase in beta-amyloid, a protein in the brain associated with impaired brain function and Alzheimer's disease.'[4]

From work done with BSE ('mad cow disease', which is also a protein cancer like CJD), there appear to be two phases. After the build-up of prions (amyloid), there then appears to be an autoimmune phase in which the body suddenly recognises this protein as being foreign. This causes inflammation against the prion material in an attempt to get rid of it. The inflammation accelerates the prion damage, so the disease progresses faster. In BSE this is often triggered by a stressful event, such as a calving or very cold weather.

Where do prions come from?

It is biologically plausible that prions represent the biofilm behind which infectious microbes hide. This explains why some are known to pass from inoculation and/or blood contact. So, for example, an epidemic of CJD followed a group of patients being treated with ECT ('electric shock treatment') at the same clinic. We know prion diseases are associated with many factors, including chronic infection (see our book *The Infection Game – life is an arms race*), heavy metals, pesticides and natural toxins.

Table 18.1: Prion disorders and associated risk factors and triggers

Disease	Implicated prion	Associated with:
Alzheimer's disease	Amyloid beta protein	Aluminium poisoning[‡] (as, for example, in dialysis dementia) See link below
		Mercury poisoning (as, for example, in the Mad Hatter in *Alice in Wonderland* – hat making traditionally involved the use of mercury)
		Infectious organisms including: borrelia (Lyme disease), toxoplasmosis, herpes virus 1 (cold sores), herpes virus 2 (genital herpes), cytomegalovirus, cryptococcus, cystercercosis, mycoplasma, syphilis, HIV, CJD (the infectious particle here is uncertain); possibly *Helicobacter pylori* and *Chlamydia pneumoniae*; fungal infection

[‡]**Footnote**: Wang et al (2016) in a systematic review of chronic exposure to aluminium and risk of Alzheimer's disease (AD) which considered eight cohort and case-control studies (with a total of 10567 subjects) concluded that: 'Results showed that individuals chronically exposed to aluminium were 71% more likely to develop AD.'[6]

Disease	Implicated prion	Associated with:
Parkinson's disease	Alpha synuclein	Manganese poisoning (miners in South Africa)
		Organophosphate pesticides
		Infectious organisms including: Helicobacter pylori, borrelia, mycoplasma, Erhlichia, anaplasma
Motor neurone disease	Copper-zinc superoxide dismutase (SOD1 – an antioxidant enzyme)	Manganese poisoning
		Cycad poisoning (MND is a natural toxin from cycad beans; 10% of deaths on the island of Guam were due to MND from cycad[§5])
		Infectious organisms including: polio virus, retrovirus, mycoplasma, borrelia and herpes virus 6 (HHV6)[l]
Multi-system atrophy	A variant of alpha synuclein	Pesticide exposure, especially to organophosphates. (Be aware glyphosate ('Round-up'), the most used pesticide today, is also an organophosphate)
Creutzfeld-Jacob disease (CJD)	PrP[Sc] (scrapie isoform of the prion protein)	Organophosphate pesticides
		Manganese poisoning
	Inoculation with PrP[Sc]	Blood transfusion or surgery Theoretically through vaccination
Familial fatal insomnia	PRNP (PRioN protein)	Genetic mutation that runs in families and is thankfully very rare.

Conventional medicine currently has no effective drug treatments for prion disorders. Even ecological medicine is struggling. This is why prevention is so important. Indeed, a common theme of this book is, as the old English proverb goes, that 'Prevention is better than cure.' (Benjamin Franklin expanded on this idea when he said that: 'An ounce of prevention is worth a pound of cure.')[**]

§**Footnote:** For more on this see Peter Spencer who stated that: 'Surveys conducted in the early 1950s demonstrated that about 10 per cent of deaths among adult Chamorros resulted from ALS (amyotrophic lateral sclerosis), frequencies about 100 times those recorded for the population of the continental United States.'[5]

l**Footnote:** HHV6 is associated with a number of nasties including motor neurone disease. Interested readers should see 'What is HHV6?' on the HHV6 Foundation's website for more detail on other conditions associated with this virus.[6]

Historical note: Benjamin Franklin (17 January 1706 – 17 April 1790), polymath and one of the Founding Fathers of the United States, was talking about fire prevention to fire-threatened Philadelphians in 1736, but his comments ring as true for disease prevention.

References

1. Challa HJ, Uppaluri KR. *Paleolithic Diet.* StatPearls Publishing, Treasure Island, FL, USA (2019) https://www.ncbi.nlm.nih.gov/books/NBK482457/

2. Forster L, Forster P, Lutz-Bonenge S, Wilkomm H, Brinkman B. Natural radioactivity and human mitochondrial DNA mutations. *Proc Natl Acad Sci USA* 2002; 99(21): 13950–13954. (www.ncbi.nlm.nih.gov/pmc/articles/PMC129803/)

3. Kearns CE, Apollonio D, Glantz SA. Sugar industry sponsorship of germ-free rodent studies linking sucrose to hyperlipidemia and cancer: An historical analysis of internal documents. *PLOS Biology* 2017; https://journals.plos.org/plosbiology/article?id=10.1371/journal.pbio.2003460

4. Shokri-Kojori E, Wang GJ, Wiers CE, Demiral SB, et al. β-Amyloid accumulation in the human brain after one night of sleep deprivation. *Proc Natl Sci USA* 2018; 115(17): 4483-4488. www.ncbi.nlm.nih.gov/pubmed/29632177

5. Spencer PS. *Behavioral Measures of Neurotoxicity: Report of a symposium.* National Academy of Sciences, 1990. www.ncbi.nlm.nih.gov/books/NBK234978/

6. HHV-6 Foundation. What is HHV-6? https://hhv-6foundation.org/what-is-hhv-6 (accessed 5 December 2019)

Chapter 19
Genetics and epigenetics

Q: How do you tell the difference between a male chromosome and a female chromosome?
A: Take down their genes

Genetics have been blamed for a great many ills. I often hear this as an excuse for people not to put in place the difficult lifestyle changes that I am asking them to make: 'There's no point....my mum had it, my dad had it, so I'll get it too...'. However, the World Health Organization tells us that the overwhelming majority of problems arise from gene-environment interactions – that is to say, if the environment can be put right, then the gene problem can be overcome. So, for example, I see many patients with myalgic encephalitis (ME) and chronic fatigue syndrome (CFS) and a central player here is poor mitochondrial function. Mitochondria have their own genes, which are different from the cell's own nucleic genomic DNA. However, if that gene defect happens to be related to a problem with endogenous production of co-enzyme Q10 (coQ10), then that can be fixed simply by administering coQ10 as a supplement. Indeed, I am coming to the view that as we age we all become less good at producing

coQ10 and maybe we should all be taking a supplement of at least 100 mg daily in order to protect our mitochondria and slow the ageing process.

Just because a patient has a genetic lesion does not mean that nothing can be done for them.* Dr Henry Turkel[1] specialised in treating Down's syndrome. Many of these patients were hypothyroid. Correction of this together with diets and other standard techniques of nutritional medicine (Groundhog Basic (page A1), in other words) resulted in patients functioning at a higher physical and intellectual level. (For a quick review of Turkel's work in this area please see www.doctoryourself.com/turkel.html – Down Syndrome: The Nutritional Treatment of Henry Turkel, M.D. and also the Case history in Chapter 77.)

Tests for genetic risk factors

SNPs
Single nucleotide polymorphisms or SNPs (pronounced 'snips') are the most common type of genetic variation among people.

---

*Linguistic note on the 'double negative': This is a grammatical construction where two forms of negation are used in the same sentence. In some languages (English included, except African American and vernacular English), double negatives 'cancel one another out' and produce an affirmative; in other languages, double negatives intensify the negation. Languages where multiple negatives affirm each other are said to have 'negative concord'; these include Spanish, Russian and Afrikaans. Some English teachers (including Craig's) hate double negatives with a vengeance!

Identifying SNPs may indicate susceptibility to certain diseases, but I never do this test – it is rather expensive and rarely has implications for management of illness. This is because it does not tell us exactly what is wrong but only what we may be susceptible to. Most potential problems are covered by Groundhog Basic and all by Groundhog Chronic.

DNA adducts

I am extremely fortunate to be able to work very closely with Dr John McLaren Howard of Acumen Laboratories, who is the most brilliant biochemist. His brilliance arises because he applies cutting-edge technology to clinical problems. A most useful test that he makes available is DNA adducts. This is a measure of what is stuck onto DNA. Of course, it should be pristine – DNA is the genetic blueprint. Having something stuck on to it (such as a toxic metal, pesticide or volatile organic compound or mycotoxin) is bad news for obvious reasons – the genetic code cannot be accurately read. Furthermore, Acumen can identify which gene the adduct is stuck on to – this may block this gene or activate it; both outcomes are undesirable because normal gene expression is upset.

Acumen Laboratories go on to do further analysis using a technique called 'microassay', which allows a more detailed view of DNA and how it is expressed. This brings us on to epigenetics – the DNA may be intact, but cannot be accessed normally, perhaps because of poor methylation. We need this biochemical tool to translate the DNA code into action.

If governments were serious about cancer prevention, then DNA adducts would be used as a routine screening test. There is no more powerful wake-up call to make Groundhog interventions than the discovery of a toxin stuck onto a cancer gene – that is, a premalignant lesion!

Epigenetics

We used to believe that anything we did within our life was not reflected in the genes we passed on to the next generation. We know now this is not true. Epigenetics reflects changes, not to the basic DNA, but to how that DNA is expressed. This is further reason to follow Groundhog ... so as not to mess things up for future generations. Get it right for your kids – see Chapter 55.

Reference

1. www.doctoryourself.com/turkel.html – Down Syndrome: The Nutritional Treatment of Henry Turkel, M.D

PART IV
What to do – the basics

*The tools of the trade to prevent disease
and the starting point to treat all disease*

PART IV

Chapter 20
Start with Groundhog Basic

The starting point for preventing and treating all chronic disease of Westerners is exactly the same. We are on a journey which has already taken us down the wrong route. We must return to square one where Mother Nature meant us to be. We must hope that we have not yet got to the point of no return. I spend more time talking about this subject – nutrition – than all others put together. This is because for many, Groundhog Basic is all that they have to do to recover, and if not, it represents the foundation stone on which all other therapies are based. Groundhog Basic is non-negotiable.

The good news is that this sustainable, ecological medicine can be used to treat all diseases and it is within the power of us all to do such. The bad news is that it is difficult. It means changing the habits of a lifetime, recognising that one is an addict, flying in the face of current medical and social norms and spending precious reserves of money and energy selfishly. During the early days of Groundhog Basic one may even get worse. This is why a clear understanding of the 'whats' and the 'whys' is essential to provide the intellectual imperative and the sheer bloody-mindedness necessary to stick to one's guns. I now know there are no short cuts and, believe me, I too am an addict and have tried them all!

What is Groundhog Basic?

Groundhog Basic (called 'Groundhog' because I repeat it to patients and readers every day) consists of these essential elements:

Paleo-ketogenic (PK) diet supplemented with a few essential micronutrients to compensate for the deficiencies of modern agriculture

Sleep – of good quality and quantity

Exercise – the right sort

Sunshine and light

Reduction of the chemical burden

Sufficient physical and mental security to satisfy our universal need to love and care, and be loved and cared for

Avoidance of infections and treating them aggressively – when they arise – with Groundhog Acute (see page A3).

---

*Historical note: Interested readers can digest the whole speech at this link: www.ibiblio.org/pha/timeline/410209awp.html

There is a summary of the Groundhog Basic whats and whys in Appendix 1 (page A1).

We then end this chapter with another double negative, this time from the pen of F Scott Fitzgerald, written in 1936 to his daughter 'Scottie' upon her enrolment in High School: 'Nothing any good isn't hard.'[†]

[†]**Historical note 2**: Scottie (26 October 1921 – 18 June 1986) was christened Frances Scott 'Scottie' Fitzgerald while her father (24 September 1896 – 21 December 1940) was Francis Scott Key Fitzgerald. You can read the letter he sent her here: www.brainpickings.org/2013/01/08/f-scott-fitzgerld-on-writing/ along with other letters of fatherly advice.

Chapter 21
The paleo-ketogenic diet

> *The cure is in the kitchen.*
> Dr Sherry Rogers,
> environmental physician

In this chapter we look at the first elements of Groundhog Basic – the paleo-ketogenic (PK) diet and essential micronutrients: multivitamins, minerals and essential fatty acids so that you will be armed with what to eat and which supplements to take.

As I said in the previous chapter, the PK diet is non-negotiable. I spend more time talking about diet and cooking than all other subjects put together. Changing one's diet is the most difficult, but the most important, thing one needs to do for good health. There is much more detail on the 'why' and the 'how' in our books *Prevent and Cure Diabetes – delicious diets not dangerous drugs* and *The PK Cookbook – go paleo-ketogenic and get the best of both worlds*. Please do use them – they are born out of bitter experience.

Remember outside of autumn, primitive man (and woman!) ate a paleo-ketogenic diet and this would largely have been comprised of raw meat and/or raw fish and shellfish depending on where he lived. That was it. You may think this a boring diet, but boredom is secondary to survival. For some of the sickest patients, we have to return to this very primitive diet to allow them to recover. Natasha Campbell McBride describes this diet in her book *The GAPS Diet*. An essential part of it is to access bone marrow. Perhaps this is what drove primitive man to using tools to smash open this treasure chest of fat and micronutrients and so the clever ones survived? Neanderthal man had a larger brain than modern man. As my patients often hear in the consulting room: '…my job is to get you well, not to entertain you.' (Some say that quoting oneself shows a lack of humility. It is a good job then that Craig wrote that last sentence.)

Guess what? I am not going to live my life eating raw meat and raw fish just so that I can live to a great age. We all have to work out a compromise diet that gets us the best of both worlds. And that is going to be different for everyone and will change with age. For me, greed gets in the way – I love good food. So, we all need a starting set of rules which can then be relaxed or tightened up depending on our age and disease state. Younger, healthy, physically active people can take more liberties than old sick ones. I find myself in the old, healthy category and so I am still no paragon of virtue.

What to eat

The following is a reasonable starting point for most people. You can have as much as you like of:

- Fats – saturated fats for energy, such as lard, butter (or, ideally, ghee so long as you are sure you are not allergic to it; I am…. Dammit!), goose fat, coconut oil, palm oil.

- Oils – unsaturated fats which are also fuels but contain essential omega-3, -6 and -9 fatty acids. Hemp oil is ideal as it contains the perfect balance of omega-6 to omega-3 fatty acids – that is, 4:1. These must be cold-pressed and not used for cooking or you risk 'flipping' them into toxic trans fats. Only cook with biochemically stable, saturated fats. (See our books listed above for more on good and bad fats.)
- Fibre – this is often included in the carb count of foods and leads to some confusion.

And also as much as you like of foods that contain less than 5% carbohydrate, of which the most important are:

- linseed (See *The PK Cookbook* for a great recipe for linseed bread which looks and behaves like a small Hovis if you cook it in a hot enough oven; it also makes a great base for muesli and porridge)
- coconut cream – the Grace coconut milk is head and shoulders above all others with a 2% carb content and is a great alternative for dairy
- Brazil and pecan nuts
- salad vegetables (lettuce, cucumber, tomato, pepper etc), avocado pear and olives (phew – I love them both)
- green leafy vegetables
- mushrooms and fungi – while a difficulty with this diet is eating enough fat, these foods are great for frying as they mop up delicious saturated fats
- fermented foods (sauerkraut, kefir) since the carb content has been fermented out by microbes.

You will need to take care with:

- meat, fish, shellfish and eggs – do not eat too much of these as excessive amounts of protein can be converted back to carbohydrate via a process called 'gluconeogenesis' (see *The PK Cookbook* for details again – ho! ho! You are going to have to buy that now!)
- Salt – 1 tsp (5 grams) daily (Ideally use 'Sunshine salt' as described below)
- coffee and tea – drink only in moderation.

Then further care will be needed with foods that are 5-10% carbs (see *The PK Cookbook* for more):

- berries
- some nuts: almonds
- herbs and spices – these do have some carb content but in the small amounts normally used these are not going to spike your blood sugar levels.

Avoid foods that are more than 10% carbohydrate as they switch on addictive eating. I know. I too am an addict, or have been. So avoid:

- all grains and pulses
- all fruits and their juices
- many nuts and seeds
- junk food, which is characterised by its high-carb content and additive potential; this includes crisps*(sorry, Craig!)
- all dairy products except ghee (see Chapter 18 for the why)
- all sweeteners, natural or artificial, which simply switch on the physical and psychological cravings.

Micronutrients and supplements

You will need to take micronutrient supplements for life to compensate for the deficiencies resulting from modern food production methods.

First, you will need a good multivitamin and multimineral. We need these simply because with Western agriculture there is a one-way movement of minerals from the soil, to plants, to animals and then to us humans. We throw them away.

This lack of recycling means we are all deficient in such. (Once again, we discuss this in much more detail in *The PK Cookbook*, with referenced studies showing the result of this 'one-way' traffic.)

I have got to the stage in my medical practice where I know exactly what must be done so I am now trying to make this as easy and inexpensive as possible. Consequently, I have formulated 'Sunshine salt' which contains all essential minerals, from sodium and selenium to magnesium and manganese, together with vitamin D 5000 iu and B12 5 mg per 5 g (1 tspn) dose. This does make life much easier. It tastes like a slightly piquant sea salt, can be used in cooking and means the rest of the family can get a dose without even realising it (especially that man who believes he is immortal!).†

Secondly, but just as important, take vitamin C: 5-15 grams (yes, I mean 5000 to 15,000 mg, and no, that is not a big dose) daily. Go to Chapter 31 (about vitamin C) to find out why.

Timing

Primitive man did not eat three regular meals a day, neither did he snack... unless the opportunity presented itself with a happenchance of berries or the like. Consultant neurologist Dale Bredesen reverses dementia with a PK diet but insists all daily food is consumed within a 10-hour window of time.[1]

Once keto-adapted you may feel a bit peckish and deserving of a snack, but the good news is that you will not get the associated 'energy dive' experienced by the carb addict who must eat according to the clock. Carb addicts feel a sudden loss of energy and *have* to feed their addiction to get rid of this awful feeling. The keto-adapted do not experience this. A weekly 24-hour fast is also good for the metabolism. It may be counter-intuitive, but the fact is that this enhances mental and physical performance.

If you have decided to go ahead with this diet, then believe me it is a bumpy ride. There is a whole new language to be learned. You will have to identify the glycogen sponge, anticipate the metabolic hinterland, get keto-adapted and prepare for detox and Herxheimer reactions (see Chapter 28). I simply cannot write all the nitty gritty detail here for this successful transition without losing the plot of this book; *The PK Cookbook* will hold your intellectual hand through this difficult transition. Or just do it....

Once established on the PK diet

The word 'doctor' comes from the Greek for 'to teach'. I can show you the path, but you have to walk it. You have to become your own physician. All diagnosis starts with hypothesis. We know the PK diet is the starting point to treat every disease and that is non-negotiable. Stick with this diet for life and it may be that this is all you have to do. Once PK is established you have to ask yourself

---

*Explanatory note: Before becoming 'PK-adapted', crisps were my addiction. I ate at least six normal-sized bags of ready-salted crisps each and every day. (See how, even now, I try to rationalise this addiction by the use of the phrase 'normal-sized' as though I am saying to my inner self, 'It wasn't that bad!') I even had a stash of 12 bags in my wardrobe, 'just in case'. I gave up crisps overnight. One Monday, I threw away all 'my' crisps, stashed in various rooms of our house, and I have not eaten even a single crisp since then. I know that eating even one packet will trigger the addiction and so I simply never eat them.

†Footnote: It is a shame that *'ichor'* (the 'blood' of the Greek Gods which was said to retain the qualities of ambrosia, the food or drink of the gods, which gave them immortality) does not seem to exist. And so, until *ichor* is found, or formulated, and made non-toxic to mortals, I shall 'eat PK', take my supplements and openly sprinkle Sunshine salts over my food.

if you are functioning to your full physical and mental potential. Only you can know this.

If you are functioning to your full potential, then you can take the occasional liberty with your diet. Primitive man surely did. He did so in the autumn, although not with the high-carb foods that we can now access. Alcohol is a peculiar problem – it is addictive, high carb and stimulates insulin directly. But I love alcohol; the jokes are so much funnier with a glass of cider on board, and so I enjoy this occasional liberty at this stage in my life. (I have to because Craig keeps sending me bottles of the most delicious cider... and I do not have the will power to tell him to stop! Craig: 'Then I shall carry on. Luckily, in return, I get delicious joints of pork and bacon.')

If you are not functioning to your full potential, then you must stick with the PK diet and read on. Even if you do not experience immediate benefits you will greatly increase your chance of a long and healthy life. It is a great consolation for me to be able to tell my CFS and ME patients that their best years are ahead of them.

> *The Chinese do not draw any distinction between food and medicine.*
> Lin Yutang, Chinese writer, 1895 – 1976,
> in *The importance of Living*,
> Chapter 9, section 7

Reference

1. Bredesen DE. Reversal of cognitive decline: A novel therapeutic program. *Aging* 2014; 6(9): 707-717. http://www.drmyhill.co.uk/drmyhill/images/0/07/Reversal-of-Cognitive-decline-Bredesen.pdf

Chapter 22
Sleep

– common reasons for poor sleep
– how to fix them

Homer, the (legendary) author of the epic poems, *The Odyssey* and *The Iliad*, knew that sleep was vital: 'There is a time for many words, and there is also a time for sleep.'*

Just as the PK diet is non-negotiable, so too is sleep. Should you hesitate to believe this, or scoff at the suggestion, re-read chapter 14. Then see below for what you need to do to achieve the quantity, quality and timing of sleep for optimal health. I know I do not know all the answers to poor sleep (another steep learning curve) but you may find some below. Recently I have learned the importance of thyroid and adrenal hormones for good quality sleep. Am I not lucky? I am on such a journey of interesting of questions I know I shall never be bored.†

1. Tackle the causes of poor sleep

First we need to think about what is disturbing sleep. In order of likelihood consider:

- Adrenalin
- Sleep apnoea
- Hormones
- Inflammation
- Detoxing
- Unpleasant symptoms.

Adrenalin

The commonest cause of disturbed sleep in Westerners is nocturnal hypoglycaemia because as blood sugar levels fall, adrenalin levels spike. Anyone who is PK-adapted (running on ketones rather than glucose for energy) can run a blood sugar level as low as 1 mmol/l and suffer no symptoms of hypoglycaemia. This is because once PK-adapted, the brain happily runs on ketones and does not panic if sugar is not available. My friend Michelle eats PK. She breast-fed and weaned baby Robyn onto a PK diet – since four weeks of age Robyn has never failed to sleep 11 hours and at two months of age she slept a solid 13 hours at night.

*Footnote: Homer was born sometime between the 12th and 8th centuries BC, possibly somewhere on the coast of Asia Minor. Very little is known about him, even whether he was really the author of these two poems. In fact, Homer may not even be a single person, but we digress. I agree with Homer about the importance of sleep. (Homer agrees with you, Sarah. Craig)

†Footnote: The Odyssey is about a 'journey'. It is the second-oldest extant work of Western literature, The Iliad being the oldest, and as such it lays the foundation for much of Western thinking. A key point is that we are all on our own individual journeys of discovery.

Sources of adrenalin include:

- mimics such as caffeine and chocolate
- stress: see Chapter 50: Psychiatry (page 50.1).
- alcohol: one of the most powerful disturbers of sleep. A large slug may get you off to sleep, but this triggers hypoglycaemia, adrenalin is poured out and you wake in the middle of the night, wide awake, often unable to drop off again. Sigh, I love alcohol, but it is sleep loss that stops me drinking the lovely stuff!
- the upper fermenting gut: fermentation of carbs, and to a lesser extent protein in the upper gut creates many toxins, including alcohol, which have the potential to disturb sleep. The last meal of the day needs to be in the early evening, should be modest with no carbs and low protein but high in fibre and fat. Many find that fasting improves sleep quality. I do… dammit!

Sleep apnoea syndrome

Stopping breathing is stressful and – surprise, surprise – wakes you up. You may stop breathing because:

- your airway is blocked, in which case breathing is noisy, often with snoring (obstructive sleep apnoea) OR
- your brain forgets to trigger a breath (so-called 'central sleep apnoea').

Causes of obstruction, and so snoring, include:

- obesity ('Pickwickian syndrome'[‡])
- oedema due to allergy or hypothyroidism
- undershot jaw with narrowing of the airways.

Causes of central sleep apnoea include:

- poisoning by mycotoxins
- poisoning by chemicals
- addictions (see Chapter 8: Poisoning and deficiency)

Disrupted or declining hormones

Hormones decline with age and parallel worsening sleep. It is melatonin that drives our sleep/wake cycle. It is produced in response to lack of light and switched off by its presence. Its production has a momentum of its own which explains why it takes a week to adjust to jet lag. Melatonin does not make us sleepy, but we cannot sleep without it. With age, our ability to make melatonin declines and, with that, sleep quality declines in parallel. One intervention known to extend life span is restricting calorie intake – this also stimulates melatonin production. To live longer, given the choice between living half-starved and taking melatonin at night… well, for a foodie[§] like me, it is a no-brainer.

Melatonin is additionally a good antioxidant. By mopping up free radicals, this slows

---

[‡]**Historical literary note**: Pickwickian syndrome is named after the character Joe (the 'fat boy') from Charles Dickens's novel *The Pickwick Papers*. Joe displayed all the characteristics of obstructive sleep apnoea. The first time that the term 'Pickwickian syndrome' was used is thought to have been in a 1956 medical paper by Burwell et al.[1]

[§]**Linguistic note**: It is thought that the term 'foodie' was first coined (in print) by *New York* magazine's food critic, Gael Green, in an article dated 2 June 1980. There are also several London-based citations of 'foodie' in 1982 and it appears that these were independent of Green. This feature of 'things happening simultaneously and independently' appears in science and is known as 'multiple discovery', or 'simultaneous invention', the hypothesis being that many scientific discoveries are made independently and nearly simultaneously by many scientists. The idea is that the conditions are right for such a discovery and that this leads to many people 'having the same thought' at roughly the same time. This hypothesis is at odds with the 'heroic theory' of invention and discovery, which contends that individuals usually come up with new ideas totally 'on their own'. Interested readers are directed to 'Multiple discovery' on Wikipedia where, amongst others, the case of the near simultaneous discovery of Calculus by Newton, Leibniz and others is quoted.

the ageing process and protects against cancer. Melatonin triggers the release of TSH (thyroid stimulating hormone), which spikes at midnight, so thyroid hormones are produced at the proper time, with T4 spiking at 4 am and T3 at 5 am. These kick the adrenals into life, with adrenal hormones and testosterone spiking at 6 am; this warms us up and wakes us up. There can be other vicious cycles here because poor sleep results in poor hormone production.

Melatonin (slow-release) 3-9 mg at night, is best. Some people just need 1 mg. I suspect the need for melatonin is what I call an 'acquired metabolic dyslexia' – as we age, we may all benefit from additional melatonin at night. The pathway for melatonin production starts with trypto-phan, which is converted to 5HTP (5 hydroxy tryptophan), then to serotonin and melatonin. Of proven benefit for sleep is tryptophan 1-3 g and/or 5HTP 300 mg. So, to correct the hormo-nal environment:

- First take tryptophan 1-3 g and/or 5HTP 100-300 mg and/or melatonin 3-9 mg at night
- Then sort out the thyroid – see Chapters 13 and 30
- Then sort out the adrenals – see Chapters 13 and 30
- Consider testosterone glandular 1-3 g in the morning (Note, too much may worsen sleep).

Inflammation

Inflammation occurs when the immune system is active for reasons of allergy, autoimmunity and infection. We all recognise the disturbed sleep of acute flu. The immune system and the brain are remarkably similar – the only difference is that the brain is contained within a bony anatomical box whereas the immune system is located throughout the whole body, including the brain. Much inflammation starts with the fermenting gut (see page 44.2), and where there is upper fermenting gut there is also 'fermenting brain' – that is, microbes in the gut may also be present in the brain, where they ferment neurotransmitters into, amongst other things, amphetamine-like substances.[2] See Chapter 36 for ways to counteract this.

Detoxing

During sleep, the 'glymphatics' of the brain (the brain's fluid drainage system) open up to allow the brain to clear the accumulated junk that is inevitably generated by daily use (see Chapter 14). I am not sure why this should disturb sleep, but it is so obvious clinically as part of detox reactions as discussed in Chapter 28.

Unpleasant symptoms

Not surprisingly, unpleasant and worrying sensations also disrupt sleep, including pain, shortness of breath, palpitations and reflux (see individual relevant chapters and Chapter 6: Pain).

2. The physical essentials

In addition to identifying and redressing the causes of poor sleep you must get the physical essentials for good sleep in place. Knowing what may be causing the problem is essential to knowing what to do, but we must then actually do that. As the saying goes: 'Actions speak louder than words.'[1]

---

[1]**Footnote**: This phrase possibly has its origins in the book of John in the Bible, where it is stressed that merely saying that you love someone is not the same as doing things for them. But in the form as above, it is attributed to Abraham Lincoln (President of the United States, 1861–1865, born 12 February 1809 and assassinated 15 April 1865) in 1856. Personally, I (Craig) prefer the version attributed to English statesman John Pym (1584 – 8 December 1643), who said in 1628: 'A word spoken in season is like an Apple of Gold set in Pictures of Silver, and actions are more precious than words.'

These essentials are:

1. A comfortable bed – we have been brainwashed into believing a hard bed is good for us and so many people end up with sleepless nights on an uncomfortable bed. Do whatever you need to distribute your weight evenly and avoid pressure points – memory foam mattresses are often helpful, or water beds.

2. A dark room – the slightest chink of light landing on your skin will disturb your own production of melatonin (the body's natural sleep hormone). Have thick curtains or blackouts to keep the bedroom dark; this is particularly important for children. Do not switch the light on or clock watch should you wake.

3. A quiet room – do not allow a bed fellow who snores; you need different rooms.

4. Temperature control – core body temperature falls at night and this is an essential part of triggering sleep. Indeed, the mechanism that wakes us up is an increase in body temperature and that is driven by a spike of thyroid and adrenal hormones, as described above. Core body temperature is controlled by blood flow to the skin, and heat is lost through sweating of this 'shell'. Wear pyjamas that 'wick' (absorb)** sweat away from the skin to facilitate this. Cotton is the best material. With no pyjamas, sweating leaves the skin icy cold; this may be painful and that disturbs sleep. Falling body temperature is a powerful and essential trigger for sleep. This may explain why a warm bath helps – once out of the bath, heat is rapidly lost through the 'shell', so core temperature follows, and sleep is induced. Do not exercise hard before sleep – you get too hot and stay hot. However, to complicate matters, a Dutch sleep study used a thermosuit to increase skin temperature by 0.4°C (core temperature was unaffected) and this greatly improved sleep quality in the young, the elderly and insomniacs.[3] The point is to experiment with heat and cold and, if not obvious from how you sleep, use a sleep app to give feedback as to whether you are winning or losing the battle,

5. Exercise/activity – your day needs the right balance of mental and physical activity. Expect to sleep better after a physically active day (note that this is not possible for CFS/ME patients). Do not take problems that keep you awake to bed but remember that during REM sleep we problem-solve – you may wake in the morning with the answer.[††]

6. Avoid stimulants such as caffeine or adrenalin, inducing TV, arguments, phone calls, family matters or whatever soon before bed time.

7. Restrict fluids in the evening if your night is disturbed by the need to pee.

8. Get the timing right – as the day progresses a 'pressure to sleep' builds up so the longer we stay awake the greater is the need and desire to sleep. Over and above this sleep pressure throughout the 24 hours, we also have a 90-minute sleep cycle. Learn to recognise this because you will have a much better chance of dropping off if you ride the

---

**Linguistic note: The word 'wick' can be a noun or a verb. As a verb it means to absorb or draw off (liquid) by capillary action.

[††]**Footnote:** Jacques Hadamard wrote a book called *The Psychology of Invention in the Mathematical Field*. He gives several examples of famous mathematicians dreaming about solutions, including Poincare. Poincare was called the 'Last Universalist' because it was said that he excelled in all fields of mathematics as it existed during his lifetime. (Jacques Hadamard, French mathematician, 8 December 1865 – 17 October 1963.)

sleep wave. You may well feel such a sleep wave during the evening – perhaps feeling dozy whilst watching TV? It will come at the same time each evening. In winter, I eat supper at 6:30-ish, then watch telly. I feel dozy at 8:15 pm, take Nancy (the terrier) out ratting at 8:45 pm, am in bed by 9:15 at the latest, read, feel the sleep wave coming on at 9:45, light out, sleep dream (see below) in place... and I am gone. I have an alarm set for 6:00 am but it rarely goes off because I wake a few minutes prior. Remember, we hibernate in winter and need more sleep than in summer.

9. Have a regular rising time – because of artificial lighting our internal clock runs late so there is a tendency is to wake later every morning. If we allow this to happen, we end up rushing and skipping breakfast in order to get to work on time. Disaster! Breakfast is the most important meal of the day. It is well recognised that a good (but counterintuitive) way to improve sleep quality is to set the alarm clock for 30 minutes earlier than your usual ring time and maintain such. I think this helps to mitigate the effects of artificial light.

3. The sleep dream

The third thing to do is to get your brain off to sleep with a sleep dream. Getting the physical things in place is the easy bit. The hard bit is getting your brain off to sleep. If you go to bed thinking about the previous day and planning the next day then you have little chance of dropping off. But the brain can be trained because, throughout life, it makes a million new connections every second. This means it has a fantastic ability to learn new things.

Getting off to sleep successfully is all about developing a conditioned reflex. The best example of such is Pavlov's dogs. Pavlov was a Russian physiologist who showed that when dogs eat food, they salivate. He then 'conditioned' them by ringing a bell whilst they ate food. After two weeks of conditioning, he could make them salivate simply by ringing a bell. This of course is a completely useless conditioned response, but it shows us the brain can be trained, by association, to do anything.

Applying this to the insomniac, firstly one has to get into a mind-set (sleep dream) which does not involve the immediate past or immediate future. That is to say, if you are thinking about reality then there is no chance of getting off to sleep. In the words of Dr Seuss (1904 – 1991): 'You know you're in love when you can't fall asleep because reality is finally better than your dreams.'

I do not pretend this is easy, but to allow one's mind to wander into reality when one is trying to sleep must be considered a complete self-indulgence. Treat your brain like a naughty child. It is simply not allowed to free-wheel.

Find a sleep dream that suits you. As I have said, if you think about real events then there is no chance of dropping off to sleep, so you have to displace these thoughts with a sleep dream. It could be a childhood dream, or recalling details of a journey or walk, making up a story, or whatever. It is actually a sort of self-hypnosis. What you are trying to do is to 'talk' to your subconscious. This best done with images, not with spoken language since your sub-conscious deals with emotions and feelings. I dream that I am a hibernating bear, snuggled down in my comfortable den with one daughter in one arm and the other in the other. Outside the wind is howling and the snow coming down and I am sinking deeper and deeper down...

Learning a sleep dream is a bit like riding a bicycle – it looks impossible at a distance but with a bit of practice becomes easy. Your brain will try to convince you that a sleep dream is not working – but that is just because the brain likes to free-wheel, especially if you are naturally hyper-vigilant.

If you do wake in the night, do not switch the light on and do not get up and potter round the house or you will have no chance of dropping off to sleep. Once again, use your sleep dream.

4. If you need more help

Fourthly, if you cannot get the sleep dream to work then reinforce this conditioning with a hypnotic. The idea here is that you take a sleeping pill *and* do the sleep dream – in other words, you apply the two together for a period of 'conditioning'. This may be a few days or a few weeks. The brain then learns that when it gets into that particular mindset, it will go off to sleep. Use of the medication should become unnecessary. Of course, I sometimes prescribe hypnotics, but it is a condition of such that all the above directions are followed. Yes, even I do blackmail‡‡ occasionally.

I instinctively do not like prescribing drugs. However, I do use them for sleep, in order to establish the above conditioning and to restore a normal pattern of sleep, after which it should be possible be tail off or keep medicine for occasional use. However, viruses can cause neurological damage (for example, polio) and this could involve damage to the sleep centre. Some people are constitutionally hard-wired for hyper-vigilance and may need medication for life to allow them to sleep. Do see PTSD in Chapter 50 for techniques to tackle this.

Sleep can break down during times of stress and a few days of medication may be required to reinforce the conditioned response. But it is vital to use the correct 'mind-set' every time the medication is used, or the conditioning will weaken.

Medication for sleep

These are the alternatives I consider to help build the sleep conditioning response:

- Nytol (diphenhydramine 50 mg). This is a sedating antihistamine available over the counter. The dose is ½ -2 tablets at night. It is long acting – don't take it in the middle of the night or you will wake feeling hung-over.
- Valerian root 400 mg 1-4 capsules at night. This is a herbal preparation which is shorter acting and can be taken in the middle of the night.
- Kava kava. I used to find it very useful but unfortunately it has now been banned in the UK; it is still available in the USA.

If there is no improvement with a combination of the above, then I would go on to a prescribed drug. I usually start with:

- one of the sedating antidepressants, such as amitriptyline 10-25 mg. I would start with 5 mg initially. Most ME/CFS patients are made worse and feel hung-over with 'normal' doses.
OR
- Some people need prescription tranquillisers, such as zolpidem 10 mg (short acting), zopiclone 3.75-7.5 mg (medium acting), nitrazepam 5 mg (long acting) or clonazepam 0.5-2 mg (long acting).

---

‡‡**Linguistic note:** The origins of the word 'blackmail' are linked to a practice of the chieftains in the border region between England and Scotland in the 16th century and part of the 17th century, whereby said chieftains ordered landholders to pay them in order to avoid being pillaged. The 'mail' in the word meant 'tribute, rent' and was derived from an old Scandinavian word, *'mal'*, meaning 'agreement'. The 'black' in blackmail is thought to be an ironic comment on 'white money', the term for the silver coins with which tenant farmers traditionally paid their legitimate rent.

It is vital to combine the above prescriptions with a good sleep dream and all the above interventions. Do not let the medication work without, otherwise tachyphylaxis (a decrease in drug response) will result and the medication will become ineffective.

I am always asked about addiction. My experience is that this is rare, especially if drugs are used as above to develop a conditioned reflex or to treat pathologically awful sleep. One has to distinguish between addiction and dependence. We are all dependent on food, but that does not mean we are addicted to it. We are all dependent on a good night's sleep for good health and may therefore become dependent on something to achieve that. This does not inevitably lead to addiction. Addiction is a condition of taking a drug excessively and being unable to cease doing so without other adverse effects. Stopping your hypnotic may result in a poor night's sleep but hopefully little more than that. This is not addiction but dependence.

We know that taking prescription hypnotics for years is a risk factor for dementia. But then so is insomnia. I am not sure where the balance lies. But if it were me? ... Well, I would take the sleeping pills and put in place all else to protect against dementia. For me, sleep is an essential, not a luxury.

Table 22.1: Common causes of disturbed sleep and how to tackle

Symptom	Mechanism	Treatment
'I just wake up as if it is morning but it's 2:00 am'	Adrenalin from nocturnal hypoglycaemia (adrenalin is the usual stimulus for normal waking)	PK diet
	Alcohol is a major cause of hypoglycaemia since it stimulates insulin release directly	Take care with alcohol Treat the fermenting gut or 'auto-brewery syndrome'
	The adrenalin of post-traumatic stress syndrome/disorder (PTSD)	See Chapter 50: Psychiatry Block this with propranolol
	Inadequate hormones or poor timing of their release	As above: melatonin, thyroid, adrenal, testosterone glandulars
	May be a detox reaction	See DDD reactions, Chapter 28
Sleep apnoea: obstructive	Metabolic syndrome, obesity Allergy Hypothyroid Undershot jaw	PK diet – low carb for weight loss Low allergen Correct the thyroid See a good osteopath
Sleep apnoea: central	From neurological damage: mycotoxins, pesticides, VOCs toxic metals	See Chapter 8
Too hot – hot flush and sweating	Menopausal	Do not take female sex hormones Testosterone is much safer Work on temperature control All above help greatly to mitigate flushes, but cure not guaranteed

Symptom	Mechanism	Treatment
	The body trying to run a fever to deal with chronic low-grade infection	Read our book *The Infection Game*
Symptoms such as pain, wheeze, itching, restless legs	Allergy to food and/or gut microbes	See Chapters 6 and 7 PK diet
Gut symptoms such as reflux, indigestion	Fermenting gut	PK diet Vitamin C to bowel tolerance
Constitutionally hard-wired for hyper-vigilance	Previous psychological trauma e.g. childhood bullying or abuse	Use hypnotics (No I do not like these but, yes, you must sleep!) Counselling
Neurological damage... which may or may not also cause central sleep apnoea	Past head injury Poisoning by chemicals Pathology: ischaemia (stroke, dementia), prion disease, tumour	Do all the above Use hypnotics Tests for toxic load followed by appropriate detox regimes Read *The Infection Game*
Depression and many other brain conditions	I think depression is more often the result of poor sleep, not a cause of it	See Chapter 50: Psychiatry More reason to try tryptophan

And so to bed.
Expression often used by Samuel Pepys at the end of his day's diary entry.
Samuel Pepys, English MP and famous diarist, 23 February 1633 – 26 May 1703

References

1. Burwell CS, Robin ED, Whaley RD, Bickelmann AG. Extreme obesity associated with alveolar hypoventilation – a Pickwickian syndrome. *Am J Med* 1956; 21: 811– 818. www.sciencedirect.com/science/article/pii/0002934356900948

2. Nishihara K. Disclosure of the major causes of mental illness—mitochondrial deterioration in brain neurons via opportunistic infection. www.drmyhill.co.uk/drmyhill/images/d/dc/NISHIHARA.pdf

3. Ryamann RJE, Swaab DF, van Someren EJW. Skin deep: enhanced sleep depth by cutaneous temperature manipulation. *Brain* 2008; 131: 500-513, https://watermark.silverchair.com/awm315.pdf

Chapter 23
Exercise

Humans, along with other mammals, evolved living physically active lives. This probably meant long hours of sustained activity, such as walking, but there would have been occasions when maximal energy output was needed – for example, to fight an enemy or bring down prey. Internal metabolism is fully geared to physical activity and without this we cannot be fully well. One needs exercise as one needs food and water – in just the right amount.

> *A bear, however hard he tries, grows tubby without exercise.*
> *Winnie-the-Pooh* by A A Milne,
> 18 January 1882 – 31 January 1956

Too much risks injury and muscle damage; too little, and we degenerate. To maintain optimal fitness, we need steady sustained exercise combined with outbursts when we push to our limits. Just as with food, the type of exercise and the amount are critical. We do not want to do so much that we wear out our body (this is what happens with so many athletes – most professional ballet dancers are carrying injuries) but when we do exercise it must be effective to improve cardiovascular fitness. This approach is explained by what we already know about energy delivery mechanisms, which are, to recap, the combined effects of diet, mitochondria, thyroid and adrenal function.

The underlying principles

We are taught that there are two types of fitness – namely, muscle power and cardiovascular fitness. However, I think these are inseparable. When muscle strength is used to its full capacity, it creates a powerful stimulus to the energy delivery mechanisms for muscle. The heart has to increase output to supply the oxygen and fuel for muscles to work. The heart is also completely dependent on good energy delivery mechanisms. This means that if muscle strength is correctly developed, this automatically translates into cardiovascular fitness. Getting fit is simply about gearing up energy delivery mechanisms so that there is the potential to delivery energy in response to future demands. This also works the other way round – being physically fit is a great test of energy delivery mechanisms. You do not need expensive tests – just get out and exercise!

Different types of muscle fibres

We have different sorts of muscle fibres to further gear energy demand to energy delivery. The body has to gear its energy use very carefully in order to ensure that energy is used most efficiently. To help achieve this there are four types of muscle fibre, with slow twitch, fast twitch and intermediate fibres between the two. Usain Bolt must be all fast twitch. Red Rum would be largely slow twitch.*

Slow twitch fibres are used when power demands are low. This makes them very efficient; they use small amounts of energy and give good endurance so that we can use them for a long time. They are rather weak fibres but are slow to fatigue and quick to recover. They are the fibres we use for walking or pottering about when we do not need much power.

If we work a bit harder, we start to recruit intermediate twitch fibres.

Fast twitch fibres are employed when power demands are high – for example, when we are working flat out to catch prey. They occupy much more space and give us big muscles. They require a lot of energy to cope with high power demands, fatigue very quickly and take a long time to recover once fatigued. During fast twitch we also move into anaerobic metabolism with the production of lactic acid. Lactic acid is painful and, as it builds up in the short term, inhibits mitochondrial function – so this sort of exercise is not sustainable. But it makes the difference between a successful or unsuccessful (depending on your view point) predator-prey interaction. A sprinter can sprint 100 metres but not a mile. Lions are clearly made up largely of fast twitch fibres.

> *A lion's work hours are only when he's hungry; once he's satisfied, the predator and prey live peacefully together.*
> Chuck Jones[†], 1912 – 2002

But the important point about lactic acid is that it provides a powerful stimulus to our energy delivery mechanisms which is to expand our muscles because it stimulates mitochondria to grow and divide. Symptomatic of this is big muscles. This is another useful clinical test. So, to improve energy delivery mechanisms it is also a case of 'no pain, no gain'. The good news is that the pain is only short-lived.

The principles of exercise to get fit

- You just need to do enough to cause a lactic acid burn but not cause any strain or injury. Enough to make you puff and pant and get your heart rate up. A rough rule of thumb for maximum heart rate is to subtract your age from 220. For me, aged 60, that is 160 beats per minute (bpm).
- The exercise has to be very slow but powerful – this prevents damage to muscles and joints.
- It must be powerful enough for the muscles being worked to burn with lactic acid and weaken – that is to say, the exercise cannot

*Footnote: Email exchange between Sarah and Craig:
From Craig: My athletics master once called me Wottle... I was school standard at 100 metres, but then got worse as the distance got longer... but I was 'famed' for an 800-metre school victory where he reckoned I did the final 100 metres in around 14 seconds. Well, now I know why I was capable of short bursts only!
(Readers who are interested in US athlete Dave Wottle (born 7 August 1950) should view this YouTube: https://www.youtube.com/watch?v=nhixMwfBL7Y)
From Sarah: You have fast twitch. My style was the first 100 metres in about 18 seconds... and all the others in 18 seconds! Deffo slow twitch. That is a great video! I will remember Wottle.

†Footnote: If you have ever watched a *Looney Tunes* or *Merrie Melodies* cartoon you will have appreciated Chuck's work, although perhaps he should have been referring to lionesses rather than lions?

be sustained any longer. What makes muscles fatigue is not lack of muscle filaments, but inability to supply energy to them.

- You may be tired at the end of the day, but you should be completely recovered the next day. Poor recovery points to overtraining. This is a feature of my CFS/ME patients and so they must pace activity very carefully until energy delivery mechanisms are restored

These principles make perfect evolutionary sense. I do not see badgers and foxes trotting round my hill every morning to get fit. Most of the time, wild animals are in hiding or pottering around feeding quietly. Once a week there will be a predator-prey interaction, when the predator must run for his life to get his breakfast and the prey must run for his life to avoid becoming breakfast. In so doing, both parties will achieve maximum lactic acid burn. This is what is required to get fit and stay fit.

What do I do?

Time is always at a premium and anything you do must be incorporated into a busy life in a way that is sustainable in the long term. To increase and maintain fitness I do two things: as part of my dog walks, I go up a hill as fast as I can two to three times a week to get my pulse up to 160 bpm. Once a day I do 20 press-ups, 50 sit-ups and 20 squats to standing. That makes me puff and pant too. Although in theory one only has to do these exercises twice a week, I find if I do not do them daily then I forget. It is frightening how much of life is done subconsciously! If you cannot do one press-up then change the angle – start against a vertical wall, then as you get stronger reduce the angle to 45 degrees and eventually horizontal.

After I broke my neck a second time, I found I had mashed my C5/6 vertebral bone and disc and as a result had neurological weakness in my right arm. It took four months before I could do one press-up on the horizontal. (Yes, 'mashed' is a medical term. Craig) All else, such as riding, walking or gardening, is just for fun.

If you are an athlete

If you are an athlete you must pay particular attention to Groundhog Basic (page A1), not just to optimise performance but also to protect yourself from disaster. In 2005, four runners, including a 28-year-old man, dropped dead during the Great Northern Run half marathon. Conditions were unusually warm and sunny. No pathological cause for death was ever found. I think it is likely this occurred due to acute magnesium deficiency. Deficiency in the general population is common, but for every mile run about 10 mg of magnesium is lost in sweat and urine, and more in heat with excessive sweating. One needs calcium to contract heart muscle and magnesium to relax them, so deficiency may cause the heart to stop in systole (its contracted state). By post mortem, minerals have leaked out of cells and the diagnosis would be missed. For intensive exercise, it is important to rehydrate with an electrolyte mix that contains multi-minerals. Salt alone is not enough. After any sweating I recommend two grams of my Sunshine salt in one litre of water to rehydrate.

Note: If you suffer from CFS/ME, please do read our book *Diagnosis and Treatment of Chronic Fatigue Syndrome and Myalgic Encephalitis – it's mitochondria, not hypochondria* for advice on exercise specific to your condition.

Chapter 24
Sunshine and light

It is never difficult to distinguish between a Scotsman with a grievance and a ray of sunshine.

PG Wodehouse, English author and humourist, 15 October 1881 – 14 February 1975

Evolution takes advantage of every free lunch and sunshine is a vital freebie. It is highly desirable, and we spend fortunes on holidays chasing it. Who does not feel well after sunshine? Why so?

Sunshine improves energy delivery mechanisms

This is because we receive heat from the sun in the form of far infra-red; such free heat means we do not have to generate so much heat from our own mitochondria. This too has survival benefits as an energy conservation method. Indeed, the mitochondria of native Africans run slower than do those of Caucasians and much slower than those of Inuit Indians living within the Arctic circle. The latter have a high metabolic rate and are excellent at fat burning, which is essential to deal with the cold. They need abundant food to fuel this demand. By contrast, because the mitochondria of native Africans run slow, this makes them much more susceptible to metabolic syndrome and all its complications. They are metabolically highly efficient.

All enzyme systems speed up with heat. Energy generation, including mitochondrial function, is dependent on such. This is why athletes warm up before competing. At the London Olympics, the velodrome was kept at 29°C and so more Olympic records were broken than ever before. Many of my CFS patients feel much better in warm weather.

Improving energy delivery mechanisms makes us happy. This is further enhanced by full-spectrum light. Sunshine deficiency can result in SAD (seasonal affective disorder).

Enzyme activity

In fact, enzyme systems speed up until an 'optimal temperature' is reached (see the dotted line in Figure 24.1) and after that they denature, but the temperature at which they denature is so high that we can ignore this for our purposes.

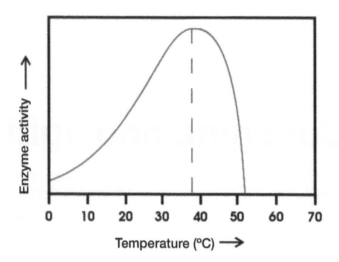

Figure 24.1: The relationship between enzyme activity and temperature

Extraneous heat reduces friction in connective tissue which relieves the symptom of stiffness

Hypothyroidism, in which sufferers run cold, often causes people to complain of muscle stiffness. Sunbathing feels wonderful and we rise from such feeling well. The mechanism of this may have much to do with the fourth phase of water. In the presence of external radiation, water molecules align themselves in an organised 'graphite-like' way to provide a frictionless layer between biological surfaces. Reducing friction further improves athletic performance.

Full-spectrum sunlight establishes our circadian rhythm

All living creatures have time-dependent natural rhythms that are essential for good health and survival. The most obvious is day-night. It is light that triggers a sequence of neurological and hormonal events which allow us to live and sleep efficiently. Without sleep, healing and repairing are impaired. So too are energy delivery mechanisms during wakefulness. Without light we have crepuscular* days and nights – half asleep by night and half awake by day.

*__Linguistic note__: 'Crepuscular' means 'resembling or relating to twilight' or 'of an animal that is active during twilight'. It derives from the Latin *crepusculum*, meaning 'twilight, dusk', derived in turn from *creper*, meaning 'obscure, uncertain'.

Heat and light kill microbes and so reduce our infectious burden

We all carry an infectious load which increases though life. (See our book, *The Infection Game*, for much more detail.) Ultraviolet light kills all microbes. It penetrates flesh by several millimetres, which is enough to irradiate the blood. Any microbes carried there will be killed. Dr Aguste Rollier's records of 1129 surgical tuberculosis cases showed that heliotherapy (sunshine therapy) cured 87% of 'closed cases' and 76% of 'open cases'.[1]

Heat reduces our burden of toxic chemicals

Warming the skin and subcutaneous fat literally 'boils off' volatile organic compounds and pesticides which, because we live in a toxic world, are invariably present in the fat of all organisms, especially those at the top of the food chain (i.e. us). Some can be exhaled, some move onto the lipid layer on the surface of the skin whence[†] they can be washed off, some are mobilised into the bloodstream with an acute poisoning (see Chapter 34: Tools for detoxing).

Ultraviolet light allows us to make vitamin D

Western cultures have become phobic about any exposure of unprotected skin to sunshine. Indeed, the US Environmental Protection Agency advised that ultraviolet light, and therefore sunlight, is so dangerous that we should 'protect ourselves against ultraviolet light whenever we can see our shadow'. That advice is just nuts! The best source of vitamin D is sunshine – not so much that the skin burns, but enough for it to tan. One hour of whole-body exposure to Mediterranean sunshine can produce 10,000 to 20,000 iu of vitamin D. We need at least 5000 iu daily, and probably more for optimal health. No studies have shown any toxicity in doses up to 10,000 iu daily. Further excellent information can be found at www.vitamindcouncil.org/

I use high-dose vitamin D routinely in the treatment of any condition associated with inflammation (allergy, infection, autoimmunity) and degeneration (such as osteroporosis and arthritis). Anybody living without one hour of daily sunshine and who does not take vitamin D supplements will be deficient. Note that the normal blood levels for NHS labs are set very low, at 30-60 ng/ml. I like to see levels between 100 and 200 ng/ml. Groundhog Basic demands a daily dose of vitamin D3 of 5000 iu. This further protects against cancer, dementia and heart and arterial disease.

What about skin cancer?

There are three types of skin cancer. Basal and squamous cell cancer are relatively benign, easily treated (see Chapter 48: Dermatology) and rarely cause problems. They only occur with sunshine over-dose where there has been inflammation and burning. The really nasty skin cancer is melanoma but there is increasing evidence that sunshine is not a risk factor for this. If it were, then this tumour would have the same distribution as other skin tumours. It does not.[2]

[†]**Linguistic note**: 'Whence' is a glorious word, meaning 'from where'. So, one should never write or say 'from whence did you come?' because that would mean 'from from where did you come?'. Instead 'whence did you come' is perfect! We also have 'whither' meaning 'to where' and the associated 'hence' (from here), hither (to here), thence (from there) and thither (to there). Collectively these are known as 'locative adverbs', and there is an (even more) archaic one – 'yonder' meaning 'to that' and deriving from 'yon'.

Because vitamin D is so protective against cancer, all studies show that sunshine reduces the risk of all cancers, from breast and bowel to leukaemia and lymphoma. There is no evidence to show that sun-tan lotions reduce the risk of skin cancer. Indeed, the toxic chemicals are hormone mimics and possibly carcinogenic. The key is to sunbathe intelligently:

- Get as much sunshine as life permits – build up exposure at a rate to allow tanning not burning
- Do not sunbathe so much as to burn (you will know that evening if you have over-done things)
- Do not use sun-screens.
  In the absence of daily sunshine:
- Take vitamin D at least 5000 iu daily
- Keep warm
- Use bright, if possible full-spectrum, lights during the day.
  Sunshine is great stuff… as Spike explains…

We reach a secondary road and – here comes the bonus – we pass the Temple of Neptune and Cerene, at Paestum, both looking beautiful in the sunlight. Strung from the Doric columns‡ are lines of soldiers' washing. At last they had been put to practical use. If only the ancient Greeks had known.

Spike Milligan, British comedian and author, 16 April 1918 – 27 February 2002

References

1. Sorenson M. Superbugs, sunlight, sanitoria and infectious diseases: the superbugs are among us – should we return to the use of sanatoria. 19 March 2018 Sunlight Institute. http://sunlightin-stitute.org/tag/tuberculosis/
2. Christophers AJ. Melanoma is not caused by sunlight. *Mutat Res* 1998; 422(1): 113-117. www.ncbi.nlm.nih.gov/pubmed/9920435

‡**Historical note**: Doric columns were developed in the western Dorian region of Greece in about the 6th century BC and they were used until about 100 BC. They are easily recognisable because of their lack of ornament and crucially the shaft is wider at the bottom than the top – one can sound so well-educated merely by stating that latter fact.

Chapter 25
Reduce the toxic chemical burden

– we are all poisoned
– what you can do to minimise exposure

This is not a new problem, but it is now vastly worse than at any time in human history due to our exponentially increasing use of toxic chemicals, of which more below. The Ancients knew how to poison those competing for the same throne – Cleopatra was especially skilled – but perhaps less well known is that the fumes in lead, silver and gold mines were recognised as being poisonous – the miners became ill and died young.

We are inevitably exposed to toxic stress. So, to reduce our body burden we must *avoid* that which we can (Table 25.1) and *detox* as much as is possible.

Table 25.1: What we must AVOID in order of importance. (This list is far from comprehensive, but you can scan down to make sure you have the addressed the big issues.)

What	How	Notes
Social drugs: smoking	Direct damage from toxins in burnt tobacco smoke, tar, toxic metals (cadmium), free radicals, nitrosamine, toxic gases	Nicotine is probably the safest part of smoking and so vaping is preferable
alcohol	Directly toxic to all cell membranes (it dissolves them) Energy delivery mechanisms are impaired Disrupts blood sugar control Buggers sleep (sorry... not sure of all the mechanisms here!)	The liver can cope with a certain amount of alcohol. So, drink occasionally and in moderation – I find this makes my jokes much funnier. Craig sends me cider when I fail to make him laugh... and Sarah sends me books in return... fair exchange is no robbery!

What	How	Notes
cannabis, etc...	At present there is no scientific evidence that cannabis is less harmful than either tobacco or alcohol. The opposite may be true. For any patient with an acute psychosis, drug addiction is the assumed cause	Just don't do it. For very occasional medicinal use only in advanced pathology for humanitarian purposes, when all else fails
Prescription drugs	My greatest hates are the Pill and HRT, Ro-Accutane (for acne), statins and pesticides used to treat insect infestations such as headlice (just comb them out!)	Also see Chapter 58: Prescription drugs, for drugs and their side effects
	All such increase the toxic load and so increase the toxicity of other chemical burdens. This is because they all use the same detoxification pathways which then become overloaded	Most drugs simply suppress symptoms and do not address disease causation. Work out the 'why?', put in place the 'how?' and tail the drugs off
Vaccines	Contain toxic metals which poison directly	Children should be allowed to get childhood infections. This trains the immune system and protects against later disease
	Contain adjuvants which may switch on the immune system inappropriately to cause allergy and/or autoimmunity	Once switched on, it is very difficult to switch off the immune system
	Contain animal tissue that may be contaminated with other viruses, such as simian virus 40 (which, with asbestos, drives mesothelioma) or xenotrophic murine retrovirus (a cause of prostate cancer and probably ME)	See Chapter 51: Immunology, allergy and autoimmunity, and our book *The Infection Game* for more detail
Dental work: Fluoride	The 'therapeutic' dose is very close to the toxic dose Knocks out the thyroid gland Carcinogenic Disintegrates collagen.	
Dental amalgam (includes mercury, silver, tin, cadmium, lead, antimony, copper and zinc)	Most are toxic and immuno-toxic. Mercury is the most toxic element known to man apart from the radioactive elements; it leaks out of amalgam from the day it is inserted	No-one should be carrying any dental amalgam or, indeed, any metals in their mouth

Braces, wires, mixed metals in the mouth	When two different metals are in contact in the wet environment of the mouth there is a 'small battery' effect which increases the release of metals into the saliva	Metals in the mouth dissolve in saliva and are swallowed. Where these is a fermenting upper gut, hydrogen sulphide may be produced. This may convert an insoluble inorganic metal into a soluble organic metal which is much better absorbed and bio-accumulates in the body – typically in the heart, brain, bone marrow and kidneys.[1]
Other dental materials e.g. palladium, titanium, gold, platinum, cobalt, stainless steel, chromium nickel	Ditto above	Yes, dentists are as dangerous as doctors. Also, see Chapter 45: Dentists and their tools
Cosmetics: Deodorants	Contain aluminium	...which drives prion disorders as such as Alzheimer's
Hair dyes	I often see hair dyes in toxicity tests such as DNA adducts and translocator protein studies; they cause genetic damage and block energy delivery mechanisms	Hair dressers have an increased risk of cancer
Perfumes and smellies	Solvents disrupt biological membranes; all who use become 'glue sniffers' Many are carcinogens	Invariably a problem for patients with chemical sensitivity[2]
Cleaning agents	Disinfectants contain triclosan (I often see this stuck onto DNA or mitochondrial membranes) Carpet cleaners use perchlorethylene. Polishes contain phenol as well as nitrobenzene Mould removers may contain formaldehyde	There are plenty of safe alternatives, but these may need more elbow grease. For example, use baking soda, vinegar, lemon juice, olive oil, essential oils and borax. Also Ecover, Akimie and Tincture London produce many good non-toxic products
Invasive procedures: Tattoos	Nanoparticles contain phthalocyanines, azo dyes and heavy metals such as titanium, aluminium, chromium and nickel	Drive cancers and prion disorders One can sensitise to metals – nickel allergy is common
Piercings	Often contain nickel	Ditto

What	How	Notes
Silicone implants	Including breast ('boob jobs' – boob in more ways than one!), testicular implants, mesh for hernia repair, tubes and pipes, body contouring, contraceptive depot devices	Silicone leaks out of implants from the day they are inserted and drives autoimmune conditions such as lupus and multiple sclerosis. 50% of breast implants rupture after 12 years and this accelerates the immuno-toxicity.*[3,4]
Surgical metal work: plates, rods, screws and stents	Comprised of toxic metals such as stainless steel…	…which may cause toxicity directly or act as a nidus for infection. Bone infections are very difficult to clear with antibiotics when a foreign material is present
Food: All foods	Pesticide residues, especially glyphosate	In August 2018 Monsanto were ordered to pay $289m to Dewayne Johnson, as a jury ruled glyphosate cause his non-Hodgkin lymphoma. The jury further found that Monsanto 'acted with malice or oppression'[5]
Genetically modified food	This may be due to as yet untested and unknown direct toxicity from modifying the food as a result of allergic response, differences in nutritional content, possible gene transfer and other effects but also from indirect effects – crops are often genetically modified to be resistant to pesticides and this allows farmers to use more pesticides on these crops and so accumulation of pesticides in GMO crops is often higher	Rats fed GM corn developed leaky gut, inflammation and pre-malignant lesions in the gut wall
Food additives such as colourings, flavourings, preservatives	These can be directly toxic to many cells. For example, see Sharma et al, 2018[6]	

*Footnote: In fact leakage of silicone could be worse than that: Dr Edward Melmed, a plastic surgeon from Dallas, told an FDA (the US's Food & Drug Agency) panel that by 10 years after patients get them, 50% of silicone implants have ruptured; by 15 years, 72% and by 20 years, 94%. Meanwhile the US's Institute of Medicine has reported that 'Prevalence of rupture differing by brand of implant has been reported by Feng (IOM Scientific Workshop, 1998), and Peters and Francel have reported major differences in rupture for silicone gel implants of different vintages, up to 95% at 12 years' implantation with thin shelled, 1972-mid 1980s-implants.'[3,4]

Food wrapping such as plastics (contain phthalates) and aluminium	Aluminium: see comments elsewhere in this Table Phthalates: endocrine and hormone disruptors	Phthalates are amongst the top Dirty Dozen of all human produced volatile organic compounds[7]
Water	All water will contain some VOCs and toxic metals. Most drinking water has additives such as fluorides and chlorines or worse, chloramine.	At the very least all drinking water should be filtered
Indoor air pollution Air fresheners Paint solvents	Air fresheners and paint solvents contain VOCs and other toxins – for example, acetone, ethanol, d-limonene, pinene and acetate are all contained in some air fresheners	If you can smell it, it is in your brain. Interested readers should see Anne Steinemann's paper 'Volatile emissions from common consumer products' which found 156 VOCs emitted from 37 fragranced consumer products[8]
Carbon monoxide (CO)	CO toxicity is due to its effect on oxygen binding to the haemoglobin molecule. CO binds to haemoglobin forming carboxyhaemoglobin (COHb) with a 220% greater affinity to haemoglobin than oxygen; this reduces the oxygen-carrying capacity of haemoglobin and leads to cellular hypoxia	Acute CO poisoning can lead to death. Chronic low level CO poisoning leads to various symptoms, such as headaches, fatigue, malaise, nausea and vomiting, numbness, unexplained vision problems, sleep disturbances and impaired memory and concentration[9]
Insect repellents	May contain pesticide	If it can kill the fly it can kill you
Fire retardants	New carpets and soft furnishings may contain fire retardants such as polybrominated biphenyls (PBBs)	PBBs are particularly 'good' at causing hypothyroidism
Pet treatments	Pesticides are used for flea control	

What	How	Notes
Outdoor air pollution: Pollution from industry	The late Dr Dick van Steenis did more for the Health of the Nation than any other doctor through his campaigning work against polluting industry. He demonstrated increased risks of cancer, heart disease, respiratory disease, and birth defects close to and downwind of such. Many industries discharge pollutants directly into the local air, water and soil. For more see Dr van Steenis's obituary in the *Times*[†10]	The worst offenders are power stations which burn toxic waste, manufacturing industry and chemical industry. Power stations often burn 'secondary liquid fuels'. This is where the spent, dirty oil drained from your car during its service may end up. These toxins are emitted into the atmosphere as tiny particulate matters (e.g. PM 1) which cannot be seen or filtered out by your lungs. They go straight into the bloodstream and drive heart disease, cancer and dementia. God only knows what they do to the poor kids. I suspect diesel fuel is being used as a smokescreen to hide the damage from other causes. Blame the car-driver, not polluting industry!
Herbicides, pesticides etc	Spray drift from agriculture	
Garden pollution[11]	Pesticides	Children with leukaemia or lymphoma are twice as likely to come from households using grass lawn treatments.[‡] As above, in August 2018 Monsanto were ordered to pay $289m to Dewayne Johnson, a golf-course groundsman, as a jury ruled glyphosate caused his non-Hodgkin lymphoma.

[†]**Footnote:** Here we refer to the newspaper which Indian and American readers may refer to as 'The London Times' or 'The Times of London' to distinguish it from the equally esteemed newspapers, *The Times of India* and *The New York Times*. Perhaps not well known is that the font 'Times New Roman' was developed specifically for *The Times* for 'legibility in body text'. It was conceived by Stanley Morison (6 May 1889 – 11 October 1967), a self-taught English typographer, who was fascinated by typefaces of the past and was instrumental in re-introducing some of these to modern usage.

[‡]**Footnote:** Once again it may be worse than a 'twice the risk' factor. See the 'toxicsaction' document[5], which references 573 medical papers and includes these comments, with respect to children. The statistics for household pets are even worse:
- A University of Southern California study showed that children whose parents used garden pesticides were 6.5 times more likely to develop leukaemia.
- According to EPA's Guidelines for Carcinogen Risk Assessment, children receive 50 per cent of their lifetime cancer risks in the first two years of life.
- Children with brain cancer are more likely than normal controls to have been exposed to insecticides in the home.
- Children in families that use professional pest control services are at higher risk of developing leukaemia than children in families that don't use pesticides.

Craig spent a very sobering hour reading this 47-page document.

Occupational	Agricultural workers (spray drift, livestock shed fumigations, greenhouse fumigations, milking parlour) Vets (glutaraldehyde and other disinfectants, hazardous drugs, farm pesticides and waste anaesthetic gases) Firemen (fumes from burning plastics) Military (chemical warfare, insect control in hot climates) Building industry (solvents, timber treatments, cavity wall insulation) Airline pilots and cabin crew (aerotoxic syndrome) Hairdressers (as above) …and many others	Use your brain to work it out!
Electromagnetic pollution (EMFs)	An increasing problem with huge potential to disrupt the body's electrical status quo. The worst offenders are mobile phones, cordless phones and wi-fi. This problem can only get worse – the impending introduction of '5G' presents new potential for harm.[12]	You can hire a detection meter from Healthy House to measure the EM stress (www.healthy-house.co.uk/electro/meters-and-monitors)

Having done your best to *avoid*, then do your best to *detox*. You may not know you have a toxic burden unless you test, and details of testing can be found in Chapter 15 (page 15.1). A good grounding is given in Appendix 3: Groundhog Chronic (page A4.1), but for details of more intensive regimes see Chapter 34: Tools for detoxing.

References

1. New World Encyclopedia. Hydrogen sulphide. www.newworldencyclopedia.org/entry/Hydrogen_sulfide (accessed 5 December 2019)

2. Campaign for Safe Cosmetics and Environmental Working Group. Not so Sexy – the health risks of the secret chemicals in fragrances. 12 May 2010. www.ewg.org/sites/default/files/report/SafeCosmetics_FragranceRpt.pdf (accessed 5 December 2019)

3. Francel TJ. Silicone-gel implant longevity (Abstract) In: *Proceedings of 67th Annual Scientific Meeting of the American Society of Plastic and Reconstructive Surgeons*, 1998.

4. Peters WJ, Smith D, Lugowski S. Failure properties of 352 explanted silicone gel implants. *Canadian Journal of Plastic Surgery* 1996; 4(1): 55-58. www.pulsus.com/scholarly-articles/failure-properties-of-352-explanted-siliconegel-breast-implants.pdf

5. Bellon T. Monsanto ordered to pay $289 million in world's first Roundup cancer trial. Reuters. 10 August 2018. www.reuters.com/article/us-monsanto-cancer-lawsuit/monsanto-ordered-to-pay-289-million-in-worlds-first-round-up-cancer-trial-idUSKBN1KV2HB (accessed 5 December 2019)

6. Sharma M, Rajput A, Rathod C, Sahu S. Food Chemicals Induces Toxic Effect on Health: Overview. *UK Journal of Pharmaceutical and Biosciences* 2018; 6(4): 33-37. www.ukjpb.com/pdf/UKJPB_SuperAdmin_1_401_1535524591.pdf

7. Johansen BE. *The Dirty Dozen – Toxic Chemicals and the Earth's Future* Praeger, 2003.

8. Steinemann A. Volatile emissions from common consumer products. *Air Quality Stmosphere & Health* 2015; 8(3): 273-281. doi: 10.1007/s11869-015-0327-6

9. Carbon Monoxide Poisoning: what is it? Harvard Health Publishing, January 2019. www.health.harvard.edu/a_to_z/carbon-monoxide-poisoning-a-to-z (accessed 5 December 2019)

10. Dr van Steenis: Campaigning GP who showed the link between air pollution and respiratory conditions. *The Times* 16 April 2013. www.thetimes.co.uk/article/dr-dick-van-steenis-sv-vcbz97tcf (accessed 5 December 2019) and www.big-lies.org/dick-van-steenis/asthma-cancer-orimulsion.htm

11. Wilson M, Rasku J. Refuse to use ChemLawn: Be truly green – why lawn care pesticides are dangerous to your children, pets and the environment. Toxics Action Center, March 2005. https://toxicsaction.org/wp-content/uploads/refuse-to-use-chemlawn.pdf

12. Electromagnetic Sense Ireland https://es-ireland.com/5g-5th-generation-greater-dangers/ which includes this YouTube by Dr Martin Pall – Dr Martin Pall To The NIH: 'The 5G Rollout Is Absolutely Insane' www.youtube.com/watch?v=kBsUWbUB6PE

Chapter 26
To love and to be loved

**– sufficient physical, mental and financial security to satisfy our universal
need to love and care and be loved and cared for**

Modern Western society has 'hijacked' the word 'love' primarily to mean 'romantic love'. But love is so much more than that. Depending where you do your research, the Ancient Greeks had between four and eight (or even more) words for love. Without wishing to labour the point, it is worth attempting a 'definition' of the various types of love. These are by their nature inadequate definitions and may well be disputed by some:

Eros – sexual desire, love of the body

Philia – love of the mind, brain, 'the person'; deep friendship between 'equals'

Ludus – playful love; that which we feel when having fun

Pragma – longstanding love, companionship

Agape – love of the soul; variations exist in interpretation here especially – often religious love

Philautia – love of self

Storge – love of the child, often your child; love of the parent.

It is beyond the scope of this book to discuss the psychological and spiritual imperatives that we must fulfil for optimal physical and psychological health and I am no expert. I am deeply grateful for a loving carefree childhood with a mum who was a brilliant cook. This love flowed further to my two gorgeous daughters, Ruth and Claire, but as they became more independent my affections embraced my pets – horses and more recently my lovely Patterdale terrier, Nancy. Pets are far more emotionally intelligent and sensitive than humans! I think it is essential for anyone living alone, or in an emotionally lacking relationship, to have a loving pet. You will make mistakes…

The voice of Love seemed to call to me, but it was a wrong number.
PG Wodehouse, English author and humourist, 15 October 1881 –
14 February 1975

My horizons are constantly changing. When my girls were little, my hobby was watching them have fun. Most recently I want my house, which is too big for one, to become the 'Marigold Hotel' for horse and dog lovers so I now have four lodgers, including Tony who will be 97 this year. Humans evolved to live in tribes, certainly not to live alone and probably not just within a single family. A complex social life is vital to good mental health.

> *Marriage is not a process for prolonging the life of love, sir. It merely mummifies the corpse.*
>
> PG Wodehouse, English author and humourist, 15 October 1881 – 14 February 1975

Simply identifying the above needs is often helpful to patients. Knowing what they need, they then come up with innovative solutions.

We all have skeletons in the cupboard which have the potential to haunt us. But having good energy delivery mechanisms and a complex social environment in which we feel emotionally safe solves much. Those with persistent skeletons, a sort of PTSD, may be helped by tools of the trade detailed in Chapter 50: Psychiatry. And those who know my contempt for psychiatrists will tell you that you do not have to be mad to enjoy this chapter!

To end with a personal note from Craig: When I was devastatingly ill with ME, and bedridden for months on end, I became very frustrated and bitter and, being a slow learner, it took me years to work out why I felt like this. The simple fact was that I was grieving for my lost ability to give love and care for something or someone. So fundamental was the drive to give love and 'care' and 'look after' that this was the single most significant loss that I felt – greater than my loss of being able to stand, or walk, or bear daylight, or listen to music. I had learnt that love, whichever form it takes, is a two-way street. I think Lao Tzu (sometimes also known as Laozi or Lao Tze, Chinese Philosopher, born 601 BC, died sometime in the Zhou dynasty) knew this when he said: 'Being deeply loved by someone gives you strength, while loving someone deeply gives you courage.'

But the final, final words are left to AA Milne (18 January 1882 – 31 January 1956) when he has Pooh say to Piglet:

> *If you live to be 100, I want to live to be 100 minus one day so I would never have to live without you.*
>
> From *Winnie the Pooh*

Chapter 27
Acute infection is inevitable

– be prepared so you can treat aggressively and get rid of quickly

Acute infections are not just an inevitable part of Life, but desirable and for at least two reasons.

- Immune training – 'Practice makes perfect':* Acute infections give our immune system a training for dealing with novel viruses and other microbes like MRSA which will inevitably evolve. Think of this as training an army – which will be much better placed to deal with an invasion given a few prior practice sessions. We know for certain that mankind will be afflicted with an infectious pandemic which will kill millions. I want my personal standing army in a fit state to fight such.

- Cancer prevention: we now know that getting an acute febrile illness as a child reduces overall cancer risk, and the more often this occurs the better. At the very least children should get rubella and chickenpox (vaccination is no substitute) which are the most protective against cancer, but so too are infections with measles, mumps, pertussis and scarlet fever. Indeed, it is increasingly my view that vaccination is unnecessary and positively harmful (see Chapter 51).[1] Hoption Cann et al (2006) conclude that:

> 'Infections may play a paradoxical role in cancer development with chronic infections often being tumorigenic and acute infections being antagonistic to cancer.'[2]

Jane Smiley (born 1949), American novelist and winner of the Pulitzer Prize for Fiction in 1992 for her novel *A Thousand Acres*, puts it well:

> A child who is protected from all controversial ideas is as vulnerable as a child who is protected from every germ. The infection, when it comes – and it will come – may overwhelm the system, be it the immune system or the belief system.

***Footnote**: The phrase 'Practice makes perfect' has a long history. Perhaps one of the earliest verified versions is: *'Uor wone maketh maister'* (Ayenbite, 1340). This phrase is found in *The Ayenbite of Inwyt* —literally, the 'again-biting of inner wit', a confessional prose text written in a Kentish dialect of Middle English. It is a 'translation' of a French original and is 'famous' for its incompetence in such translation. However, it is a valuable record of Kentish pronunciation in the mid-14th century. For example, words are often translated as compounds rather than 'finding' a single word to 'fit'. The title *'Ayenbite'* is one example – 'again-bite' – but also, we have 'amen' translated as *'zuo by hit'* ('so be it'), immediately giving insight into how words were actually 'said'.

However, I do not want my children, my patients or myself to suffer the misery of an acute infection. Neither do I want a microbe to get into our bodies and make itself at home, thereby driving other pathology. The studies above concluded that chronic infections are often tumorigenic. The answer to acute infection is Groundhog Acute, which gives the immune system a huge leg up by reducing the numbers of invaders. Remember, by taking vitamin C to bowel tolerance (see Chapter 31: Tools: vitamin C) and using iodine (see Chapter 32: Tools: iodine), symptoms can be abolished within a few hours. This means I can be greedy and get the best of both worlds: immune training and freedom from misery.

The features of Groundhog Acute to apply immediately, at the first symptom or sign of any infection, in order of importance, are:

- Vitamin C to bowel tolerance. This means taking 10 grams of vitamin C every hour until you get diarrhoea (half the dose for children). People seem astonishingly reluctant to do this. However, I would far prefer to have a good shit (and it is!) than suffer the misery of a cold or flu and risk all the long-term consequences of chronic infection. Also, people seem more than willing to 'drown their sorrows' during an infection by eating hundreds of grams of chocolate or other such 'comfort food', though, with all its sugar, this is feeding the infection, let alone giving rollercoaster hormone effects. (See our book *Prevent and Cure Diabetes* for much more detail on this.)

- Iodine for any respiratory symptoms. Use a salt pipe with 2 drops of Lugol's iodine 15% drizzled into the mouthpiece to sniff every hour until the iodine smell passes. This contact-kills all microbes in the upper and lower airways. If you do not have a salt pipe, put Lugol's iodine 12% 2 drops in a small glass of water and drink this every hour until the symptoms resolve. Swill it round your mouth, gargle, sniff and inhale the vapour. Then go and purchase a salt pipe for the future!

- Iodine for any skin infections (or potential infections i.e. skin breaches). Use iodine oil or pure Lugol's iodine applied directly. (Also see Chapter 48: Dermatology.)

- Do not suppress symptoms with drugs (for all the reasons given in Chapter 7: Inflammation).

- Stop eating, but drink water with 5 grams of Sunshine salt (a teaspoonful) per one litre, so providing a 0.5% solution. Drink this ad lib.

- Rest and keep warm.

- Sleep.

Be prepared! Stock up now with ascorbic acid (this is the cheapest and the best) 500 grams, Lugol's iodine 15%, iodine oil (100 ml of coconut oil mixed with 10 ml of Lugol's iodine 15%), a salt pipe and Sunshine salt. (See Appendix 2: Groundhog Acute.)

References

1. Zandvliet HA, Wel E van der. Science: Increase in cancer cases as a consequence of eliminating febrile infectious diseases. Nederlandse Vereniging Kritisch Prikken, Zandvliet and Wel, www.wanttoknow.info/health/cancer_link_vaccination_fever_research.pdf (references 54 medical papers)
2. Hoption Cann SA, van Netten JP, van Netten C. Acute infections as a means of cancer prevention: opposing effects to chronic infections? *Cancer Detect Prev* 2006; 30(1): 83-93. Epub 2006 Feb 2. www.ncbi.nlm.nih.gov/pubmed/16490323

Chapter 28
Diet, detox and die-off reactions

– Expect to get worse
– See this as a good sign
– Why this happens
– What to do about it

'The darkest hour is before dawn'
Old English Proverb
now universally used*

Expect to get worse before you improve. This may be demoralising but it depends how you see it... and I am an optimist so I see progress in the right direction. Such reactions are a well-recognised phenomenon and are given comforting names such as a 'healing crisis'. Symptoms can be very severe. Often when patients are so ill, they cannot afford to become any worse. I have great sympathy but no easy answers. Understanding the mechanisms may help. You must be a patient patient.

Also expect a bumpy ride – die-off reactions do not follow a smooth course. Be prepared for something more like this:

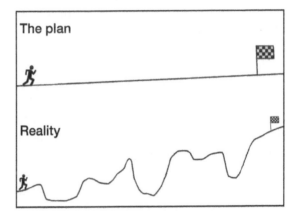

*Footnote: The English theologian and historian, Thomas Fuller (19 June 1608 – 16 August 1661), is perhaps the first person to commit this phrase to the printed word. His religious travelogue, *A Pisgah-Sight Of Palestine And The Confines Thereof,* 1650, contains this sentence: 'It is always darkest just before the Day dawneth.' Meant metaphorically, this phrase is not 'actually' true although it can be said that it is coldest before dawn. (Please see https://davidson.weizmann.ac.il/en/online/askexpert/sky-darkest-just-dawn for more detail on this.) Sometimes, just before sunrise, the sun casts a shadow of the earth into the visible sky and this gives an impression of a sweep of darkness, much akin to that experienced in a total solar eclipse. It could be that this sweep of darkness gave a 'physical' truth to this phrase and led to its common use.

We are fighting a war, but this is composed of many battles. Battles are fought by the macrophage foot soldiers and the lymphocyte officers of our immune system. They can be activated by infections, allergies and toxins. The army throws it all at the invaders and kills them with cytokine bullets. The inflammatory friendly fire that results makes us feel ill. Then the immune armies rest and recover (we feel a bit better) before attacking again – I told you it was a bumpy ride! Then the immune system sweeps up the mess – the parts of dead microbes look like the parts of live ones and this explains 'Herx' reactions (see below).

Diet reactions – there are three common players

1. The metabolic hinterland

The transition from burning carbs to burning fat is difficult and takes time – usually one or two weeks. The body has been used to running on carbs and there is an inertia in the system – it is as if it takes time to 'learn' to burn fat. During this window of time the body cannot get fuel from carbs (because they have been cut out of the diet) so it uses adrenalin to burn fat. To the patient this gives some of the symptoms of low blood sugar because adrenalin is partly responsible for such. We call this 'keto flu', but it is also given the dreadful and confusing name of 'ketogenic hypoglycaemia'. It was first described in the 1960s in children treated for epilepsy with a ketogenic diet. Let me explain further.

We experience the collective symptoms of low blood sugar not only for reasons of low blood sugar, but also for the hormonal response to such:

- fatigue, foggy brain and (indeed for some, especially diabetics on medication) loss of consciousness due to poor energy delivery caused by low blood sugar
- feeling 'hyper', shaky, anxious, possibly with palpitations and fast heart rate, due to adrenalin release
- feelings of hunger and the need to eat, due to gut hormones.

If all is well with the metabolism, the body switches into fat burning mode (as I've said, it takes one to two weeks for this to happen) and all the above symptoms, which we associate with low blood sugar, disappear. If all is not well with the metabolism, then these symptoms do not disappear and the clinical picture which results is called 'ketogenic hypoglycaemia'. I suspect two causes: lack of carnitine (easily corrected with 2 grams daily) and, more commonly, lack of sufficient thyroid hormone to burn fat . That clinical picture is characterised by:

- normal or (even better) low and stable blood sugar levels
- ketosis (confirmed by blood and urine tests)
- the body is burning fat to produce ketones, but it does not have sufficient thyroid hormone to do so efficiently – it relies on extra adrenalin to fat burn
- BUT the adrenalin release gives us nasty symptoms of being 'hyper', shaky, anxious, possibly with palpitations and fast heart rate
- AND INDUCE gut hormone release – which 'follow' adrenalin release – that is, feelings of hunger and the need to eat
- Clinically, this feels like hypoglycaemia.

Analyse your symptoms. We know keto-adapted athletes improve their performance and the foggy brain clears… despite perhaps feeling dreadful in other respects.

To treat ketogenic hypoglycaemia I recommend: acetyl L carnitine 1 gram daily, and sort out the thyroid problem. But we have to go gently here. In the short term, thyroid and adrenal hormones have very similar actions – that is, to speed things up. If one is still in the metabolic hinterland you may still be spiking adrenalin as your body has yet to 'learn' to use thyroid to burn fat. If you add thyroid hormones to this mix you will end up with the combined effects of thyroid hormones and adrenalin and feel constantly 'hyper'. Chapter 30: Tools to improve energy deficiency, explains how to do this.

2. Addiction reactions

We use addiction to mask unpleasant symptoms such as fatigue, foggy brain and/or pain. Stop the addiction and those symptoms return. Ghastly in the short term, great in the long. Obviously sugar and starch addiction are illustrated by the metabolic hinterland[†] but chocolate, caffeine, alcohol, nicotine, cola and other such all have the potential to cause 'train spotting' pain.

3. Allergy reactions

Allergy and addiction seem to be two sides of the same coin. I once had a patient who, before I was allowed to introduce myself, declared that when he died, he would like to take a cow to heaven with him to ensure a supply of his favourite food. The diagnosis was not difficult. I am not sure of the mechanism by which allergy has this addictive effect, but it is very real.

Detoxification reactions

In the short term, the body can deal with a spike of some toxins by stuffing these into fat and thereby out of harm's way. When I do fat biopsies, results come back in milligrams per kilogram. By contrast, blood results come back in micrograms per kilogram. This alone tells us toxic levels in

fat are a thousand-fold higher than in blood. Losing weight, heating fat or perhaps even physical massage may mobilise these toxins into the bloodstream and cause an acute poisoning. These toxins, especially pesticides and volatile organic compounds (VOCs), 'boil off' through the skin with heating regimes and cause rashes as the skin reacts allergically to them passing through. The commonest include urticaria and acne-like rashes. The clue can be found in the skin reaction to organochlorine poisoning, so called 'chloracne'. I have seen several patients who have been chemically poisoned develop acne whilst detoxing with heat treatments (such as sauna-ing), persist with treatment regardless and eventually find their acne reaction resolved. I can explain this only by a reaction to toxins as they are excreted through the skin.

Some patients being treated with vitamin B12 by injection and/or iodine also get an acne reaction. Both B12 and iodine are good at mobilising toxins from the body. Again, this resolves with time if the sufferer is prepared to put up with the acne in the short term.

Heavy metals stick to proteins and bioconcentrate in organs, particularly the brain, heart, kidneys and bone. They can be mobilised by techniques described in Chapter 34: Tools for detoxing, and this too may result in detox reactions.

Mobilising such chemicals is akin to throwing a handful of sand into a finely tuned engine – this may produce almost any symptom. In the very short term, energy delivery mechanism will be impaired. Many toxic metals and chemicals are immuno-toxic – that is, they switch on inflammation.

[†]**Independent film note by Craig**: One of my favourite films is *Hinterland* (not to be confused with the BBC series of the same name). This film is an independent British feature, written and directed by Harry Macqueen. You can watch it here: www.amazon.co.uk/Hinterland-Harry-Macqueen/dp/B00VA61A34. It is the story of an old friendship rekindled, and of self-discovery and heartbreak. Yes, I know – I am such a soppy git! Craig

Die-off reactions ('Herx' or 'Herxheimer')

Die-off reactions were first described by two immunologists, Drs Jarisch and Herxheimer, in patients with syphilis treated with antimicrobials. They are partly due to endotoxin-like products released by the death of micro-organisms within the body and partly by immune activation. (I think of this as 'allergy to dead microbes', which may explain why Herx reactions are not universal.) Such reactions are potentially very serious and must always be taken as such by at least reducing the dose of any antimicrobial employed and relaxing the regimes that may have triggered the reactions. In the treatment of chronic infection with antimicrobials, I suggest starting with a tiny dose and building up slowly over a few days.

Symptoms of diet, detox and die-off

In practice I have found one can experience:
- Inflammation:
  - systemic symptoms (fever, malaise, aches and pains, depression and fatigue) or local symptoms (acute cold, cough, catarrh, diarrhoea, cystitis etc). See Chapter 7 for symptoms of inflammation.
  - local symptoms: it seems to be characteristic of sniffing with an iodine salt pipe that there is an initial increase in mucus and catarrh production; I suspect that as the iodine kills the microbes the body recognises them as invaders and sweeps them out with snot.
- Fatigue: when the immune system is active it takes all our energy, so there is none available to spend physically.
- Foggy brain: the inflamed body is paralleled by the inflamed brain and symptoms of poor energy delivery to the brain result, in particular, with foggy brain, depression and malaise.
- Sickness behaviour: 'Leave me alone. I just wanna go to bed!' This is an energy-saving strategy.

Table 28.1: Summary: getting worse with Groundhog regimes when they should be making you better

Problem	Mechanisms	Action
Metabolic hinterland with ketogenic hypoglycaemia...	Adrenalin is high	Stick with the PK diet. Do not cheat (many do without realising it) or you will never exit the metabolic hinterland. Wait two weeks
...if this persists	Hypothyroidism	Sort the thyroid (Chapters 13 and 30). T3 is the fat burner
	Lack of carnitine	You need acetyl L carnitine to burn fat. I suggest 2 grams daily for two months, then a maintenance dose of 500 mg daily (but with a good PK diet, this should not be necessary in the long term)

	'Glycogen storage disorder'[‡]	This may be associated with poor adrenal function – work out the cause. Other than testing for poor adrenal function via an Adrenal Stress Profile Saliva Test (available from Medichecks via www.naturalhealth-worldwide.com) further investigations, including blood tests to check blood glucose levels, abdominal ultrasound to look for enlarged liver, or tissue biopsies to directly measure the level of glycogen enzymes may be necessary
Detox reactions	Acute poisoning as chemicals are mobilised from fat	Heating regimes bring toxins out through the skin and this reduces the poisoning effect
Consider zeolite clays which adsorb (not absorb) fat soluble toxins in bile to pull them out in faeces		
Addiction withdrawal symptoms in response to withdrawal of social, recreational (this really is a misnomer) and/or prescription drugs	Addiction masks unpleasant symptoms	If too awful then take a tiny dose of your addiction and wean yourself off slowly. Confession time – I love caffeine; consumption waxes and wanes, with detox windows when I avoid it completely.[§]
Allergen withdrawal, typically grains or dairy	Do not know for sure – many possibilities	Stick with the PK diet
Symptoms as micronutrient status improves	Mobilising and excreting toxic metals	Consider zeolite clays which adsorb (not absorb) fat-soluble metals in bile to pull them out in faeces
Symptoms from heating regimes and/or weight loss	Mobilising pesticides and VOCs from fat	Difficult – slow the regimes down to a point that is bearable
Symptoms from reducing microbial loads with Groundhog Acute or antimicrobial drugs	Herx reactions	Relax the regime and then once tolerated, get up to speed again

[‡]**Footnote**: GSD is a metabolic disorder caused by enzyme deficiencies. It can affect glycogen synthesis, glycogen breakdown or glycolysis – glucose breakdown – and it typically occurs with muscle and/or liver cells. It can be genetic or acquired.

[§]**Footnote**: regarding caffeine from Craig – Sarah is not alone in her love of caffeine. I drink green tea every day and I make a cup of coffee for my wife, Penny, first thing in the morning every day too. Figures show that 89% of Americans consume some caffeine every day of their lives.[1] According to new research, humans have been drinking caffeinated beverages since at least 750 AD.[2]

Problem	Mechanisms	Action
Adrenalin spiking with high blood sugar, blood pressure and/or loss of sleep	Any one of the above is a stress and the body responds with adrenalin	Stick with it and hang on to your hat![l]
Skin rashes – urticaria, itching, acne	'allergic' reactions to toxins coming through skin	Stick with it! It will pass and as it does so other symptoms will improve

All the above illustrates the point that time is a vital part of the diagnostic and therapeutic process. I expect patients to get to this stage after an initial consultation with me that usually concludes with me saying, 'You may love me now, but in a week's time you will hate me.' It is no consolation to tell them that I too have been on the same journey and been equally grumpy about the whole process... I am sure Craig has experienced the same. (Craig: Indeed, I have but I have never 'hated' Sarah! When going through these DDD reactions, I always have Penny on hand to remind me, 'This is just what Sarah said might happen!')

References

1. Fulgoni VL 3rd, Keast DR, Lieberman HR. Trends in intake and sources of caffeine in the diets of US adults: 2001-2010. *Am J Clin Nutr* 2015; 101(5): 1081-1087.
   doi: 10.3945/ajcn.113.080077.
2. Cueto E. How old is coffee? *Bustle* 16 Sept 2015. www.bustle.com/articles/110861-how-old-is-coffee-the-first-caffeinated-beverages-might-be-1200-years-old-so-heres-a (accessed 24 March 2020)

[l]**Footnote:** This expression may derive from the need to do just this on rollercoaster rides – according to lexicographer Eric Partridge (Colloquial; first half of 1900s). This rather suits our 'Reality' graphic above. Eric Honeywood Partridge (6 February 1894 – 1 June 1979) was a New Zealand–British lexicographer of the English language, particularly of its slang.

PART V
The bolt-on extras

The therapeutic tools of the trade to tackle established pathology

Chapter 29
Bolt-on extra tools of the trade

– when things get complicated you need extra tools

We now move on to the bolt-on extra 'tools of the trade'. As I get older, and perhaps wiser (although my daughters doubt such), my medicine becomes more simple. The basic things done really well get you a long way. Furthermore, I try to use tools which are within everyone's grasp. Yes, we may occasionally need the 'atomic bombs' of prescription drugs, but much can be achieved before that stage. You can progress and achieve without doctors getting in the way. Furthermore, tools of the trade multi-task and interact with each other in positive ways. Patients want a simple one-symptom, one-tool approach so beloved of conventional medicine. But it just ain't like that. We are complex machines with huge potential for things to go wrong. We have to find tools that are safe for the long term, multi-task and enhance each other. Even without a full diagnosis (which may entail prohibitively expensive tests) much can be achieved with the multi-tasking tools below.

Always start with Groundhog Basic (page A1) and then to enhance this add extra tools from Table 29.1.

Table 29.1: The bolt-on extra tools and what they contribute

Bolt-on extra tools...	...and the jobs that these tools can help with:					
	Helps energy delivery	Tackles fermenting gut	Reduces the useless inflammation of allergy and autoimmunity	Supports detox	Aids healing and repair	Fights infection
Groundhog Basic	Yes	Yes	Yes	Yes	Yes	Yes
Mito regimes (page 30.1)	Yes		Yes	Yes	Yes	Yes
Glandulars (page 30.2)	Yes		Yes	Yes	Yes	Yes
Vitamin C (page 31.1)	Yes	Yes	Yes – mops up the mess created by inflammation	Yes	Yes	Yes
Iodine (page 32.1)	Yes	Yes	Yes	Yes	Yes	Yes
Vitamin B12 (page 33.1)	Yes		Yes – mops up the mess created by inflammation	Yes – via methylation	Yes	Yes
Detox tools (Chapter 34, page 34.1)	Yes	Yes – mop up the mess	Reduce the triggers	Yes	Reduce the damage	Yes – mop up the mess
Heal and repair tools (Chapter 35, page 35.1)	Yes	Repair the gut defences	Yes	Yes	Yes	Yes – mop up the mess

Chapter 30
Tools to improve energy delivery

– the PK diet
– mitochondrial engine
– thyroid and adrenals

Allowing the body to heal from any condition is like conducting an orchestra. Not only do we need to know who all the players are, but these players also need to be playing the right tune at the right time. Then you get a melody. Eric Morecambe, when he famously stood in for the missing concert pianist, knew this when it came to playing Grieg's Piano Concerto:

> Andre Previn: 'Mr Morecambe – you are not playing the right notes!'
> Eric Morecambe (in confident mode): 'Mr Preview, I can assure you I am'
> ...and (slightly bashful)... 'I am playing all the right notes... but not perhaps in the right order!'[1]

This is particularly the case with chronic fatigue syndrome (CFS) and myalgic encephalitis (ME). (Remember from earlier: CFS = poor energy delivery mechanisms; ME = CFS + inflammation.)

With respect to energy delivery mechanisms, I think there are four key players that must be addressed in the following order:

1. Start with the fuel in the tank (PK diet) – you have read enough of that! (See Chapters 11 and 21.) It is an essential part of Groundhog Basic. Then move on to
2. the mitochondria (engine)
3. the adrenals (gear box) and finally
4. the thyroid (accelerator pedal).

The mitochondrial engines

Almost always these are going slow in CFS. We know this from our first paper, 'Chronic fatigue syndrome and mitochondrial dysfunction', published in 2009.[2] As importantly, our third paper, 'Targeting mitochondrial dysfunction in the treatment of Myalgic Encephalomyelitis/ Chronic Fatigue Syndrome (ME/CFS) – a clinical audit', published in 2013,[3] showed that when the necessary nutritional supplements are in place, together with the detox regimes, then mitochondrial function improves reliably well. This means that although mitochondrial function tests may be desirable, they are not essential for recovery. (For much more detail see our book *Diagnosis and Treatment of Chronic Fatigue Syndrome and Myalgic Encephalitis – it's mitochondria not hypochondria*.)

In order of likely need, the daily supplements to deal with the common rate-limiting steps are as follows, taken daily:

co-enzyme Q10 100-200 mg

niacinamide 1500 mg slow-release (or 500 mg taken three times daily)

magnesium 300 mg (Sunshine salt with 5000 iu of vitamin D is a great start and may be all that is required)

acetyl carnitine 500-1000 mg (a PK diet supplies the necessary meat protein and good gut function, so a carnitine supplement is rarely needed in the long term)

D ribose 5-15 g daily – this is a sugar and so must be part of your PK diet allowance for carbohydrates. It is often helpful as a rescue remedy at the end of a day in which you have overdone things, to prevent delayed fatigue.*

Mitochondria may be going slow because they are blocked. This blocking may be caused by products of the fermenting gut, toxic stress (pesticides, VOCs, toxic metals or mycotoxins) or because of poor antioxidant status. Chapter 15 gives the likely offenders and how to test for them. Chapter 34 gives the 'tools of the trade' to get rid of them. Yes – there are short-cuts.

Remember, every engine needs servicing and mitochondria need eight to nine hours of quality sleep, taken at the right time in every 24 hours to heal and repair the metabolic damage of every day. You must be as disciplined, possibly more disciplined, about sleep as you are about diet.

The thyroid accelerator pedal and the adrenal gearbox

Just like a car, the accelerator (thyroid) and gearbox (adrenals) work together in order to precisely match energy delivery to energy demand. Optimal use of energy is a critical survival mechanism – energy wasted is a survival loss. But how to do this well?

Blood tests for thyroid function and saliva tests for adrenal function give us a rough guide. Bloods can be easily done on a DIY finger drop sample through Natural Health Worldwide (https://naturalhealthworldwide.com). The main reason for this is to make sure that the thyroid is not over-active. Adrenal function can be assessed with saliva samples as an 'adrenal stress profile', also accessible through Natural Health Worldwide and interpreted as shown in Table 30.1.

---

*Note from Craig: I use D Ribose as a more immediate rescue remedy as well. I dissolve around 5 grams in some mineral water and then keep it in my battered old hip flask. I do this if I am going out and think that I may need a 'rescue' at some point. For example, I used this method to help me through my father's funeral, only to be accosted by an old school friend afterwards, who thought it rather disrespectful of me to be swigging 'whisky' during my father's eulogy!

Table 30.1: Interpretation of the adrenal stress profile

Test finding	Mechanism	Action
High levels of cortisol through the day	Cortisol follows adrenalin. High cortisol means high adrenalin	Identify the cause of the stress: the commonest is the adrenalin of falling blood sugar that is part of metabolic syndrome. It's the PK diet again! Psychological stress
Low cortisol (note reference ranges fall with age – I rely on a youthful reference range)	The adrenal gland is fatigued	Start adrenal glandulars
Flat throughout 24 hours ('circadian')	Suggests hypothyroidism	Thyroid stimulating hormone (TSH) spikes at midnight; this is followed by spikes of T4 and T3 which kick the adrenals into life and wake us up
High dehydro-epiandrosterone (DHEA)	DHEA follows cortisol – in response to any stress (physical, psychological, mental or whatever) the adrenal gland will pour out the required hormones to cope. For short-term stress (seconds to minutes), the hormone is adrenalin; for medium-term stress (minutes to hours) we need cortisol; and for long-term stress (hours to days), DHEA. In this sense DHEA follows cortisol as a response to longer-term stress.	Identify the cause of stress as above
Low DHEA relative to cortisol	The adrenal glands are starting to fail	Identify the cause of the stress Start taking adrenal glandulars and 'fine tune' the dose using core temperature as explained below

Interpretation of thyroid blood tests

The most important reason for doing a thyroid blood test is to exclude thyrotoxicosis – a thyroxin level that is too high. In this event, the TSH level would be very low and the free T4 and free T3 levels well above the reference range.

With adequate replacement therapy it is common to see the TSH level be very low and the T4 and T3 levels at, or even a little above, reference range. However, so long as the patient is clinically euthyroid (i.e. showing no signs of thyrotoxicosis) then no matter. The point here (see Chapter 41) is that blood tests are notoriously misleading and should not be relied upon wholeheartedly.

The clinical input is more important than the biochemistry. In this respect, the prescribing of thyroid hormones has come full circle. When hypothyroidism was first described in the late 19th century, it was diagnosed using clinical tools and treated with dried pig thyroid glands. My view is that this remains the best management plan. Let's use the best of both worlds. Blood tests may provide the 'coarse tuning' but this needs further refinement.

Fine tuning

We now need to add in some clinical fine tuning, as in any good car service. The best and cheapest measure of overall energy generation in the body is the core temperature. Core temperature has often been used just to diagnose an underactive thyroid, but it is actually a measure of the combined effects of diet, mitochondrial function, thyroid and adrenal function. This is why it is so important for the PK diet to be established and the mitochondrial lesions corrected. Core temperature then reflects combined thyroid and adrenal function.

The 'at rest' core temperature should be 37° Centigrade and, with the patient at rest, *stable*. This makes perfect sense – all enzyme systems in the body are temperature dependent – if temperature fluctuates you get a 'now we are working well' to a 'now we are going slow' change of states. This is inefficient. Ask any factory production manager – the more constant the supply of raw materials and environment the more efficient is production.

What is so interesting is that the adrenal and thyroid hormones manifest on core temperature in different ways and this allows us to tease out what is a thyroid and which is an adrenal issue. Broadly speaking, thyroid hormones 'base load' for the coarse tuning of body temperature and so we are warm by day and cool by night. Adrenal hormones are responsible for the 'fine tuning' over the seconds, minutes and hours, and they do this in response to environmental demands. An outpouring of adrenalin in response to a stressful demand will double the output of mitochondria in seconds; this would allow me to run the fastest 100 metres ever if faced by a sabre-toothed tiger.[†] Over minutes this allows me to feed my horses and pigs. Over the hours it allows me to work physically and mentally.

Conversely, when we are resting or sleeping, we do not need so much energy. If we run too hot, we waste energy, so we have less energy to spend on life; it is like tearing up £10 notes.

The practical details

To fine-tune the engine we need to use the techniques of Dr Bruce Rind.[4]

Get yourself a digital thermometer which records to an accuracy of at least 0.1° Centigrade (or 0.18° Fahrenheit). The most accurate reading is rectal temperature – but this is not convenient! I suggest you measure rectally once and compare this with the temperature under your tongue. I recommend doing oral first and then go for your bottom. Expect to see a difference of about 0.4° Centigrade between the two. The point here is that the average core rectal temperature should be 37° Centrigrade – so the average under the tongue temp should be 36.6°.

Record your temperature in exactly the same

[†]**Note from Craig re sabre-toothed tigers:** Of course, the real test is whether Sarah can run faster than whoever she is with at the time. She doesn't have to run faster than the sabre-tooted tiger, just faster than any other prey that happens to be in the vicinity!

way several times through the day, but do not take your temperature after a hot drink, hot meal or activity, for obvious reasons. What we need is a 'video' of your temperature, not a snapshot.

Interpretation of the results

Work out the average temperature and the wobble, which will be easy to interpret if done in the format shown in Table 30.2.

Table 30.2: An example of the results from a four-day tracking of temperature – averages and ranges

Day	Oral or rectal, at least 6 measurements in a day, more if very wobbly	Average temperature (reflects thyroid)	Temperature range (the wobbles reflect adrenal function)	Wobbles by	Extra notes
Mon	Oral x 8	36.0	35.7-36.6	0.9	
Tues	Oral x 7	36.3	35.5-36.7	1.2	
Wed	Oral x 9	35.9	35.5-36.7	1.2	
Thurs	Oral x 8	36.3	35.8-36.8	1.0	

The average temperature is the total of each day divided by the number of readings. In the example in Table 30.2, the average was below 36.6, suggesting that this person needs thyroid glandulars (see below).

The temperature range is the difference between the lowest in the day and the highest in the day. In the example in Table 30.1, there is a wobble of more than 0.6, suggesting that this person needs adrenal glandulars (see below).

Nutritional support with thyroid and adrenal glandulars

Thyroid and adrenal glandulars provide the most physiological support when these glands are wanting. What this means in practice is that the proverbial 'man on the Clapham omnibus' can access safe and effective support directly.

The general rules for glandular therapy are:

If the temperature range is above 0.6° Centigrade:

Start with adrenal glandular at a low dose e.g. 62.5 mg

Wait two weeks for this to take effect, then repeat the core temperature measurements.

If the wobbles still exceed 0.6° Centigrade, increase the dose in 62.5-mg increments every two weeks.

Most people need 250-750 mg to stabilise the wobble.

If your readings do not stabilise, then this suggests another cause (such as poor mitochondrial function, not doing the PK diet, ovulation, or inflammation going on somewhere that is driving a fever).

If the average temperature is low:

First, recheck to make sure this reflects rectal temperature.

If it does, start with thyroid glandular 15 mg daily taken sub-lingually on rising.

Wait two weeks for this to take effect, then repeat the core temperature measurements.

If the average temperature is still below 36.6° Centigrade, increase the dose in 15-mg increments (split the dose: 15 mg on rising; 15 mg midday) every two weeks until the temperature is normal.

Again, if your readings do not normalise, then this suggests another cause (such as poor mitochondrial function, not doing the PK diet or not eating sufficient calories).

If you are not sure, then repeat the blood test to make sure you are not overdosing.

At all times, monitor your pulse and blood pressure (BP): your pulse should not exceed 90 beats per minute (bpm) and BP should not exceed 130/80 mm Hg. (Failure to do a PK diet is the commonest cause of high blood pressure.)

Most people need 60-150 mg to feel well.

As you increase the doses of either of the glandulars, use the temperature readings to guide you to adjust the thyroid or adrenal glandular dose. Wait two weeks on each occasion for these to take effect. Then repeat the core temperature test over four days, further adjust, wait two weeks… and so on, until the core temperatures are normal and stable. If they continue to wobble despite 750 mg of adrenal glandular, this may reflect the body trying to run a fever so you will need to look for a chronic infection.

Clinical worsening may occur as a result of detox and Herxheimer reactions (see Chapter 28). If that is the case, make the changes more slowly.

Conclusion

Once done (all in the right order) you should be able play just as Previn wanted and not as Morecambe delivered (Khatia Buniatishvili plays Grieg's Piano Concerto – www.youtube.com/watch?v=e1CMsIXBSss)

References

1. Playing all the wrong notes: THAT iconic Morecambe & Wise sketch. www.dailymail.co.uk/video/news/video-1009121/Playing-wrong-notes-THAT-iconic-Morecambe-Wise-sketch.html
2. Myhill S, Booth NE, McLaren-Howard J. Chronic fatigue syndrome and mitochondrial dysfunction. *Int J Clin Exp Med* 2009; 2: 1-16. www.ijcem.com/files/IJCEM812001
3. Myhill S, Booth NE, McLaren-Howard J. Targeting mitochondrial dysfunction in the treatment of Myalgic Encephalomyelitis/Chronic Fatigue Syndrome (ME/CFS) – a clinical audit. *Int J Clin Exp Med* 2013; 6(1): 1-15. www.ijcem.com/files/IJCEM1207003.pdf
4. Rind B. Track your temperature: a quick and easy way to determine metabolic health. www.drrind.com/therapies/metabolic-temperature-graph (accessed 26 October 2019)

Chapter 31
Tools: vitamin C

– learn to use this vital tool well
– the key is getting the dose right

Vitamin C is an unsurpassably useful tool and in recent years has revolutionised my practice. It is the starting point for treating the upper fermenting gut (page 44.2) and all infections, acute and chronic, and therefore any condition involving inflammation. It multi-tasks to improve detoxing, is an essential antioxidant, and is vital for healing and repair. It kills all microbes (bacteria, viruses and fungi) and is toxic to cancer cells. In healthy people it slows the ageing process; in the acutely and chronically sick, vitamin C to bowel tolerance is an essential part of Groundhog Acute (page A2) and Chronic (page A3). In achieving all this, vitamin C is completely non-toxic to human cells. (There is much more detail in our book *The Infection Game – life is an arms race*.)

Vitamin C was the final tool that allowed me to tell my patients that vaccination is redundant since we have a far more effective, and far safer, tool in vitamin C. With vitamin C we get the best of both worlds. Children can safely experience viral infections without risking complications of such, but receive the vital,

live-virus immune programming needed to protect against disease later in life, particularly cancer. The only vaccination I now recommend is tetanus,* but this should be postponed until the child is at risk of stabbing a muck-caked pitchfork through her foot. And yes, I have done that too!

The key to vitamin C is the dose. We simply do not take enough of the stuff. The reason is to be found in Nature – all other animals (except guinea pigs, fruit bats and dry-nosed primates) can synthesise their own vitamin C.[1] Furthermore, the amount generated is matched to requirements – vitamin C synthesis is hugely ramped up to deal with infection. Goats, for example, may generate 15 grams a day on demand. We humans have lost this essential biochemical function but instead we have our brains. So we need to use them!

Thankfully, we have a mechanism to determine the dose we require. This will need to be varied from day to day because the body absorbs what it needs and leaves the excess in the gut. This allows us to adjust the dose according to our

---

*__Note from Craig__: My 'tetanus moment' was whilst climbing a tree at my nan's. I was reaching to a bird's nest and fell. A strategically placed rusty nail (holding a swing) ripped down my chest from just under the neck to near the tummy button. If you look carefully, you can still see a scar. It is only the second time I ever saw my nan cry. We went to the hospital for the vaccination. I was over the moon because I had a scar to show off to my school friends.

guts. Turn this logic on its head – the dose required to achieve bowel tolerance is a reflection of our total infectious load, the extent to which we have a fermenting gut as well as our toxic load and possibly other issues. In other words, our bowel tolerance of vitamin C is a measure of our health.

Lower bowel tolerance => lower infectious load

Higher bowel tolerance => higher infectious load

How to take vitamin C to bowel tolerance

First of all, do the PK (paleo-ketogenic) diet as vitamin C is much better absorbed in the absence of sugar and/or starch. There is no point killing microbes with vitamin C if you are feeding them with sugar at the same time.

Take ascorbic acid (vitamin C in its most basic, effective – and cheapest! – form) at least twice daily (and it could be more often). It dissolves much better in warm water. Add fizzy water to produce a rather delicious drink. The ascorbic acid helps to sterilise the upper gut and prevents fermentation of food. Any microbes inadvertently consumed with food are killed. Acid further helps digest proteins and also helps the absorption of essential minerals, such as iron and zinc.

If ascorbic acid is not tolerated, then use a neutral preparation, such as sodium or magnesium ascorbate. Once you are PK– and vitamin-C-adapted, you should tolerate ascorbic acid well. The cheapest form of ascorbic acid is fermented from corn but those with an allergy to corn may not tolerate this at all. Failing that, one can get ascorbic acid from sago palm.

Start with 2 grams twice daily and increase at the rate of 1 gram every day. You will start to get foul-smelling wind. This occurs initially as microbes in the upper gut are killed, swept downstream and fermented by microbes in the lower gut. Later it occurs as you start to kill some of the friendlies in the lower gut. This is likely to need more than 10 grams of vitamin C per day. Keep increasing the dose until you get diarrhoea. Hold the dose at this level for 24 hours. At this point you should have a clean, digesting (non-fermenting) upper gut, with low levels of microbes in the lower gut.

Adjust the daily dose in the longer term. The idea is to find a dose of vitamin C that kills the grams of unfriendly microbes in the upper gut but does not kill the kilograms of friendly microbes in the lower gut. This will depend on several variables that you will have to work out for yourself, vis:

- A dose that allows you to pass a normally formed daily turd
- No smelly farting
- A dose that stops you getting coughs, colds and flu when all around are succumbing
- A dose that reduces, gets rid of or reverses any disease symptoms that you may be suffering from. These may be symptoms of the upper fermenting gut or of chronic infection. As you can see from the Cathcart link below, you have to get to 90% of bowel tolerance to reverse the symptoms of any disease process.

At the first hint of any infection, such as a tickle in the throat, a runny nose, sneezing, coughing, feeling unwell, headache, cystitis... well you know what from bitter experience:

Immediately take 10 grams of vitamin C.
(Half this dose for children, according to body weight.)
If this does not produce diarrhoea within one hour...
Take another 10 grams
If this does not produce diarrhoea within one hour...
Take another 10 grams...
and so on.

Some people need 200 grams to get a result. Whilst this may seem like a huge dose, compare this with sugar – four bars of milk chocolate would provide a similar dose of sugar, and vitamin C is legions safer than sugar.

Some people are appalled at the idea of vitamin C causing diarrhoea, but I have to say I would rather have a jolly good bowel emptying crap than suffer the miserable symptoms of flu or a cold for the next two weeks. Indeed, I have not suffered such for 35 years thanks to vitamin C. (My father used to say, 'You can't beat a good shit, shave and shampoo.')

Adjust the frequency and timing of subsequent doses to maintain wellness. Remember the dose is critical. You cannot overdose, you can only under-dose. Just do it!

I am not alone in this advice.

Dr Robert Cathcart

Dr Robert Cathcart was a similar advocate of high-dose vitamin C. Some helpful clinical details can be seen at:

http://vitamincfoundation.org/
www.orthomed.com/titrate.htm

Key points of the Vitamin C Foundation paper are:

- Everyone's bowel tolerance dose is unique to them. It will vary through time with age, diet and infectious load. You have to work it out yourself and it will not remain constant.
- You must get to 80% of your bowel-tolerance dose for vitamin C to relieve symptoms. This is another useful clinical tool as you can feel so much better so very quickly if you use vitamin C properly.

Cathcart details many diseases that are improved with vitamin C. Interestingly, this includes many cases of arthritis. I suspect this illustrates one mechanism of arthritis which is that it is often driven by allergy to gut microbes.

Correct this and the arthritis goes. For example, we know ankylosing spondylitis is an inflammation driven by klebsiella in the gut, and rheumatoid arthritis is driven by proteus mirabilis.

Dr Paul Marik

From the Eastern Virginia Medical School in Norfolk, Virginia, Marik added intravenous vitamin C to his normal antibiotic protocol for treating patients diagnosed with advanced sepsis and septic shock in his intensive care unit. Before using vitamin C, the mortality was 40%. Mortality is now less than 1%.[2] Had this been a novel antibiotic it would have made headline news.

Dr Marik offered the following observations:

In the doses used, vitamin C is absolutely safe. No complications, side effects or precautions. Patients with cancer have safely been given doses up to 150 grams – one hundred times the dose we give. In the patients with renal impairment we have measured the oxalate levels; these have all been in the safe range. Every single patient who received the protocol had an improvement in renal function.

(Please note that anyone receiving *intravenous* vitamin C must be first checked for glucose-6-phosphate dehydrogenase deficiency. High-dose vitamin C in these people may cause a haemolytic anaemia. I can find no evidence of this being an issue for oral vitamin C.)

Lots more good science and practical detail can be found at 'AscorbateWeb': http://seanet.com/~alexs/ascorbate/index.htm#Rev-Ed and www.orthomolecular.org

And if nothing else, please do remember that vitamin C is Spanish for 'vitamin Yes'!

References

1. Drouin G, Godin J-R, Page B. The genetics of vitamin C loss in vertebrates. *Current Genomics* 2011; 12(5): 371-378. doi: 10.2174/13892021179642973

2. Levy TE. Vitamin C and sepsis – the genie is now out of the bottle. *Orthomolecular News Service* 24 May 2017. www.orthomolecular.org/resources/omns/v13n12.shtml

Chapter 32
Tools: iodine

– another vital multi-tasking tool that should be
a household word
– keep in every first-aid box

Iodine* is another tool that has revolutionised my practice. Like vitamin C, it contact-kills all microbes. It is the only agent that is consistently active against gram-positive and gram-negative bacteria, mycobacteria, spores, amoebic cysts, fungi, protozoa, yeasts, drug-resistant bacteria (such as MRSA) and viruses. In the doses below, it is non-toxic to the immune-system cells responsible for healing and repair. Indeed, studies show it enhances healing.[1, 2, 3, 4] This is why the surgeons love it. Skin painted with iodine before incision does not get infected and heals perfectly. (Again, there is much more detail in our book *The Infection Game – life is an arms race.*)

Furthermore, iodine is volatile and so it can get to areas that vitamin C cannot. Even if it cannot be applied directly to the infected area, it will penetrate flesh easily and is carried in the air to be inhaled.

This way, infection can be hit from within by vitamin C and from without by iodine. I use it in two ways to deal with infection and, indeed, Lugol's iodine, a salt pipe and coconut oil should be an essential part of your first aid box.

To treat all conditions of the mouth and airways

These infections include: gingivitis (gum disease), pharyngitis, tonsillitis, rhinitis, sinusitis, laryngitis, bronchitis, chest infections and bronchiectasis.

- Use a salt pipe. This is simply a clay pot filled with sea salt that can be used as an inhaler. Drizzle Lugol's iodine 1-4 drops (whatever is tolerated) into the mouth-piece – sniff this through the nose and exhale

Historical note: Iodine was discovered by the French chemist Bernard Courtois (8 February 1777 – 27 September 1838) in 1811. It exists as a purple black solid or sublimes to a violet-coloured gas and so it was named after the Greek ιώδης (*iodes*), or 'violet-coloured'. Although they did not know why, as far back as 1600 BC, Chinese writers described goitre treatment using burnt seaweed and sponge, as did European physicians, including Roger of Palermo and Arnold of Villanova in the 12th and 13th centuries. There are also records of the ancient Chinese using such burnt seaweed and sponge as antimicrobials. Of course, the seaweed and sponge were delivering iodine which was supporting the enlarged thyroid (goitre) and fighting infections. This is a classic example of 'science catching up with clinical experience'. Those early Chinese doctors knew that the seaweed and sponge worked, weren't sure why, but carried on anyway.

through the mouth. (You will find that the salt pipe has a mouthpiece for inhaling. You can either use this mouthpiece by inhaling through the nose directly or inhale through the mouth and blow out through the nose, using the valsalva manoeuvre to blow the iodine into the middle ear and sinuses whilst doing so – see https://goflightmedi-cine.com/clearing-ears/)

- Also use the valsalva manoeuvre to blow the iodine vapour into your middle ear and sinuses: pinch your nose and blow into the pipe so your ears pop (see http://goflight-medicine.com/clearing-ears/).
- Keep going until the iodine smell is gone (about 20 sniffs).
- Do this at least three times daily, but as often as you can according to the severity of the infection.
- In the short term, expect to see more catarrh as your body sweeps out the dead microbes.

For a child who cannot manage a salt pipe, smear the nostrils and lips with a coconut oil/iodine mix. The volatile iodine will be inhaled. You will have to think of a good joke to explain the necessity for a yellow nose and mouth!

Iodine to treat all skin conditions and superficial pathology

These infections include: infected spots, chicken pox, cold sores, swollen lymph nodes, nail infections, ear infections, cradlecap, skin fungal infections (tinea, ringworm, acne, boils) scabs and bruises.

> Take 100 ml of coconut oil and place the pot in a warm place so the oil just melts.
> Stir in 10 ml of Lugols 12% [15%] iodine to give you a 1.5% mix.[†]
> Apply ad lib.

Nobel Laureate Albert Szent-Gyorgyi, who discovered vitamin C in 1928, agreed: 'When I was a medical student, iodine in the form of KI (potassium iodide) was the universal medicine. Nobody knew what it did, but it did something and did something good. We students used to sum up the situation in this little rhyme: "If you do not know where, what and why, prescribe ye then K and I".'

[†]**Footnote:** Here is your real 'medicinal compound' as advocated by 'Lily the Pink' (but they got the recipe wrong – see Historical note[‡]). Coconut oil is additionally beneficial as this contains the fuel that powers the immune system, also further helping the healing and repair process.

[‡]**Historical note re Lily the Pink:** The 1960s hit song *Lily the Pink* was based on an American folk song, *Lydia Pinkham* or *The Ballad of Lydia Pinkham*. This original song was inspired by Lydia E Pinkham's Vegetable Compound. It was originally supposed to relieve menstrual and menopausal symptoms. From 1876 onwards, the compound was mass-marketed in the US. It is thought that the song 'travelled' over to Europe when Canadian WWI POWs sang their version in camps:

> Have you heard of Lydia Pinkum,
> And her love for the human race?
> How she sells (she sells, she sells) her wonderful compound,
> And the papers publish her face?

Lydia Estes Pinkham (February 9, 1819 – May 17, 1883) was the inventor and marketer of the herbal-alcoholic 'women's tonic' for menstrual and menopausal problems. You can still buy a (slightly changed) supplement version or the compound here: www.numarkbrands.com/products/#product_lydia-pinkham-supplement

Just like the Chinese thousands of years before them, no one knew how it worked but they could see with their own eyes that it did work, and so they used it! Just like vitamin C, the key is in the dose. Iodine can only kill if present. You know it is present because you can see the yellow colour. You must apply it as often as is necessary to keep the relevant area stained yellow/orange/brown.

Iodine to treat other infections

- Lymph node swelling (often called 'glands' but they are not) – as one may see in acute tonsillitis, glandular fever, local skin infections.
- Parotitis (for example, mumps) – I saw one case of mumps disappear overnight with topical ad lib iodine oil. Yes, the iodine stain made her look like a victim of wife beating but she felt so much better. I have yet to try this with a mumps orchitis, but I can hardly wait for the opportunity!
- Vaginal and perineal infections – warm your iodine oil so it melts and steep tampons in it. Allow these to cool so the oil solidifies. Use at least twice daily, possibly more often. This has the potential to contact-kill any vaginal infection and possibly viruses occupying the cervix also.
- Eye infections (for example, blepharitis, conjunctivitis, iritis etc) – do not put the iodine oil into the eye, but smear it over the eyelids and the iodine will evaporate and get into the eye.
- Wounds, ulcers or broken skin – any such must be kept still to allow the immune system to build new flesh. This is where pain is such a vital symptom because that ensures such. The wound should be fully debrided (cleaned and damaged tissue removed), comfortably dressed in non-sticky gauze and a bandage. Keep this dressing undisturbed for at least a week, but drizzle pure Lugol's

12-15% onto the outside of the dressing. The volatile iodine will keep the wound infection free so it can heal without disturbing the rebuilding process. (I have to say this works very well with dogs and horses too.)
- Warts and veruccas – put a spot of pure Lugol's 12-15% iodine directly onto the lesion. Keep it stained brown. It will kill the virus causing the wart/verucca, but you must keep applying it for several weeks until the skin has grown out the lesion.

Finally, be mindful that it is possible to be allergic to iodine. This is very rare. It is only a real problem when iodine is injected intravenously by a radiologist for imaging. But as with all treatments, start with a low dose and build up.

Iodine multi-tasks too

Iodine has other essential benefits:
- an essential raw material to make thyroid hormones and oxytocin (the love hormone).
- detoxes and greatly increases the excretion of mercury, lead, cadmium, aluminium, fluoride and bromine (see Chapter 34).
- deficiency is associated with cysts, such as of the breast and ovaries. I do not know the mechanism of this.
- clinically it has also been used with good results to treat:
  - cardiac dysrhythmias (indeed, it may be this is the mechanism by which the iodine-containing drug amiodarone is effective)
  - thyrotoxicosis.

Iodine to treat fatigue

Just like vitamin C, many patients with fatigue

respond well to large doses of iodine. They reported improved overall wellbeing when prescribed a 90% urinary-tolerance dose.[5,6] Again, the dose is critical. Drs Flechas and Brownstein used up to 50 mg (8 drops of Lugol's 12%) a day of iodine.[7] They did this by measuring urinary iodine excretion and increasing the dose until 90% was excreted, by which means they could infer body stores were saturated. They did this for 4000 patients over three years and saw no cases of allergy or Woolf Chaikoff effect (see below). They commented that iodine sufficiency was associated with a sense of overall wellbeing, lifting of brain fog, feeling warmer in cold environments, increased energy, needing less sleep, achieving more in less time, experiencing regular bowel movements and improved skin condition. In some subjects who were overweight or obese, this ortho-iodo ('correct dose') supplementation resulted in weight loss, decreased percentage body fat and increased muscle mass. Iodine is multitasking here to improve energy delivery mechanisms, correct hormone receptor resistance issues, detox, treat the upper fermenting gut and reduce any infectious load.

My guess is one could safely do this without the need for urine testing. Start low and build up slowly by one drop every three days. You may well see detox and die-off reactions (as per Chapter 28); do not be put off by such. Read more at www.optimox.com/iodine-study-8

Take vitamin C away from iodine – they work in different ways and combining them reduces the effectiveness of both.

The Wolff–Chaikoff effect

The Wolff-Chaikoff effect is a reduction in thyroid hormone levels caused by ingestion of a large amount of iodine. It is a protective mechanism against iodine overdose whereby the blood supply to the thyroid is temporarily reduced and, in consequence, the output of thyroid hormones.

It is often quoted as a reason not to take iodine, but the fact is the thyroid quickly adjusts and so normal function is restored. Again, this is further reason to build the dose of iodine up slowly.

References

1. Selvaggi G, Monstrey S, Van Landuyt K, Hamdi M, Blondeel P. The role of iodine in antisepsis and wound management: a reappraisal. *Acta Chir Belg* 2003; 103(3): 241-247. pubmed 12914356
2. Derry D. Iodine: the Forgotten Weapon Against Influenza Viruses. *Thyroid Science* 225 2009; 4(9): R1-5. (www.thyroidscience.com/reviews/derry/Derry.flu.iodine.9.19.09.pdf accessed 5 October 2019)
3. The Cure Zone. Iodine is by far the best antibiotic. (www.curezone.org/blogs/fm.asp?i=1413057 – accessed 11 February 2018)
4. Bigliardi PL, Abdul S, Alsagoff L, El-Kafrawi HY, Pyon J-K, Wa CTC, Villa MA. Povidone iodine in wound healing: A review of current concepts and practices. *International Journal of Surgery* 2017; 44: 260-268. www.sciencedirect.com/science/article/pii/S1743919117305368
5. Abraham GE. The historical background of the Iodine Project. Optimox. www.optimox.com/iodine-study-8
6. The Iodine Project: Treating symptoms, not masking them. https://theiodineproject.webs.com
7. Abraham GE, Brownstein D. Validation of the orthoiodosupplementation program: a rebuttal of Dr Gaby's editorial on iodine. *The Original Internist* 2005; Winter: 184-194. iodineonmymind.com/weather (accessed 24 March 2020)

Chapter 33
Tools: vitamin B12

For:
- energy
- detoxing
- switching off inflammation
- healing and
- repair

Vitamin B12 also goes by the name 'cobalamin', which is a portmanteau of 'cobalt' and 'vitamin'. Cobalt is found at the centre of the 'ring' B12 molecule.* It is an essential trace element for humans and is additionally found in a range of other co-enzymes, also called cobalamins.

B12 was the first multi-tasking tool I stumbled across in my medical career. Both my grandparents were GPs and used vitamin B12 injections as a first-line treatment for fatigue. Again, like vitamin C and iodine, B12 multi-tasks. It also has no known toxicity and can be taken to urine tolerance – that is, when you start to pee pink then you have saturated body stores.

The only way you could kill yourself with B12 is to drown in the stuff.
Dr Chris Dawkins, environmental physician (and good friend)

The problem with vitamin B12 is getting enough of the stuff into the body. Although it is water soluble, it is poorly absorbed. Absorption requires an acid stomach, the presence of intrinsic factor (produced by the parietal cells in the stomach lining) and a healthy ileum (the section of the gut where it is actually absorbed into the bloodstream). All of these are eroded by the Western diet and fermenting guts. My view is deficiency (by which I mean not having enough for optimal health, not simply enough to avoid

*__Historical note__: It was the British chemist, Dorothy Hodgkin (12 May 1910 – 29 July 1994), who, in 1956, described the structure of the B12 molecule, for which she received the Nobel Prize for Chemistry in 1964. In 1934, at the age of 24, Hodgkin began experiencing pain in her hands and rheumatoid arthritis (RA) was diagnosed. The disease progressed and in her last years, Hodgkin spent a great deal of time in a wheelchair, but she remained scientifically active always. Dr Alan Ebringer has done work suggesting that rheumatoid arthritis is allergy to the *Proteus mirabilis* bacterium.[12] Maybe this was the cause of Dorothy's RA. (RA is another example of a clinical description masquerading as a diagnosis.)

pernicious anaemia) is pandemic in Westerners. Groundhog Basic supplies 5000 mcg daily; the recommended daily intake is a laughable 2.4 mcg. The best form is methylcobalamin, though other forms will still be effective.

What vitamin B12 does

Vitamin B12 multi-tasks to:
- improve energy delivery mechanisms – patients often comment that their foggy brains and low moods are much improved. Indeed, patients have to be warned to stop B12 injections if they feel they are going 'hyper'
- improve detoxing via the methylation cycle (page 34.3)
- facilitate protein synthesis through the 'reading' of DNA (methylation is how genes are switched on and off)
- kill viruses – it is often helpful in herpes virus-driven pathologies, such as myalgic encephalitis (ME) and multiple sclerosis (MS). It is of proven benefit in hepatitis C[1]
- be anti-inflammatory. Professor Martin Pall has looked at the biochemical abnormalities in patients with ME and shown that sufferers have high levels of nitric oxide and its oxidant product peroxynitrite. These substances are produced when the immune system is activated by whatever cause – such as microbial inflammation or toxic inflammation. B12 is important because it is the most powerful scavenger of nitric oxide and will therefore reduce the symptoms of inflammation regardless of the cause. So often inflammation becomes self-perpetuating, like a pro-inflammatory fire, and B12 helps to quench such.[2, 3, 4, 5, 6, 7, 8, 9, 10]

To achieve the above effects, for some people high-dose sublingual vitamin B12 is sufficient (about 6% is absorbed). I also use transdermal B12 with DMSA as a carrier. I don't know the percentage of B12 that is absorbed but for some this works better. There is no point measuring blood levels as whatever the result, it does not change management. Knowing the levels does not predict who will and who will not benefit from B12 in high doses. You just have to 'suck it and see'. The clinical 'how do you feel?' feedback is the most important.

Vitamin B12 by injection

B12 by injection is often a really good tool. Do not be put off by the prospect of injection. I too am a wimp and would not advocate anything I could not do. I recommend the same technique that insulin dependent diabetics employ – that is, a 0.5 ml syringe with needle attached. Fill this with B12 and inject into the roll of fat that everyone gets around their midriff when they sit down. (The needles can be snipped off with a needle cutter and the rest of the syringe recycled with household plastic.[11])

I suggest a daily injection of 0.5 mg initially. Sometimes there is immediate benefit, in which case adjust the frequency of injections accordingly. If there is immediate benefit, then patients should experiment with how frequently to inject, ensuring that they continue to feel the benefit. This will involve trial and error, getting to a frequency that is 'just right' to maintain the benefit – more frequent injecting than this will not cause any harm, but will be more expensive! If there is no obvious immediate response, then I suggest a daily 2.5 mg for two months. This allows time for all the above benefits to be realised. It is possible for some people to maintain wellness with sublingual or transdermal B12, but many of my patients continue to inject themselves with B12 for the long term because this allows them to feel well. The name of the game is to arrive at a frequency of dose that maintains the benefit but which is not more frequent than is 'necessary' to maintain that benefit.

References

1. Rocco A, Compare D, Coccoli P, Esposito C. Vitamin B12 supplementation improves rates of sustained viral response in patients chronically infected with hepatitis C virus. *Gut* 2013; 62(5): 766-773. doi.org/10.1136/gutjnl-2012-302344; https://gut.bmj.com/content/62/5/766

2. Pall ML. Elevated, sustained peroxynitrite level as the cause of chronic fatigue syndrome. *Medical Hypotheses* 2000; 54: 115-125.

3. Pall ML. Elevated peroxynitrite as the cause of chronic fatigue syndrome: Other inducers and mechanisms of symptom generation. *Journal of Chronic Fatigue Syndrome* 2000; 7(4): 45-58.

4. Pall ML. Cobalamin used in chronic fatigue syndrome therapy is a nitric oxide scavenger. *Journal of Chronic Fatigue Syndrome* 2001; 8(2): 39-44.

5. Pall ML, Satterlee JD. Elevated nitric oxide/peroxynitrite mechanism for the common etiology of multiple chemical sensitivity, chronic fatigue syndrome and posttraumatic stress disorder. *Annals of the New York Academy of Science* 2001; 933: 323-329.

6 Pall ML. Common etiology of posttraumatic stress disorder, fibromyalgia, chronic fatigue syndrome and multiple chemical sensitivity via elevated nitric oxide/peroxynitrite. *Medical Hypotheses* 2001; 57: 139-145.

7. Pall ML. Levels of the nitric oxide synthase product citrulline are elevated in sera of chronic fatigue syndrome patients. *J Chronic Fatigue Syndrome* 2002; 10 (3/4): 37-41.

8. Pall ML. Chronic fatigue syndrome/myalgic encephalitis. *Br J Gen Pract* 2002; 52: 762.

9. Smirnova IV, Pall ML. Elevated levels of protein carbonyls in sera of chronic fatigue syndrome patients. *Mol Cell Biochem* 2003; 248(1-2): 93-96..

10. Pall ML. NMDA sensitisation and stimulation by peroxynitrite, nitric oxide and organic solvents mechanism of chemical sensitivity in multiple chemical sensitivity. *FASEB J* 2002; 16: 1407-1417.

11. www.cc.nih.gov/ccc/patient_education/pepubs/subq.pdf

12. Wilson C, Rashid T, Ebringer A. Worldwide Links between Proteus mirabilis and Rheumatoid Arthritis. *Journal of Arthritis* 2015; 4: 142. doi:10.4172/2167-7921.1000142 www.omicsonline.org/open-access/worldwide-links-between-proteus-mirabilis-and-rheumatoid-arthritis-2167-7921.1000142.php?aid=37117

Chapter 34
Tools for detoxing

How to get rid of:
- toxic metals
- pesticides
- VOCs
- mycotoxins

Step 1 in getting rid of these nasties is Groundhog Basic – diet, supplements, sleep, exercise, sunshine, love. Indeed yes – Groundhog multi-tasks.

Good nutrition is highly protective against toxic stress. Look at thalidomide. This drug was prescribed to women in pregnancy as a 'pregnancy-safe hypnotic' but only caused serious birth defects if taken during early pregnancy. This drug was tested in rats, none of whose offspring was abnormal. This was a mystery to researchers, until someone had the bright idea of putting the rats onto nutritionally depleted diets. When this was done, the baby rats developed the foetal abnormality of phocomelia (horribly dubbed 'flipper limbs').[1] It was a combination of toxic stress (the drug) *and* nutritional deficiency (riboflavin – vitamin B2) at a critical stage of foetal development which caused the problem to become apparent. My mother was prescribed thalidomide throughout all four pregnancies, but we all survived unscathed. Thank goodness she was a great cook.

How to reduce to the body's load of VOCs and pesticides using heating regimes

The liver cannot access VOCs (volatile organic chemicals) and pesticides to detox them because they are stuck elsewhere in the body to do as little damage as possible. The places where they end up stuck are the fat tissues and fatty organs (brain and immune system, viz bone marrow and lymphy nodes). This is where heating regimes are so helpful – they mobilise chemicals from these tissues.

Many of the pesticides and VOCs are stored in fat, much of which is subcutaneous. The idea of heating regimes is to heat up this subcutaneous fat and literally boil off the toxins. They migrate through the skin onto the surface where they dissolve in the fatty lipid layer that covers the skin. It is not essential to sweat for these regimes to be effective – the idea is to 'boil off' toxins in the subcutaneous layer of skin onto the lipid layer on the surface from where they can be washed off. The washing off is as important as the heat, or toxins will simply be reabsorbed.

Some toxins will mobilise into the blood-stream and that may cause acute poisoning. It is therefore important to start regimes with low heats and short times and build up slowly.

I have now collected data from over 30 patients who have undergone tests of toxicity both before and after these heating regimes. The tests have been chosen for particular situations but include fat biopsies, translocator protein studies and DNA adducts. The tests prove to my satisfaction that heating regimes are effective. These heating regimes include sauna (traditional and far infrared (FIR)) and Epsom-Salts hot baths. I would expect sun-bathing and exercise to be just as effective. Indeed, similar research was conducted by Dr William Rea in America and he used similar regimes of massage, gentle exercise, sauna-ing and showering to achieve very similar biochemical results. He concluded that 63% of patients decreased their levels of toxic chemicals via these regimes of massage and heating.[2]

My experience, roughly speaking, is that 50 episodes will halve the body load. One would expect chemicals to come out exponentially, so one never gets to zero but can end up in some sort of equilibrium with the environment, which is as low as reasonably possible. Indeed, because we live in such a toxic world, I think we should all be doing some sort of heating regime at least once a week. I am lucky enough to be able to exercise; I deliberately overdress to make sure I get hot and sweaty, then shower off subsequently – what a treat that is!

Furthermore, it is my view that because we live in such a toxic world we should not wait until we become ill, we should be using detox regimes on a regular basis and those regimes, in my opinion, should include heating regimes. Take advantage of what is available locally to detox your system on a weekly basis. For those people lucky enough to live in a hot climate, an hour of sunbathing followed by a dip in the sea is ideal. We British relish hot baths, and the effect of detoxification is further enhanced by adding Epsom Salts into the water. The idea here is that not only are the toxins pulled out by the heat but magnesium and sulphate pass through the skin into the body, both of which are essential co-factors to allow detoxification. This was established by a lovely study by Dr Rosemary Waring who showed that both magnesium and sulphate levels in the blood increased markedly following such hot baths, as did the excretion of magnesium sulphate in the urine. Her formula was for 500 grams of Epsom Salts in 15 gallons of water. (We British also love to mix our metric and imperial measurements! OK, OK… 15 gallons is 68 litres.)[3]

For countries with a tradition of such, sauna-ing is an excellent method of detoxifying through the skin. Indeed, I recall a case of one family who were all poisoned by organophosphate and had high levels in their fat biopsies. They decided to take themselves off for a three-week holiday in Eastern Europe at a lovely hotel which offered regular massage, sauna-ing, hot springs and mineral bath treatments. They all cycled from one treatment to the next. The results were little short of astonishing – after three weeks of treatment their toxic load of organophosphates had reduced substantially, almost to background levels.

Some people feel terrible following heating regimes, probably because of die-off reactions (see Chapter 28). It may be that such reactions are a useful clinical measure of one's combined toxic and infectious load. Should they occur, reduce the time, heat and frequency to whatever is bearable. With time, this will improve.

How to reduce the body's load of toxic metals using detox tools

There are many ways to skin a cat, as the saying goes. All the below are of proven effectiveness.

Oral chelation gets the quickest results, but some people do not tolerate this well. In practice I suggest putting in place as many of the tools below as are tolerable and affordable.

Use a chelating agent such as DMSA

The word chelation comes from the Greek, χηλή, chela, or a 'crab's claw'. DMSA literally grabs toxic metals so that they can be excreted in urine. Indeed, this is the basis of the urine test for toxic minerals (see Chapter 15). Because DMSA also chelates friendly minerals, it should be taken only once a week and one should take no friendly minerals on one's 'DMSA day', but then take good doses to rescue the situation for the other six days of the week. My experience is that most poisoned patients need at least 12 weeks of DMSA, after which the test can be repeated. This gives us two points on the graph and an idea of how much more, if any, chelation is required to reduce the body load to an acceptable level. As I have said, one can never get the body load to zero – all one can do is establish a reasonable equilibrium with the external environment.

Table 34.1: Supplements which help detox over and above Groundhog Basic

Supplement	Mechanism	Maximum dose
Zinc, selenium and magnesium	Displace toxic metals from binding sites in the body…	Zinc 50 mg Selenium 500 mcg Magnesium 300 mg – no oral maximum dose but diarrhoea if too much
Glutathione	…so the toxic metals can be picked up by glutathione and excreted	No maximum dose but 250-500 mg is usual
Vitamin C to bowel tolerance	Vital antioxidant – the final repository of free radicals	The dose is key and everyone is different
	Binds to toxic metals so they can be excreted in urine	Vitamin C also pulls out friendly minerals so it is vital to take Sunshine salt to replace the 'lost' 'good' minerals
Iodine	Binds to toxic metals so they can be excreted in urine	Lugol's iodine 15% 2-4 drops daily
High fat diet with several dessertspoons of organic hemp oil	'Washes out' the polluted fats in the body and replaces with clean. Phospholipids can be given intravenously to good effect	Oral fats and oils probably work as well as when given intravenously but the process takes much longer
Vitamin B12 and ensuing correction of homocysteine	Improves the methylation cycle – sticking a methyl group onto toxins renders them water soluble so they can be peed out	B12 is extremely safe – take at least 5 mg sublingually daily. Consider B12 injections

Supplement	Mechanism	Maximum dose
	If homocysteine low then correct with…	…Methyl B12 as above, methyl B6 (pyridoxal 5 phosphate) 50 mg and methyltetrahydrofolate 800 mcg daily
Adsorbent clays	See below	

Whichever technique is used, retest to make sure it is working. If not, consider the possibility that there is unrecognised ongoing exposure. For example, is the mercury coming from incomplete amalgam removal? Or fish in the diet?

How to reduce the load of mycotoxins

First you need to identify the source of production, which may be outside the body or inside. The main source outside is water-damaged buildings.

From within the body think either:

- fungi fermenting in the gut (see Chapter 31: Vitamin C), and/or
- fungi in the airways (see Chapter 32: Iodine).

Then use clays to mop up mycotoxins from the gut.

Adsorbent clays to get rid of toxic metals and mycotoxins

Many fat-soluble toxins, such as VOCs and pesticides, are excreted in the fatty bile salts, only to be reabsorbed lower down in the intestine. This is called the 'enterohepatic circulation'. However, clays will adsorb (not absorb – yes, I am a pedant) such toxins so they can be excreted in faeces. This is a benign way to remove toxins since they are not mobilised into the bloodstream and so do not cause detox reactions.

Clays will also remove friendly minerals. Thus, I suggest taking them away from food and supplements – for example, last thing at night. There are many clays with good potential, but I tend to use zeolite 3-10 grams stirred into water and swallowed. As a guide, 3 grams is about a heaped teaspoonful. It does not taste too bad – elephants seek out and love river clay* and I am very happy to be compared to an elephant.

*Historical note: Geophagia is the word used to describe the deliberate consumption of earth, soil or clay. It has been widely regarded as a psychiatric disease. Indeed, the standard reference guide for psychiatrists — the fourth edition of the *Diagnostic and Statistical Manual for Mental Disorders (DSM-IV)* — classifies geophagia as a subtype of 'pica', an eating disorder in which people consume things that are not food, such as cigarette ash. But studies of animals and human cultures suggest that geophagia is not necessarily a madness. The behaviour is prevalent in more than 200 species of animal, including parrots, deer, elephants, bats, rabbits, baboons, gorillas and chimpanzees. It is also well documented in humans, with Pliny (Gaius Plinius Secundus, 23 – 79 AD) describing the popularity of *alica*, a porridge-like cereal that contained red clay as: 'Used as a drug it has a soothing effect... as a remedy for ulcers in the humid part of the body such as the mouth or anus.'[4] Maybe this is another example of the Ancients not knowing why this practice worked but forging ahead anyway, on the strength of the clinical results.

Improve energy-delivery mechanisms

All the above functions are greatly demanding of energy. The liver uses 27% of all the energy generated by the body and much of this is consumed by detox enzymes. The kidneys demand constant energy delivery – they do not tolerate anything less. So, for example, a patient who becomes acutely ill with very low blood pressure may damage their kidneys irreparably with kidney failure.

The gut too requires energy to function – indeed, in its ability to absorb essential nutrients and reject the rest. The gut, biochemically speaking, is comparable to a giant nephron.[†]

References

1. Friedman L, Shue GM, Hove EL. Response of Rats to Thalidomide as Affected by Riboflavin or Folic Acid Deficiency. *The Journal of Nutrition* 1965; 85(3): 309–317. https://academic.oup.com/jn/article-abstract/85/3/309/4777256

2. Rea W, Md YP, Faaem ARJ do, Ross GH, Md HS, Fenyves EJ. Reduction of Chemical Sensitivity by Means of Heat Depuration, Physical Therapy and Nutritional Supplementation in a Controlled Environment. *Journal of Nutritional and Environmental Medicine* 1996; 6(2): 141-148. www.tandfonline.com/doi/abs/10.3109/13590849609001042

3. Waring RH. Report on Absorption of magnesium sulfate (Epsom salts) across the skin. The Magnesium Online Library, 10 January 2004. www.mgwater.com/transdermal.shtml

4. Pliny. *Natural History*, Vol. 9, Rackham H, transl. London: Heinemann, 1972: pp 285.

[†]**Linguistic note**: The nephron (from the Greek νεφρός – *nephros*, meaning 'kidney') is the functional unit of the kidney.

Chapter 35
Tools for healing and repair

To heal* and repair we need:
- the right raw materials, together with
- good energy delivery mechanisms (since it is the immune system that does the healing and repairing and this is hard work, requiring lots of energy)
- the right amounts of movement to create the gentle forces that give direction to the healing process – 'use it or lose it' as the saying goes
- good quality sleep when the tissues are physically still to consolidate the healing process (most likely during REM sleep when muscles are paralysed)
- anabolic hormones: adrenal glandulars and testosterone

The raw materials

Groundhog Basic (page A1) but in particular work on:
- Bone broth is ideal but not convenient. Making it is easy but takes time (see our book *The PK Cookbook* for details). Any bones, tendon, gristle, trotters will do nicely. (Include the eyes because that will see you through the week – boom, boom.) For convenience, take supplements with glucosamine, methylsulphonylmethane (MSM), chondroitin sulphate and hyaluronic acid, all of which are of proven benefit.
- Keep hydrated to minimise friction – to achieve such needs not just water but minerals to hold water within cells, fat to waterproof cell membranes and heat (sunshine is ideal) for the fourth phase of water (see Chapter 17: Mechanical damage).

Then, some bolt-on extras are very useful where there is pathological pain or damage. In order of priority, try:
- Vitamin D – up to 10,000 iu daily. No studies have ever shown any toxicity at this dose. Vitamin D is highly protective against osteoporosis. It also improves muscular strength and balance, so one is less likely to fall over and break a bone. Use Vitamin D3 (cholecalciferol); the cheap vitamin D2 only has 25% of the activity of D3.

*Linguistic note: The word 'heal' most likely derives from the Old English, *hælan*, meaning 'cure', 'save', but more often *hælan* was translated as 'make whole, sound and well' because of its previous derivation from the Gothic *ga-hailjan*, meaning literally 'to make whole'. In this context, equating 'heal' with 'to make whole, sound and well' seems a good place to start.

- Boron – up to 20 mg daily. Boron is essential for normal calcium and magnesium metabolism. Rex Newnham showed how people living in boron-deficient areas were prone to arthritis and vice versa.[1] When farmers inject their cows, who are dying from grass staggers, calcium and magnesium alone are ineffective; they inject calcium magnesium boro-gluconate to prevent death.
- Niacinamide (vitamin B3) – 1500-3000 mg daily. In his book *The Common Cause of Joint Dysfunction*, published in 1949, Dr William Kaufmann carefully documented the responses of 1500 patients to such. What I found interesting was that all age groups, from children to octogenarians, responded, and the older the patient, the better the response. Furthermore, it did not matter what the cause of the arthritis was, all responded equally well. I suspect this was because NAD (derived from niacinamide) improves energy delivery systems, so healing and repair were faster. There were no side effects. Niacinamide is a precursor of the coenzyme nicotinamide adenine dinucleotide (NAD) and NAD is the substrate (reactant) for at least four classes of enzymes.
- Vitamin C to bowel tolerance – it is essential to make good quality connective tissue. Many have commented that their need for reading glasses has diminished with vitamin C; I suspect it improves the elasticity of the lenses, which can contract for near sight.
- Silica 200 mg daily (bone contains more silica than calcium) – if the efficacy of a supplement can be ascertained from its cheapness and the degree to which the discoverer of such has been persecuted then this is clearly an excellent supplement. (See *The Persecution and Resistance of Loïc Le Ribault* by Martin Walker.)

For osteoporosis – strontium 250–500 mg daily is of proven benefit and it reduces fracture risk and rates.[2] The NHS prescribable form of strontium is strontium ranelate (marketed in the UK as Protelos or Protos) – this form does not occur naturally and so can be patented. I suspect side effects relate to the fact it is a ranelate and made up with the toxic sweetener aspartame. I use natural strontium chloride or carbonate to provide 250-500 mg of elemental strontium daily. It requires an acid stomach for its absorption, but hypochlorhydria (low stomach acid) does not occur on a PK diet. Do not take doses of calcium above 200 mg daily. I never recommend supplements as there is plenty of calcium in a PK diet; what is important is how well it is absorbed and whether it is dumped in the right place. Vitamin D improves calcium absorption from the gut and its deposition in bone. Furthermore, calcium and magnesium compete for absorption and the latter is arguably more important with respect to preventing osteoporosis and certainly the commoner deficiency – taking high-dose calcium makes this imbalance even worse. Dairy products are a risk factor for osteoporosis.[3]

Good energy delivery mechanisms

Since it is the immune system that does the healing and repair, it needs an excellent energy supply. See Chapter 30 for details of how to maximise this.

The right amounts of movement

As I said earlier, to repair injury we need the right amounts of movement to create the gentle forces that give direction to the healing process.

The human body is intrinsically unstable and needs powerful co-ordinated muscles to allow it to function. Look at yourself in the mirror – most people are not symmetrical. Furthermore, they tend to tip forwards. If you are not sure, then ask an athlete, a personal trainer, a physiotherapist, Alexander Technique teacher or whoever to teach you correct posture. Learn to exercise correctly to maintain correct posture (including poise and flexibility – this is not about holding a 'correct' position rigidly) and power.

Movement, use and pressure generate such forces, which are an essential part of healing and repair. Live normally and exercise within pain limits. Indeed, the amount of exercise needed to get fit should be determined by pain. We live in a constant state of breaking down and building up. The body precisely matches demands to delivery – to do otherwise would be wasteful. If we are idle, then muscles waste and bones thin. Resting too much is dangerous. Sleep is essential for the healing and repair of the inevitable daytime wear and tear.

With pathological damage, pain is an essential symptom which tells us what is possible. That is not to say ignore pain, but listen to it. Do not use painkillers to allow you to do more. Support bandages and splints are often helpful to allow one to do more up to the same pain level. Wrappings also help keep the area warm and well supplied with blood. Complete rest is counterproductive.

The following are also useful:

- Massage and manipulation – My Patterdale terrier Nancy stretches all her muscles after rest and before exercise. We humans should do the same. After exercise she loves to be stroked and massaged, sighing with pleasure. We humans should do the same. I think of this as ironing out the mechanical and electrical irregularities and restoring the normal frictions of connective tissue. Blood supply is enhanced, and toxic wastes massaged out. There will be an outpouring of endogenous opiates from the brain. I cannot think of any medical condition that would not benefit from daily massage and the systemic anti-inflammatory, analgesic, feel-good factor that accompanies such.

- Transdermal (TD) magnesium – I was initially sceptical about the benefits of TD magnesium because I could not see how such a tiny dose could have a therapeutic effect. However, the clinical benefits are profound – so many patients see benefit. Again, remember the words of Ovid: 'The result validates the deeds.'

- Heat and light – Heat improves circulation while light penetrates the skin and further 'lines up' the healing process. Sunshine is ideal. We can explain this by the fourth phase of water (see Chapter 17: Mechanical damage).

- Spas, swimming, hydrotherapy, hot baths with Epsom salts – It is not difficult to see the benefit of giving joints, connective tissue and muscles the chance to heal and repair without gravity getting in the way. This, combined with the massaging effects of water, transdermal absorption of minerals and warmth have wonderful healing properties.

- Remapping the brain – Many physical therapies, such as Bowen therapy, are so gentle one cannot imagine how they work. I learned much from Ramachandran's remapping hypothesis. The brain has its own map of the body and may learn and remember things incorrectly. The best example is phantom limb syndrome. Ramachandran worked out how to remap his patients' brains using simple physical techniques to abolish their phantom pain.[4]

Good quality sleep

Much healing occurs during sleep. Remember the name of the game is to 'heal' – to make whole, well and sound again. As I said above, we live in a constant state of breaking down and building up.

Healing is the 'building [back] up [again]' and is crucial to good health. See Chapter 22 for the details of sleep.

Anabolic hormones: adrenal glandulars and testosterone

The anabolic hormones are essential for healing and repair; the key is the dose. Young people do not need extra help – they heal perfectly with all the above. With age our production of anabolic hormones declines, and this partly explains the loss of muscle and connective tissue that accompanies ageing. A physiological dose of adrenal glandular (see Chapter 30) and testicular glandular 1-3 grams can only do good. Both are essential for quality sleep.

References

1. Newnham RE. Essentiality of boron for healthy bones and joints. *Environ Health Perspect* 1994; 102 Suppl 7: 83-85. www.ncbi.nlm.nih.gov/pubmed/7889887
2. Cortet B.Use of strontium as a treatment method for osteoporosis. *Curr Osteoporos Rep* 2011; 9(1): 25-30. www.ncbi.nlm.nih.gov/pubmed/21120641
3. Michaëlssonc K, Wolk A, Langenskiold S, Basu S, et al. Milk intake and risk of mortality and fractures in women and men: cohort studies. *BMJ* 2014; 349. www.bmj.com/content/349/bmj.g6015
4. Ramachandran VS, Hirstein W. The perception of phantom limbs: The D O Hebb Lecture. *Brain* 1998; 121: 1603-1630. www.rctn.org/bruno/psc129/handouts/rama2.pdf

Chapter 36
Tools to switch off chronic inflammation

– treating infection, allergy and autoimmunity
– reprogramming the immune system

Chronic inflammation causes unpleasant symptoms. Something must be done. The principles of treatment are:

- identify the cause and remove it (turn off the gas to the cooker)
- extinguish the inflammatory fire (smother the flames)

but, if that is not enough,

- reprogramme the immune system (learn not to make the same mistake again; not easy as old habits die hard).

Identify the cause and remove it (turn off the gas to the cooker)

Time is of the essence and you may not be able to diagnose the cause at first. That does not matter. Acute inflammation is usually driven by infection. Apply Groundhog Acute (page A2) at the first symptom of any inflammation – at worst you can do no harm; at best you may switch off and prevent the development of chronic inflammation.

Most people come to me with established disease and established inflammation. It is as much as these patients can do to survive already using large doses of symptom-suppressing medication. They are trying to smother the flames but have not switched off the gas. The inflammatory fire is in full swing and simply sorting out the underlying cause may not be sufficient to dampen the flames. It is as if the inflammation has a momentum of its own. We have a Grenfell towering inferno* and it is killing people. We need to douse it. Urgently.

With chronic inflammation, the patient's history is vital. Our book *The Infection Game* goes into much more detail as to how to diagnose and treat this. You may need this to identify the underlying infection, but do not wait for the book to arrive – get cracking now. Many infections can be effectively treated with Groundhog interventions through improving the immune defences without having to know which microbe is involved. I know this because many of my myalgic encephalitis (ME) patients have recovered through these cheap, intellectually easy, but practically difficult, interventions.

Think about when the inflammation started. Chapter 16 gives a guide to mechanisms. Toxic

---

*__Footnote__: For our non-UK readers, the Grenfell Tower fire was a tragedy that occurred on 14 June 2017, where the re-cladding of this 24-storey tower-block served only to 'fan the flames' of a ferocious fire. Altogether 72 people lost their lives.

metals are good at switching on inflammation. There may be a time-lag of weeks to years. In order of likelihood, did the symptoms follow vaccination? Dental work? A surgical implant? Piercings? Are you having a eureka moment as you consider these questions? If you do not look, you will not see.

Extinguishing the inflammatory fire (smother the flames)

Groundhog Chronic (page A3) helps to treat many of the underlying causes. This must be done as soon as possible. But this is very difficult for sick patients with no energy, no money and, often, little help, because such interventions trigger reactions to diet, microbe die-off and detox, with clinical worsening. Often my job is to prioritise, price and pace the changes so they can be lived with and improvement achieved eventually. I have to say this is one of the most frustrating aspects of my work – knowing what to do but not having the resources to put it in place, or rendering the patient so ill that they cannot stick with the regimes.

The inflammatory fire may also be allergic or autoimmune; regardless, essentially this is 'useless' inflammation that is counter-productive either because it is against incitants that are benign (e.g. foods, pollen) or, even worse, against a part of the body. This is civil war.

In the event of civil war, we may well need to use prescription anti-inflammatories to snuff it out. In the short term, these may be highly effective, in which case the patient feels better very quickly. In autoimmune conditions like polymyalgia rheumatica and temporal arteritis (TA), results can be seen within 24 hours of steroids and, with TA, such intervention is sight-saving.

When steroids were first discovered, they were hailed as miracle drugs, instantly reversing rheumatoid arthritis, chronic asthma and inflammatory bowel disease. Consequently, they were dished out like Smarties. Then the long-term side effects became apparent. I still use steroids today in such cases, but they must be paralleled by Groundhog Chronic so the steroids can be safely tailed off. I think of this process as reprogamming the immune system.

Reprogramming the immune system

So how do we switch off an inappropriate chronic response by the immune system? Let us start from the very beginning: how are our immune cells programmed to learn what is right and what is wrong?

I suspect that the immune system learns in just the same way as all other biological systems learn – that is, on the apprenticeship model. The immature immune system that we are born with is initially programmed genetically (the innate system) and also by Mother. It is programmed to accept whatever Mother offers the baby as being safe. The biggest two factors in this are diet and gut flora. Mother should be eating a paleo-ketogenic (PK) diet, meaning that those antigens spill over into breast milk and the baby learns to accept those as the norm.

The same is true of gut flora – the foetal gut starts to be inoculated even across the placenta whilst in utero and then there is a further large inoculation at the moment of birth. Indeed, we know these first 24 hours after birth are a critical window of time for this immune education to take place. These microbes are then fed friendly foods from breast milk and so the gut is colonised with friendly bacteria. In its plastic learning state, the baby's immune system accepts all this as the norm. Weaning follows the same process – babies should be weaned directly onto Mother's PK diet. Mother chews the food to ensure it is soft, free from bones, mixed with her saliva and easily swallowed. Kissing is a useful evolutionary tool to transfer the food into the baby's mouth. Indeed, this is the evolutionary reason why kissing, and breasts, are so attractive to men – they need to know their partners can feed their offspring well. (And brains, we like them too! 'Smart is sexy'. Craig)

We now know that 90% of the immune system is associated with the gut and these mature, grown-up cells at the 'coal face' know what they must and must not react to. Immature adolescent immune cells are released on a daily basis from the bone marrow into the bloodstream and they learn from the 'grown-ups' (i.e. the already existing immune cells). They learn to tolerate the status quo, they too become mature cells and so immune memory is passed down through the generations and maintained in this way. This explains the mechanism of ongoing immune tolerance to gut microbes and food – we ignore these friendly antigens and do not react against them as if they were viruses. We have learned to distinguish friend from foe.

The problem with modern life is that it is pro-inflammatory, and much of this book is about dealing with this. So, even once we have reprogrammed the immune system, it can still be switched on again, and left unable to distinguish between friend and foe, by, for example, the wrong diet (carb and sugar based), an infection that becomes chronic and is left unchecked, vaccinations, toxic metals, pesticides and so on. We must be on our guard and stick to Groundhog Chronic.

I see a five-pronged approach to reprogramming the immune system and switching off inappropriate immune responses. In order of priority:

1. Identify possible causes – see Chapter 16: Inflammation mechanism, for a check list. Don't forget infection (see our book *The Infection Game*).

2. Detox (see Chapter 34 for the tools for detoxing) and so reduce those factors which are switching the immune system on.

3. Quench the inflammatory fire with good doses of antioxidants, especially vitamin C (see Chapter 31).

4. Put the immune system in a straitjacket[†] and stop it reacting. If this is done for a sufficient length of time (probably months – see below) then the immature cells coming along behind will learn not to react. They will again become immune tolerant.

5. Use proven methods to re-educate the immune system, such as probiotics (including *Lactobacillus rhamnosus*), micro-immunotherapy incremental desensitising injections, enzyme potentiated desensitisation (EPD) and neutralisation.

I shall now expand on steps 3, 4 and 5.

Quench the inflammatory fire with good doses of antioxidant

Inflammation generates free radicals (for the boffins[‡] these are molecules with an unpaired electron) which have the potential to stick on to any other molecule and create biochemical havoc (for example, to stick to DNA and trigger cancer). An antioxidant is any molecule that will accept such an unpaired electron and so neutralise a free radical. However, in the process of achieving such, the effectiveness of that molecule is lost. It has to be refreshed to

---

[†]**Historical note**: The straitjacket was invented in France in 1790 by an upholsterer named Guilleret, for Bicêtre Hospital, and was first known as a 'camisole de force'. Some camisole!

[‡]**Linguistic note**: The derivation of the word 'boffin' is uncertain but the term possibly derives from Nicodemus Boffin, from *Our Mutual Friend* by Charles Dickens, who is described there as a 'very odd-looking old fellow indeed'; then it was perhaps taken on by Alan Turing and colleagues who broke the Enigma code, amongst other things, at Bletchley Park during WWII. In fact, usage of this term may have been used to confuse eavesdroppers or spies.

become effective again. The body achieves this with a chain of molecules. This is akin to putting out a fire with a chain of people passing on buckets of water – we have a brave fire-fighter in the front row with second and third liners behind keeping her supplied.

So, who are these wonderful characters who grab these hot electrons and flick them back to other catchers before they are finally quenched? The front-line grabbers include:

- Inside mitochondria – co-enzyme Q10 and manganese-dependent superoxide dismutase (SODase)
- Inside cells – zinc and copper-dependent SODase
- Outside or between cells – extracellular zinc-copper-dependent SODase, glutathione peroxidase (which needs glutathione and selenium).

The intermediate catchers comprise lots of molecules, including many B vitamins, especially B12, vitamins A, D, E and K, and melatonin. All plants have their own system of antioxidants which we plant eaters make use of. This means that all fresh, organic, raw foods will have an abundance of natural antioxidants.

The final quencher of hot electrons is vitamin C.

This system of catchers and quenchers (cripes – sounds like a game of quidditch!) has a numbers dimension. We need front-liners in microgram amounts, catchers in milligrams and the final quencher – vitamin C – in gram amounts. All have to be present and correct in adequate amounts for this system to work effectively. The commonest deficiency is vitamin C. That is why the commonest treatment for any inflammation is vitamin C to bowel tolerance.

So which supplements do we need to improve antioxidant status?

Table 36.1: Supplements to improve antioxidant status

Supplement	Containing:	To improve:
Groundhog Basic multivitamins and minerals	Zinc 30 mg and copper 1 mg	Intracellular superoxide dismutase Extracellular superoxide dismutase
	Manganese 1 mg	Mitochondrial superoxide dismutase
	Selenium 200 mcg (up to 500 mcg)	Glutathione peroxidase
	Methylcobalamin 5 mg (5000 mcg)	Vitamin B12 (also see Chapter 33 – possibly by injection)
	Vitamins A 2000 iu and E 50 mg	
	Vitamin D up to 10,000 iu. If you are off dairy and taking no calcium supplements it is safe to take up to 20,000 daily AND/OR sunshine 1 hour daily	Vitamin D Some physicians use 50,000-200,000 iu daily but calcium levels must then be monitored with blood tests
	Vitamin C to bowel tolerance	Vitamin C

Glutathione 250 mg (up to 500 mg)		Glutathione peroxidase Multi-tasks to help detox
Co-enzyme Q10 100 mg (up to 300 mg)	Ubiquinol	Co-Q10
Vegetables and berries in the PK diet	Natural antioxidants	

Other anti-inflammatories, over and above Groundhog interventions, which are non-prescription, affordable and safe include:

- boron – at least 3 mg and up to 20 mg daily (in my joint mix there are 2 mg per capsule)
- turmeric 5 g daily (active ingredient curcumin)
- ginger 2 g daily (I love chewing raw ginger root)
- CBD oil – start with 10 mg; most people need up to 50 mg; some safely take and tolerate 1500 mg daily.

Put the immune system in a straitjacket and stop it reacting

If the immune system can be stopped from reacting for a sufficient length of time (probably months – see below) then the immature cells coming along behind will learn not to react. They will again become immune tolerant. Using drugs as below will also suppress symptoms, so it is vital to do all the above in addition.

Examples of immunological straitjackets, starting with the most benign and moving on to the toxic, include:

- Low dose naltrexone – This is a popular and very safe treatment for any condition associated with inflammation. The idea here is to give a miniscule dose of the opiate-blocker naltrexone (start with 1 mg at night and build up to 4 mg), which has the effect of blocking the body's own production of endogenous opiates or endorphins. The body responds to this by ramping up this production. Opiates are natural anti-inflammatories.

- Sodium cromoglicate – this is a very useful and benign drug available on NHS prescription. I most often use this for food allergy. I suggest 100 mg emptied into the mouth, swilled round and swallowed 10 minutes before food. It coats the mast cells and prevents them producing histamine.
- Antihistamines for hay fever, urticaria and other itchy rashes.
- Antimicrobials to reduce the infectious load so the immune system does not have to work so hard vis:
  - Antibiotics to treat pathology driven by bacteria
  - Antifungals to treat pathology driven by fungi
  - Antivirals to treat pathology driven by chronic viral infections

(There is much more detail of the whys and wherefores in our book *The Infection Game*).

The drugs listed next should be used rarely and only in the very short term, because of major side effects:

- Anti-inflammatory drugs such as paracetamol and non-steroidal anti-inflammatories (NSAIDs).
- Steroids for inflammatory conditions, like rheumatoid arthritis, lupus, polymyalgia rheumatica, temporal arteritis, and severe allergies, such as asthma and inflammatory bowel disease.

- In theory, immunosuppressives, such as methotrexate, entanercept and gold injections for rheumatoid arthritis, psoriatic arthritis, ankylosing spondylitis and juvenile idiopathic arthritis. However, I have never prescribed these drugs.
- Again, in theory, rituximab for CFS/ME and inflammatory arthritides. However, I do not recommend rituximab for the treatment of CFS/ME (one of the side-effects is death) but one can infer the need for immune system re-programming from the results of its use.

Use proven methods to re-educate the immune system

These include:

- **Probiotics** (such as *Lactobacillus rhamnosus*, which is of proven benefit). *L. rhamnosus* is easily grown on home cultures, which makes for an inexpensive and delicious therapy.
- **Micro-immunotherapy** – This was developed by Dr Maurice Jenaer in the 1970s and is in wide use in Germany, France, Italy, Austria and other countries. It is comprised of tiny doses of bio-identical mediators (messengers) of inflammation, namely: neurotransmitters, cytokines, growth factors, hormones and specific nucleic acids. Some combinations of specific nucleic acids interfere with viral RNA reproduction and this explains the anti-viral effects. It can be used in any condition associated with acute or chronic inflammation which may be due to chronic infection with virus (not bacteria or fungi), allergy or autoimmunity. It can be combined with other treatments and is particularly helpful for the very sick patient who is intolerant to all else. It is an effective, safe, simple intervention, non-prescription medication and that appeals greatly to me. I am training practitioners to use micro-immunotherapy and so go to https://naturalhealthworldwide.com/ to find someone to recommend the best remedy from my web page.[1] It can also be safely combined with any other treatment detailed in this book including prescription medication.
- **Incremental desensitising injections, enzyme potentiated desensitisation (EPD)** and **neutralisation** (a description of the use of these is beyond the scope of this book and all need professional help). I have been using these techniques, especially EPD, since 1985. However, these days I rarely initiate desensitising injections because I find all other interventions effective in reducing allergy problems.

But I must repeat, putting the immune system in a drug straitjacket is potentially dangerous; it may impair the normal efficient response to infection as well as impairing healing and repair, and even cancer surveillance. Any such intervention should be done for as short a time as possible.

Cautionary note

I think it is important to recognise that for the above to be effective the patient needs to be as free from inflammation symptoms as possible. If patients are experiencing such, then the immune system is active and reacting and, therefore, not being educated 'the right way' – that is, towards being less prone to inflammation. However, not all symptoms are due to inflammation. It may be symptoms are from die-off, detoxing and/or diet reactions (see Chapter 28).

Symptom suppression allows one to feel better and with that comes the temptation to spend energy and do more. This alone may promote inflammation because mitochondria generate free radicals. This means that the dose of any drug must be very carefully balanced. This fine tuning is best done by the educated patient with the support of a physician who understands symptoms and mechanisms.

> *Too much of a good thing can be a bad thing.*
> *Old English saying*
> (Deriving from *Proverbs* 25:16 – 'Hast thou found honey? Eat so much as is sufficient for thee, lest thou be filled therewith and vomit it')

The above mechanisms may not be proven but are biologically plausible and have clearly passed the Ecomed doctors' clinical test of time. It may well be that there are some years to go before the science catches up, but this is characteristic of the development of new ideas in a clinical setting. Just as the Chinese knew that seaweed and sponge helped with goitre and infections but did not know why, we move forward with our clinical tests of time.

Reference

1. www.drmyhill.co.uk/wiki/Reprogram_the_immune_system_with_micro-immunotherapy

Chapter 37
Tools to reduce benign and malignant growths

– do not switch them on
– get rid of growth promoters

Benign growths have largely nuisance value, but they are also a risk factor for malignant growths. For example, benign breast disease increases the relative risk (RR) of breast cancer to 1.56 (a normal RR is 1.0). Benign prostatic hypertrophy is also a risk for prostate cancer. It is not difficult to see why:

- Benign growths result from pure growth promotion factors
- Malignant growths result from genetic damage PLUS growth promotion.

See benign growths as an early warning symptom of cancer and put interventions in place now. Many people are not told this by their physicians. Again, it is a case of 'What a shock, what a surprise, and what bad luck!' Doctors may think they are being kind with this false reassurance but actually they are cruelly preventing their patients from taking preventive action at once. They are putting them on a path to cancer.

Treatment for benign growths

Cysts, (breast, ovarian, others) may be symptomatic of iodine deficiency. If benign lumps are disfiguring or causing pressure symptoms, then it is off to the surgeon. Surgeons are my favourite doctors.* They are incredibly skilful, good at diagnosing the battlefield and its excision.

The next job is to prevent recurrence or progression to cancer. This involves getting rid of growth promoters.

Getting rid of growth promoters

The first thing to get rid of the growth promoters is Groundhog Chronic (page A3).

Footnote: 'My favourite doctor is Sarah.' Craig. 'You can see why I have a big head.' Sarah.

Table 37.1: The most important growth promoters to get rid of

Mechanism	How to counteract
Female sex hormones are growth promoting and immunosuppressive	Stop the Pill and HRT
Carbohydrates (which trigger an insulin response) and dairy products are growth promoters	The PK diet
Organochlorine pesticides (These have been found to alter levels of hormones, enzymes and growth factors.[1])	Get rid of these with heating regimes
Iodine protects against benign and malignant growths through several possible mechanisms	Take Lugol's iodine 12%, 4 drops daily (or 15%, 3 drops daily)
Look for an infectious driver that may be treatable with specific antimicrobials – for example, endometriosis has a fungal driver. (As discussed in their 2018 paper, Cho et al note that 'in human endometriosis patients, there is high M2 macrophage polarisation' and also that 'macrophages are guided toward the M2 type of fungal cells'; the clear inference is a fungal infection is involved.[2])	See our book *The Infection Game*.
First improve the immune defences (Groundhog Chronic)	

At this point, look for toxins that may trigger cancer. It is not that getting rid of toxins will cure a cancer, but having one cancer is a major risk for a second – you can at least prevent that.

The inquisitive patient may want to do tests to look for the toxic incitant, which will be either a pesticide, volatile organic compound (VOC), toxic metal or mycotoxin. The pragmatic, experienced physician knows that common things are common and that her impoverished patient may not be able to afford investigation – precious resources are best spent on treatments. The list of common toxins is given in Chapter 25.

Then put in place the necessary detox regimes to get rid of them. These are detailed in Chapter 34. Again, one does not have to know what the toxin is for these treatments to be effective. I know from my clinical experience and data gathered that the regimes are highly effective.

Where to go from here in this book

- For treatment of malignant growths, see Chapter 53: Oncology
- For treatment of prion disorders such as Alzheimer's disease, Parkinson's, motor neurone disease, multi-system atrophy (MSA) and others, see Chapter 49: Neurology.

References

1. Gourounti K, Lykeridou K, Protopapa E, Lazaris A. Mechanisms of actions and health effects of organochlorine substances: a review. *Health Science Journal* 2008; 2(2): 89-98. www.hsj.gr/abstract/mechanisms-of-actions-and-health-effects-of-organochlorine-substances-a-review-3667.html (accessed 5 December 2019)

2. Cho YJ, Lee SH, Park JW, Han M et al. Dysfynctional signalling underlying endometriosis: current state of knowledge. *Journal of Molecular Endocrinology* 2018; 60(3): R97-R113. doi: https://doi.org/10.1530/JME-17-0227

PART VI
How to apply what we've learnt to current branches of medicine

Chapter 38

How to slow the ageing process and live to one's full potential

**– I want to live well and drop off my perch
very quickly aged 120**

Of course, we will all die eventually but my job is to optimise quantity and quality. I want my patients to live well to a high standard and then suddenly drop off the perch at home. As I write, a dear friend has recently died. He lived at home, had a great Christmas with his family during which time he enjoyed some good wines, and then on 4 January he woke at 5 am with a tummy upset and malaise, and quietly slipped away at midday. He was 96. He did not live up to Shakespeare's picture and neither shall I!

Last scene of all,
That ends this strange eventful history,
Is second childishness and mere oblivion,
Sans teeth, sans eyes, sans taste, sans
everything.
'All the world's a stage' from
Shakespeare's *As You Like It*, 1600

As we age, many disease processes result from 'degeneration'. There is a general assumption amongst doctors that this is an inevitable part of ageing about which we can do nothing. This is NONSENSE! The human body is not a passive lump that is eroded by the passage of time. It is a dynamic, exquisitely crafted object of beauty that is constantly changing in response to demands. One such example is osteoporosis. I have collected 32 patients whose thin bones have either stopped thinning or gained density with simple nutritional inputs. Remember, degeneration occurs when the rate of healing and repair cannot keep pace with damage to tissues. Attention to both sides of this equation has the potential to prevent degeneration.

- To prevent damage from inflammation, see Chapter 36
- To heal and repair we need the raw materials (see Chapter 25), good energy delivery mechanisms (Chapter 30) and sleep (Chapter 22).

Arthritis with pain is not an inevitable part of ageing

We know that the major risk factor for arthritis is metabolic syndrome.*

There is a simple mechanism to explain this: a high-carb diet results in upper fermenting gut, unfriendly microbes spill over into the blood-stream and drive inflammation at distal (faraway) sites. Inflammation results in degeneration. This has been demonstrated by the Danish surgeon Albert who has shown the presence of bacteria in joints and connective tissue driving an inflammatory process – it may well be that many cases of arthritis are actually low-grade infections. An article in *The Guardian* in 2013 extrapolated from this that antibiotics are the answer,[3] but you and I know antibiotics will not cure – they may afford temporary relief but without the Groundhog interventions the problems will return.

I know that the simple things done really well get you a long way. But these things will change as we age. We can stay just as fit and just as well, but we have to work harder at it. Life should start with Groundhog Basic (page A1.1), apply Groundhog Acute (page A2.1) for the inevitable infections and morph into Groundhog Chronic (page A3.1) as function and symptoms dictate. It is difficult. Oscar Wilde could not do it:

> *If I could get back my youth, I'd do anything in the world except get up early, take exercise or be respectable.*
> Oscar Wilde, 16 October 1854 –
> 30 November 1900,
> *The Picture of Dorian Gray*

There are no shortcuts here – no hideous portrait locked away to change and age in place of our physical selves! One has to do the 'hard yards' and one has to do them well.[†]

Table 38.1: The checklist to make sure you have covered all the bases, starting with Groundhog Basic

What	Why
The paleo-ketogenic (PK) diet	Evolutionarily correct. The starting point to prevent all diseases of Westerners
A basic package of nutritional supplements – multivitamins, multi-minerals and vitamin D	Western agriculture results in mineral-deficient soils and so deficient foods. Even organic foods are lacking
Vitamin C, 5 grams daily	Humans cannot make their own vitamin C so it must be consumed; it multi-tasks to prevent infection, to prevent cancer, as a vital antioxidant, to detox and to heal and repair

*Footnote: Cojocaru et al concluded that 'Patients with RA have a significantly higher prevalence of the metabolic syndrome (MS) compared to the general population'[1] while Courties et al concluded that 'The systemic role of metabolic syndrome in osteoarthritis pathophysiology is now better understood.'[1, 2]

†Note from Craig: But the more you do them, the less hard the yards become.

Sleep 8-9 hours between 10 pm and 7 am, more in winter, less in summer	Time for healing and repair.
Sleep protects against all diseases of Westerners	
Exercise at least once a week, when you push yourself to your limit. Your limit is defined by a pulse rate of 220 beats per minute minus your age (see Chapter 23)	We are naturally idle because we can be.
Exercise protects against all disease of Westerners	
Make sure your First Aid box is properly stocked – see Appendix 4	Deal immediately with acute infection – sweep it off the beaches before it becomes chronic. (See Groundhog Acute)
Use herbs, spices and fungi in cooking	These help with the Arms Race – they all contain natural antimicrobials, are anti-cancer, antioxidant and much more.
Increase the diversity of the gut microbiome which is protective against all diseases of Westerners	
Optimise energy delivery	Age is defined by energy. To maximise this you need PK fuel in the tank plus the mitochondrial engine, the thyroid accelerator pedal and the adrenal gear box – all need to be working well
Heat and light – get outside as much as is possible. Indoors, aim for being in natural light	To set our body clock and make us cheerful
Use your brain – you must be intelligent, disciplined and determined to, as my daughter would put it, 'Get your shit together'	We are heading for evolutionary disaster. Make sure you, your friends and family will survive – see Chapter 1

Then, with age and circumstance, move on to Groundhog Chronic (Table 38.2). Meanwhile, at the first symptom or sign of any infection, apply Groundhog Acute (see Appendix 2).

Table 38.2: Groundhog Chronic is all the above plus the following

What	Why
Glutathione 250 mg daily Lugol's iodine 12%, 4 drops daily	We live in such a toxic world we are inevitably exposed. Glutathione and iodine are helpful detox molecules
Vitamin C to bowel tolerance, including 5 grams last thing at night. Remember the dose will change with age, diet and circumstance	With age, acute and chronic infections become killers. Vitamin C is the commonest antioxidant deficiency and protects against the three common causes of blindness – namely, macular degeneration, cataract and glaucoma
Exercise within limits. By this I mean you should feel fully recovered next day. If well enough, once a week push those limits, so you get your pulse up to 220 beats per min minus your age, and all your muscles ache. It is never too late to start. Strong core muscles are essential to prevent incontinence	No pain no gain. Muscle loss is part of ageing – exercise slows this right down Exercise helps to physically dislodge microbes from their hiding places; I suspect massage works similarly
Take supplements for the raw materials for connective tissue, such as glucosamine, boron and organic silica. Bone broth is the best	With age we become less good at healing and repair
Consider 'super' herbs – our favourites are astragalus (lovely in stews), cordyceps (makes a wonderful 'chocolate' – see *The PK Cookbook*) and rhodiola (delicious herb tea)	To improve the immune defences – see *The Infection Game*
Take the mitochondrial package of supplements daily, vis: CoQ10 100 mg, niacinamide (B3) slow-release 1500 mg, acetyl L carnitine 500 mg. D-ribose 5-10 grams at night if you have really overdone things	With age, fatigue becomes an increasing issue because our mitochondrial engines start to slow. The ageing process is determined by mitochondria. Look after them
Thyroid and adrenal function declines so...	...many benefit from glandulars. A typical dose would be thyroid glandular 60-150 mg, adrenal glandular 250-750 mg and testicular glandular 1-2 grams daily‡
Review your body burden of toxins – we all have one!	Consider tests of toxic load to see if you need to do any extra detox – see Chapter 15
Check your living space for electromagnetic (EM) pollution (see Chapter 25) and minimise exposure.	We know EM radiation is carcinogenic and neurotoxic

Review any prescription medication – all such are potential toxins. Ask yourself why you are taking drugs? Read on…	Once Groundhog interventions are in place, many drugs can be stopped. Taking prescription drugs is the fourth commonest cause of death in Westerners[§]

As Pierre-Jules Renard, or 'Jules Renard' (22 February 1864 – 22 May 1910), French author and member of the Académie Goncourt, said: 'It`s not how old you are, it`s how you are old.'

And dear Reader, I invite you:

> *Grow old with me! The best is yet to be.*
> Robert Browning, English poet and playwright, 7 May 1812 – 12 December 1889

References

1. Cojocaru M, Cojocaru IM, Silosi I, Vrabie CD. Metabolic Syndrome in Rheumatoid Arthritis. *Maedica (Buchar)* 2012; 7(2): 148–152. www.ncbi.nlm.nih.gov/pmc/articles/PMC3557423/

2. Courties A, Sellam J, Berenbaum F. Metabolic syndrome associated osteoarthritis. *Current Opinion in Rheumatology* 2017; 29(2): 214-222. doi: 10.1097/BOR.0000000000000373.

3. Sample I. Antibiotics could cure 40% of chronic back pain patients. *The Guardian* 7 May 2013. theguardian.com/society/2013/may/07/antibiotics-cure-back-pain-patients

4. Light DW. New Prescription Drugs: A Major Health Risk With Few Offsetting Advantages. Harvard University Edmond J Safra Center for Ethics. 27 June 2014. https://ethics.harvard.edu/blog/new-prescription-drugs-major-health-risk-few-offsetting-advantages

[‡]**Footnote:** In addition to supporting adrenal and thyroid function in Groundhog Chronic, the use of testicular glandulars is also discussed in relation to healing and repair (Chapter 35), rheumatology and orthopaedics (Chapter 47) and women's health (Chapter 54).

[§]**Footnote:** Please see 'New Prescription Drugs: A Major Health Risk With Few Offsetting Advantages' on the Harvard University Centre for Ethics website, which states that: 'About 128,000 people die from drugs prescribed to them. This makes prescription drugs a major health risk, ranking 4th with stroke as a leading cause of death. The European Commission estimates that adverse reactions from prescription drugs cause 200,000 deaths; so together, about 328,000 patients in the U.S. and Europe die from prescription drugs each year.'[4]

Chapter 39
Infectious disease

– life is an arms race which must be fought for life
– how to win

We cannot exist without grappling with infection. You and I are a free lunch for microbes, which are constantly looking for any opportunity to make themselves at home in our delicious and comfortable bodies where they can enjoy free sex and multiply. Once in the body, many remain for life. Microbes have evolved extremely cunning techniques to dodge our highly practical and intelligent systems of defence. Only too often they win. Throughout evolution more humans have died through infection than any other mechanism. You must read our book *The Infection Game – life is an arms race* to learn that this is as true today as ever before,* with most major pathology being driven by infection. This is a game we think we have won. How wrong we are.

Our best chance of dealing with infection occurs when microbes are most vulnerable, as they enter the body. Think of a foreign army trying to invade a country – sweep them off the beaches before they can get a foothold. Our immune system switches on a range of activities to do this – obvious symptoms include coughing, sneezing, runny nose, runny eyes, vomiting, diarrhoea, frequency of micturition and other discharges. If the microbe becomes more systemic, the sphere of war moves accordingly and we develop local inflammation with local pain and swelling as the immune cells engage directly with microbes. If the attack is overwhelming, then systemic symptoms of inflammation include fever, malaise, foggy brain and prostration. All the body's energy goes to the immune system for this battle, so acute fatigue ensues.

I cannot possibly cover the treatment of infectious disease in one chapter, but there are simple principles to follow, viz:

- Symptoms are effective in reducing the size of the invading forces, so do not suppress them with drugs. Rest up, keep warm, allow,

*Historical footnote: Because of increased travel by air and sea, infectious diseases spread more easily and quickly than they ever did before. We talk about this in *The Infection Game*, but I was fascinated to read that the 'Silk Road' provided such a conduit for the spreading of diseases up to 2000 years ago. The Cambridge University Research website describes how: 'An ancient latrine near a desert in north-western China has revealed the first archaeological evidence that travellers along the Silk Road were responsible for the spread of infectious diseases along huge distances of the route 2000 years ago. Cambridge researchers Hui-Yuan Yeh and Piers Mitchell used microscopy to study preserved faeces on ancient 'personal hygiene sticks' (used for wiping away faeces from the anus) in the latrine at what was a large Silk Road relay station on the eastern margins of the Tamrin Basin, a region that contains the Taklamakan desert. The latrine is thought to date from 111 BC (Han Dynasty) and was in use until 109 AD.'[1] Interested readers can digest more in the original research paper by Hui-Yuan Yeh and colleagues.[2]

nay, encourage a fever, perhaps stop eating (stay PK – avoid fruit), stay hydrated and use your brain to reinforce your armies.

- Learn to use tools that you must always have in your first aid box. Use them properly, use them soon and they will prevent much. My difficulty is persuading people to take enough of them and soon enough. These tools are:
  - Vitamin C – see Chapter 31
  - Iodine – see Chapter 32
- If all the above, done well, does not relieve symptoms quickly, then you need professional help. That may include antibiotics, antivirals, antifungals and/or hospital care. I would not like to practise medicine without these essential tools.

References

1. Mitchell P. Ancient faeces provides earliest evidence of infectious disease being carried on Silk Road. University of Cambridge Research, 22 July 2016. www.cam.ac.uk/research/news/ancient-faeces-provides-earliest-evidence-of-infectious-disease-being-carried-on-silk-road

2. Yeh H-Y, Mao R, Wang H, Mitchell P. Early evidence for travel with infectious disesases along the Silk Road – intestinal parasites from 2000 year-old personal hygine sticks in latrine at Xuanquanzhi Relay Station in China. *Journal of Archaeological Science* 2016; 9: 758-764. https://doi.org/10.1016/j.jasrep.2016.05.010

Chapter 40
Ophthalmology

– eyes are so very precious
– get the dose of vitamin C right and prevent much

The soul, fortunately, has an interpreter – often an unconscious but still a faithful interpreter – in the eye.
Charlotte Brontë, 21 April 1816 – 31 March 1855, in *Jane Eyre*

Ophthalmologists and opticians are good doctors. They are asking the right questions and are good at diagnosing problems. However, there seems to be a general acceptance that we will lose sight with age and little can be done to prevent this.

The business of sight requires huge amounts of energy. The job of the retina is to convert the stimulus of a photon landing on it into an electrical signal that the brain can work with. The brain represents 2% of body weight but consumes 20% of all the energy generated. The retina, weight for weight, demands energy at a rate 10 times higher than the brain. No system can generate energy perfectly without some collateral damage. The units of damage are free radicals. For the chemists, free radicals have an unpaired electron – this makes them very sticky and in sticking they denature and damage other substances, causing degeneration. Indeed, this is the mechanism that results in the three major eye diseases of cataract, glaucoma and macular degeneration. To mop up these free radicals we need an excellent

antioxidant system – see Chapter 36 for how to quench the inflammatory fire with good doses of antioxidant.

Go back to Chapter 38 and put in place Groundhog Chronic interventions. When sight is the prize, motivation and determination improve. Sight is so precious. Since much eye degeneration is irreversible, prevention becomes so much more important.

A very early symptom of eye degeneration is the hardening of the lens, which results in the need for reading glasses in one's late 40s and 50s. Any such and now is the time to put in place Groundhog Chronic. Try not to use glasses unless you must – the business of trying keeps the lens more elastic. Some find visual acuity is improved with vitamin C to bowel tolerance.

Symptoms of acute eye problems

- Any loss of vision requires urgent assessment by a professional
- Any major inflammation or pain or eye injury needs the same
- Mild inflammations, such as conjunctivitis, can be effectively treated by iodine oil – see Chapter 32.

Deteriorating visual acuity

There is a general acceptance that with ageing, reading glasses become essential. This arises either because the muscles of the eye that control the thickness of the lens weaken or the lens hardens and so cannot fatten. But it is the old story – use it or lose it. Make the eye muscle work by not focusing for too long on near or distant objects. Every time you switch, the eye muscles are exercised – furthermore you can make them stronger by using less strong reading lenses. Make your eyes work! Combine this with vitamin C to bowel tolerance to keep the lenses soft and you can improve your vision. I know of several, including self, who have thrown away their reading glasses.

Chapter 41
Endocrinology

– problems are very common
– most endocrinologists are very arrogant

I have a consultant physician league of arrogance which is headed by endocrinologists. Poor practice is endemic, largely because these doctors are more interested in tests than patients.* If the test is within population reference range then the suffering patient is told, 'Nothing is wrong, nothing can be done and do not darken my door again'.

Thyroid disorders are so badly treated because endocrinologists do not take a proper medical history, do not properly examine patients (even their gender!) and rely instead entirely on blood tests to diagnose and treat. Here is a brief summary of thyroid terminology – it is necessarily incomplete but aims to give an overview:

- **TSH** – Thyroid stimulating hormone – this is the hormone that the pituitary gland secretes in order to kick the thyroid gland into life
- **Free T4, or thyroxin** – this is the main hormone produced by the thyroid gland. It is fairly inactive and has to be converted into active T3
- **Free T3 or Tertroxin** – this is the active form of thyroid hormone needed to kick

mitochondria into action
- **Reverse T3** – this is an inactive form of T3 but which fits into receptors thereby preventing T3 from working.

Thyroid problems: why the underactive thyroid is so badly treated

The standard NHS tests and interpretations of thyroid function, including normally at best only T4 and TSH levels, are inadequate for several reasons:

- **The population reference range is not the same thing as the individual's reference range.** A patient with a free T4 reading right at the low end of the reference range may feel much better running at the top end of the range, but will be told no action is necessary.
- **The population reference range has fallen with time.** Reference ranges are established

*Footnote: Craig knew of a couple, Pat and Peter, where Pat was the husband and Peter was the wife. Peter had an underactive thyroid. Pat and Peter attended an appointment with a consultant endocrinologist who spent the entire time talking to Pat because he (the endocrinologist) had simply looked at the test results, seen the name 'Peter' attached to the test result, had assumed that this was a man, and had therefore assumed that the man (Pat) was the one attending for a consultation.

by measuring levels in 'normal' people, but hypothyroidism is now so common that the reference range for free T4 levels has moved, in some labs, from 12-22 pmol/l to 7-14. Reference ranges are now decided by what the 'average' population levels currently are. This is patently absurd. Imagine using that system for obesity – we would be constantly 'adjusting' upwards what obese meant so that, say, only 5% of the population were 'defined' as obese. Medical reference ranges should be determined by what is good for health, not by what is average.

- **The threshold for prescribing thyroid hormones has risen.** In the USA, thyroid hormones are prescribed when the TSH level rises above 3.0 mIU/l. In the UK, no prescription is deemed necessary until the TSH is above 10.0 mIU/l (as stated in the current NICE Guidelines[1]). What is so illogical is that once a patient is taking thyroid medication, thyroid replacement therapy is not deemed sufficient until the TSH is below 2.0 (I like to see it below 1.0), and in pregnancy the TSH should be below 1.5. Compare these figures with the 10 that is needed to commence treatment in the first place! TSH during pregnancy is inversely proportionate to the mental development and IQ of the baby – that is, a high TSH results in low IQ. So, someone could have a level of 4.0 mIU/l and not be receiving thyroid replacement therapy (because their level is not above 10.0 mIU/l), whereas if someone was *already* on thyroid replacement therapy, a level of 4.0 mIU/l would be considered much too high and would need to be brought down to below 2.0 mIU/l, or even 1.5 mIU/l. A further absurdity is that a woman may be considered to have adequate replacement therapy, but the moment she becomes pregnant her dose would be considered inadequate.

- **Standard tests of thyroid function never include free T3.** This is despite T3 being the active hormone. Increasingly I am seeing cases of T3 hypothyroidism with normal or high T4, high TSH and low T3. These diagnoses would be entirely missed by standard NHS tests.

- **The time of day for testing is ignored.** This is despite our knowing that TSH peaks at midnight, T4 at 4:00 am and T3 at 5:00 am.

- **Standard tests of thyroid function do not include reverse T3.** Reverse T3 blocks the effect of T3 on cells, resulting in thyroid hormone receptor resistance.

- **There is no test for thyroid hormone receptor resistance.** This resistance is becoming more common for the same reasons that type 2 diabetes with insulin receptor resistance is increasing – that is, the toxic burden of Western life (see Chapter 25).

This reliance on tests means that many cases of hypothyroidism are missed, as detailed in Table 41.1.

Table 41.1: The reasons a diagnosis of underactive thyroid may be missed

Diagnosis	Missed because...
Primary hypothyroidism	TSH production is set too high
Secondary hypothyroidism (this is common in CFS)	The population reference range is set too low and/or one feels better running at the top end of reference range for T4 and/or T3 levels
T3 hypothyroidism	T3 level is not measured at all
Thyroid hormone receptor resistance (THRR)	Reverse T3 level is not measured Other causes of THRR are not considered A trial of thyroid hormones in a patient with 'normal' tests is never done
All the above	Clinical factors are ignored completely. Other clues showing poor energy delivery mechanisms are vital, including fatigue, foggy brain, low core temperature, slow pulse and low blood pressure

From a clinical perspective, blood tests are most useful simply to exclude the possibility of thyrotoxicosis (from an overactive thyroid). From a personal, selfish perspective, they also protect me from further prosecution by the General Medical Council. Increasingly I rely on clinical measurements for adequacy of replacement therapy and, indeed, this is the only way to assess adequacy of replacement in patients with thyroid hormone receptor resistance. (There is more on the diagnosis and treatment of hypothyroidism in Chapter 30.)

Causes of hypothyroidism

We then have to think about the cause of hypothyroidism – which is often autoimmune. Having one such autoimmune condition greatly increases the risk of others. Take steps now to prevent this from happening, as explained in Chapter 51: Immunology. I suspect that there are many mechanisms for thyroid damage, including viral infection, toxic damage and iodine deficiency,

and probably others. This means hypothyroidism is extremely common. Consultant endocrinologist Dr Kenneth Blanchard (one of the good ones) estimates 40% of Westerners are hypothyroid, more so with age. One should consider hypothyroidism in all cases characterised by poor energy delivery mechanisms.

Thyrotoxicosis – when the thyroid is overactive

The accelerator pedal is flat on the floor and everything is going at double speed. The brain races, ideas flow, optimism is unbounding and clinically this may look like a manic psychosis. The heart is racing, muscles are trembling (best seen by spreading the fingers of an outstretched arm), the skin may be hot to the touch, the eyes may be bulging so that the whites can be seen all around the iris with a 'Marty Feldman look'.[†] With time, weight drops off with uncontrolled fat burning. It is a potentially dangerous condition

---

[†]**Celebrity note:** Marty Feldman suffered from Graves' disease, a type of hyperthyroidism. According to rumour, a car accident at the age of 30 and subsequent corrective plastic surgery made Feldman's eyes appear even more unusual.

which demands expert medical attention.

The symptoms can be immediately controlled with beta blockers. This illustrates how similar are the functions of adrenalin and thyroid hormones – beta blockers 'work' by blocking the effects of both. But then production of thyroid hormones from the thyroid gland must be controlled. All the choices are bad (but better than the toxicosis). One has to choose between carbimazole, radioactive iodine and surgery. All have risks and side effects.

Before the advent of these treatments, the standard treatment was iodine – but in high doses. I have yet to try this for any patient, but it is worth considering since it is very safe if done with close clinical (pulse, blood pressure, tremor) and biochemical (weekly blood tests until a clear response emerges) monitoring. According to *Clinical Thyroidology for the Public* by the American Thyroid Association, the range of dose to control the thyrotoxicosis ranged from 13 to 800 mg daily. This is equivalent to Lugol's iodine 12%, 2 to 130 drops daily (1 drop contains 6 mg, with 20 drops in one ml).[1]

In parallel with treating the high levels of thyroxin one must also look for the cause (see Chapters 16 and 51). Concentrate on toxic metals, other poisonings, vaccinations, infections and mycotoxins.

Adrenal disease

Adrenal fatigue is not even recognised, let alone treated, by endocrinologists. The 'gold standard' test of adrenal function is the 'short synacthen test', during which the patient is injected with ACTH (a hormone which gives the adrenal gland a huge kick) and levels of cortisol measured before and after. This will pick up cases of complete adrenal failure (Addison's disease) but will not pick up the milder adrenal fatigue of chronic disease and/or ageing. Yet again, this

test is used as an excuse for therapeutic nihilism, and again patients are told their adrenals are functioning normally.

The most useful test is an adrenal stress profile because:
- It measures salivary levels of hormone and this gets round the problem of protein binding (which may distort blood results). Tests for serum cortisol measure both free (bioactive) and protein-bound (non-active) cortisol. The free cortisol level is the measure that we need to know for our clinical diagnosis and treatment, and the saliva test gives us exactly this.
- Measurements are made over 24 hours. This reflects normal life more closely than a single reading. One can see disturbances of circadian rhythm which may point to other problems. So, for example, a flat circadian rhythm points to hypothyroidism.
- Measurements are made of cortisol and DHEA. Since cortisol follows adrenalin this give us a handle on hour to hour stress levels experienced by the patient. DHEA reflects the production of other steroid hormones.
- This is an easy test to do, accessible to all, without reliance on doctors.

For the interpretation of this test and treatment of adrenal fatigue, see Chapter 30.

The adrenal pathology recognised by endocrinologists is largely autoimmune or degenerative, rarely cancerous. Over-production and failure of production disorders were described by Drs Cushing and Addison and bear their names. They are rare – I have dealt with two cases in my career. You need modern investigations to determine the cause, but ecological medicine to prevent and treat. Again, concentrate on toxic metals, other poisonings, vaccinations, infections and mycotoxins. Mycotoxin-driven adrenal lesions have been described in captive whooping cranes (the bird) but not in humans. Why? Because the doctors are not looking.

Growth hormone (GH)

Modern humans are now too tall and too fat – both are risk factors for cancer. This is a result of too much GH driven by insulin and growth promotors (dairy products and pollutants acting as endocrine mimics). Too little GH in children causes stunted growth (surprise, surprise). In any age group, expect slow healing and repair, which manifests with an accelerated ageing process.

Treatment is to identify and, where possible, treat the pituitary damage. This may be physical (head injury) or part of poor energy delivery mechanisms, inflammation (infection, autoimmunity) or toxicity. GH injections may be needed for replacement therapy.

Anti-diuretic hormone (ADH[‡])

This hormone, ADH, controls how hard the kidneys have to work to retain sodium. Where there is insufficient ADH, salt is lost through the kidneys and this is followed by water. Treatment is to identify and treat causes and use synthetic ADH to replace.

Reference

1. National Institute for Health and Care Excellence (NICE). Guidelines on hypothyroidism. [June 2018] https://cks.nice.org.uk/hypothyroidism

‡**Footnote on abbreviations**: I appreciate that there are several acronyms in this chapter – TSH, T3, T4, GH, ADH – but I make no apology, especially considering this webpage listing the acronyms used by the British Army: www.armedforces. co.uk/abbreviations.php#.XGZ-NfrAPIU

Chapter 42
Cardiology and vascular medicine

– the allopathic approach does not address the root cause
– diet and supplements can be highly effective
– if we all adopted Groundhog interventions, cardiologists would become virtually redundant

Metabolic syndrome: cholesterol, hypertension and diabetes

Metabolic syndrome is easily diagnosed because it is defined by the contents of the supermarket trolley. Eating carbohydrates (bread, pasta, cereals, fruit etc), results in blood sugar levels that when tested throughout 24 hours (a video as opposed to a snap shot) look like a rollercoaster. Insulin is triggered as blood sugar rises and this makes us fat. As blood sugar drops, the brain panics, 'We are running out of fuel', and so out pours the stress hormone adrenalin, which spikes blood pressure. Sugar is sticky stuff; it adheres to arteries and damages them to cause arteriosclerosis, an effect that is compounded by high blood pressure. Eventually we have permanent high blood pressure, loss of control of blood sugar, the development of insulin resistance and finally, of diabetes. (There is much more detail in our book *Prevent and Cure Diabetes – delicious diets not dangerous drugs*.)

Big Pharma makes a fortune out of metabolic syndrome: drugs for blood pressure, drugs for cholesterol and drugs for diabetes. Patients are reassured because they are receiving treatment, but this is symptom suppression – again, doctors are smothering the fire but not switching off the fuel supply. There is an inevitable progression to arterial disease, heart disease, dementia and cancer, and this provides another treasure trove of treatments for investors.

In 2014, total pharmaceutical revenues worldwide exceeded one trillion US dollars for the first time. Metabolic syndrome can be quickly reversed by Groundhog interventions. With established diabetes, you will need to monitor your blood sugar levels yourself at home so you can safely tail off and stop the drugs. With established hypertension, you will need to do the same – home monitor blood pressure and tail off the drugs.

Cholesterol

Cholesterol is a very useful tool to diagnose arterial damage; it is a symptom of damage, not a cause.

Total cholesterol is irrelevant to arterial disease but a wonderful money spinner for Big Pharma. We have been fed the intellectually risible mantra that high fat diets mean high cholesterol and so arterial disease. Worse, the doctors have swallowed this thinking and are still regurgitating and spewing this nonsense over patients. Statins are my pet hate. Through sheer good fortune they do afford mild protection against some disease, but this has nothing to do with their cholesterol-reducing power. It so happens they are vitamin D mimics, and all the benefits of statins can be ascribed to the anti-inflammatory properties of vitamin D. The real problem is that statins inhibit the body's own production of co-enzyme Q10. We know that this is a major risk factor for chronic fatigue, muscle damage and premature ageing. Dementia is an obvious risk, but the cardiologists seem not to care about that. Their vital statistics look good; it is a case of 'the operation was a success, but the patient demented'.

It is vital to realise that 'cholesterol' is not a cause of arterial disease but a symptom of it. The key measurement is the proportion of 'friendly' high-density lipoprotein (HDL), and this is easily calculated by taking the level of HDL and dividing it by the total cholesterol reading. HDL is what is used up in the business of healing and repairing arteries, so this percentage of 'friendly' cholesterol is an indirect but very useful indicator of the level of arterial damage. If the HDL percentage is low, we can infer that arteries are being damaged, and vice versa. I have been collecting HDL percentages and dietary histories for years. It is very clear that people eating carbohydrate-based diets have consistently low HDL, often below 20%, whilst those eating PK diets consistently have an HDL above 40%. My top score of 63% belongs to a 90-year-old, recently retired from running his own business having won a Queen's award for industry.

The HDL percentage is so useful because occasionally I see a low level in someone eating a good PK diet. This means there must be another cause for arterial damage and that is often homocysteine.

Homocysteine – a vital test

High homocysteine is a major risk factor for arterial disease, dementia and cancer. I do not know the mechanism for this, but we know high homocysteine is a marker of poor methylation and methylation is an essential healing and repair tool. I suspect slow healing and repair of damaged arteries means there is greater potential for thrombosis and thromboembolism.

High homocysteine is an important diagnosis for two reasons. It is easily, safely and inexpensively treated with B vitamins (which need to be in the methylated form – that is, methyl tetrahydrofolate 800 mcg, pyridoxal 5 phosphate 50 mg and methylcobalamin 5 mg daily for life). For a few people with poor methylation, correct homocysteine levels can be achieved only with injected methylcobalamin, so it is vital to monitor the response to treatment. Secondly, high homocysteine runs in families – so all first-degree relatives (siblings, parents and children) should be screened. Indeed, homocysteine is an essential screening test for anyone with a family history of these problems.

Why is this not standard medical practice? Why is homocysteine not a familiar word in our language? Follow the money and work it out for yourself – vitamins are not patented and so there is no money there for Big Pharma.

Inflammation is a major cause of arterial damage

If, despite a PK diet and normal homocysteine, the HDL percentage is still low, then look for inflammatory causes of arterial damage. Think allergy, chronic infection and autoimmunity and read Chapters 7, 16 and 36 which all deal with inflammation. Also read the chapters that relate to poisoning (Chapters 8, 15, 25), of which smoking is a major cause. Again, the starting point to treat is Groundhog Chronic and this may be all that is necessary. Recheck the HDL percentage to be sure after three months.

Arteriosclerosis

Arteriopsclerosis leads to heart attacks, TIAs, strokes, organ failures, intermittent claudication* and gangrene.

It is a healing process that repairs the damage to the lining of blood vessels created by all the above (inflammation etc). It starts with a scab over the arterial damage which matures into a patch of scar tissue. But more blood may stick to the scab and the whole lump may flick off in a process called thromboembolism. The blood supply is cut off downstream and this may result in myocardial infarction (a 'coronary'), stroke or gangrene. Thromboembolism further results from sticky blood (the commonest causes being sugar and inflammation) and poor circulation (enforced bed rest).

When thrombosis (a blood clot) forms in a vein, a piece flicking off (called an embolus) the clot may result in a blood clot in the lungs (called a pulmonary embolus). This process is called a thromboembolism.

Much, if not all, can be prevented and often reversed with Groundhog Chronic. If you have suffered any of the above then of course you need conventional medical investigations and interventions, such as clot-busters, to, perhaps, save your life. But the need for such should be a real wake-up call to do Groundhog. I can hear myself shouting: 'You are steering for the rocks.'

> *If you do not change direction, you may end up where you are heading.*
> Lao Tzu, founder of the philosophical system of Taoism (likely 6th or 4th century BC)

So, what are the symptoms and diseases that I see when all the above has been ducked?

Angina

Angina is the symptom of lactic acid burn of heart muscle. It occurs when energy demands exceed energy delivery so there is a switch into anaerobic metabolism with the production of lactic acid. As any athlete can testify, lactic acid is painful and can stop them in their tracks. It prevents them winning gold medals. Angina sufferers also know this and suffer similarly.

Cardiologists and other doctors are very familiar with the causes of poor blood supply to the heart, such as arteriosclerosis, together with all the causes of heart failure detailed below. I see many CFS patients with what is called 'atypical chest pain', but is actually angina; it too is a lactic acid burn of heart muscle, but in their case it is due to poor energy delivery mechanisms. It is called atypical because is does not resolve quickly on resting. This is because these very sick patients do not even have the energy delivery mechanisms in place to clear lactic acid, even with good blood supply. (There is much more detail in our book *Diagnosis and Treatment of Chronic Fatigue Syndrome and Myalgic Encephalitis – it's mitochondria not hypochondria*.)

I learned much about the importance of mitochondria in heart disease through the work

---

*Footnote: Claudication is a condition in which cramp-like pain occurs in the legs with exercise. The pain is the result of a reduction in the blood flow to the muscles of the legs. The word derives from the Latin stem of *claudicātiō , claudic(āre)*, to limp (itself a derivative of *claudus*, lame).

of consultant cardiologists Drs Gabriela Segura and Stephen Sinatra. Both started their careers walking the conventional path of drugs, pacemakers and surgery but moved to the ecological route. Both have become far more effective physicians, reversing disease instead of postponing the inevitable.

Heart failure

Symptoms of heart failure include fatigue, shortness of breath and angina. Very early heart failure manifests with exercise intolerance. This is further good reason to exercise regularly so that pathology can be diagnosed early before organ damage ensues. Exercise intolerance is a far more sensitive test of disease than ECG or echocardiography.

Postural orthostatic tachycardia syndrome (POTS) is the name given to when the heart beats even faster on standing. Why does it do this? Because it is harder work to circulate blood when the body is in a vertical compared with a horizontal position. If it cannot beat more powerfully then, to maintain output, it has to beat faster. This is a feature of my CFS patients who are also in a state of low cardiac output. Signs include fast pulse, low blood pressure, then bilateral (both sides) pitting ankle oedema (swelling that keeps indentation after being pressed). Other organ failures follow. POTS sufferers also experience headaches, dizziness, and sometimes fainting, amongst other symptoms.

Heart failure is a symptom with many causes, and in any patient there is likely to be more than one cause. It is a very serious diagnosis with poor prognosis so sufferers must do all the Groundhog regimes. I shall be using some further medical terms in Table 42.1 that follows; I hope that the simplified heart diagram in Figure 42.1 will help.

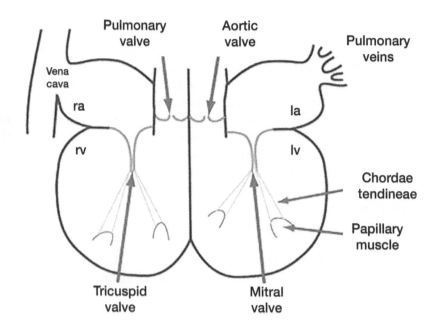

Figure 42.1: Simplified diagram of the heart

Table 42.1: Heart failure mechanisms and treatments

What is going wrong	Mechanism	Treatment – Groundhog Chronic in particular
Poor blood supply to the heart so fuel and oxygen cannot be delivered	Arteriosclerosis	Diagnose the causes: metabolic syndrome, high homocysteine, chronic inflammation? Advanced cases may need surgery to replace blocked arteries
	Anaemia	See Chapter 57: Haematology
The heart is beating too slowly	Hypothyroidism	Sort the thyroid – see Chapter 30
	Overtreatment with beta-blockers	Review need for such
The heart is beating irregularly e.g. atrial fibrillation reduces cardiac output by about 20%	This makes the heart inefficient as a pump because it may have too much or too little time to fill optimally	See above for the treatments as listed for poor blood supply See below for the treatments as listed for poisoning by heavy metals, pesticides or other such
Poor cardiac output because valves are narrowed so blood cannot flow	Aortic stenosis or mitral stenosis	Surgery – if you are not fit enough for surgery then make yourself fit with Groundhog Chronic
Poor cardiac output because valves are floppy so blood leaks back the wrong way	Aortic incompetence	Ditto
	Mitral valve incompetence – perhaps because of a damaged valve due to infection or the rupture of a heart string	Ditto
	Mitral valve incompetence because the mitral ring (see Figure 42.1) is dilated (the doorway is too big so the doors do not meet in the middle). This may result from weak heart muscle due to poor energy delivery mechanisms	See Chapter 30 – the following need attention: PK fuel, mitochondrial engine, thyroid accelerator pedal and adrenal gear box

What is going wrong	Mechanism	Treatment – Groundhog Chronic in particular
Poor energy delivery mechanisms to the heart muscle. Clinically this results in cardiomyopathy (hypertrophic cardiomyopathy (HOCM), where the heart muscle becomes thick, or – congestive cardiomyopathy, where the heart becomes stretched and weakened and is unable to pump effectively)	Cardiac muscle is 25% by weight mitochondria; muscle is only as strong as the energy available to it	See Chapter 30 – the following need attention: PK fuel, the mitochondrial engine, the thyroid accelerator pedal and the adrenal gear box
	Mitochondria lack the raw materials to function, or are blocked by toxins	Correct the mitochondrial dysfunction; this may have many causes – see Chapter 12 for the mechanisms and Chapter 30 for the treatments
	Possibly chronic infection e.g. Keshan disease[†]	Take selenium 500 mcg daily for four months Groundhog Chronic

Cardiac dysrhythmias

The symptoms of cardiac dysrhythmia (or 'arrhythmia') can include all symptoms of low cardiac output failure as detailed above. There may also be palpitations (an undue awareness of the heart beating).

For the signs, feel your pulse – at rest it should be between 65 and 75 beats per minute (bpm). Is it too fast? Too slow? Is it irregular? Dysrhythmias come in many guises, but the underlying causes are the same, as listed in Table 42.2.

[†]**Footnote**: Keshan disease is a congestive cardiomyopathy caused by a combination of dietary deficiency of selenium and the presence of a mutated strain of Coxsackie virus, named after Keshan County of Heilongjiang province, Northeast China, where the symptoms were first noted.

Table 42.2: Symtoms of cardiac dysrhythmia, their causes and treatment

Symptom	Mechanism	Treatment – Groundhog Chronic in particular
Resting pulse regular but too fast	Physically unfit (an inevitable part of CFS and ME)	See Chapter 23: Exercise (but not for those with CFS/ME)
	The adrenalin of normal life provoking anxiety	Life is not normal without some… address the work/life balance
	The adrenalin of metabolic syndrome	PK diet
	The adrenalin of pathological anxiety (e.g. PTSD)	See Chapter 50: Psychiatry
	Anaemia	See Chapter 57: Haematology
	Thyrotoxicosis	See Chapter 41: Endocrinology
	Heart failure	See above
	Supraventricular tachycardias	See below
Pulse too slow	Hypothyroidism Overtreatment with beta-blockers	See Chapter 30: Thyroid Review the need for such
Poor blood supply to the pacemaker	Arteriosclerosis	See above
Irregular pulse – ventricular ectopics (an irregular heart rhythm due to a premature ventricular contraction), atrial fibrillation, bundle branch blocks etc	Poor blood supply	See above
	Poisoning – usually by toxic metals	See Chapter 15 for diagnostic tests See Chapter 34 for getting rid of toxic metals
	Pesticides – my farmer patients with sheep dip flu commonly suffered dysrhythmias	See Chapter 34 for detoxing with heating regimes

Infections of the heart

Infections of the heart are always very nasty, should always be taken very seriously and need medical input. **Pericarditis** occurs when the covering of the heart, the pericardium, is inflamed and this is characterised by pain. It probably results from a viral infection – apply Groundhog Acute.

Endocarditis (inflammation of the heart's inner lining, called the endocardium) may accompany the above and is more severe.

Rheumatic fever thankfully is very rare. It is a very rare complication of a streptoccocal throat infection – all the more reason to apply Groundhog Acute.

Drugs to treat heart‡ disease

Remember drugs do not address the underlying causes of arterial and heart disease. They put the system into a chemical straitjacket which may postpone the inevitable but does not cure. Cure lies in Groundhog and all else described in this book. These interventions take months to fully manifest and you may see initial worsening (see Chapter 28). Only when you are past the worst of these reactions and you have objective evidence of benefit dare you slowly reduce your drug burden.

---

‡**Note by Craig**: As I read this on Valentine's Day 2019, I wonder why the heart is currently associated with love. The Ancient Egyptians and Greeks thought that the heart was the 'seat of thought, feeling and will' and this in turn may have derived from the quickening of the heart that we all feel at emotional times or even when we have faced an intellectual challenge. The great Greek, cum Roman, physician Galen (130 AD – 210 AD) put forward the idea of the heart being at the centre of emotions (the *thumoeides* or 'spirited part of the soul') because of his work on the circulatory system. According to Galen, there were two other parts of the soul – the rational (*logistikon*) or leading-part (*hēgemonikon*), which Galen located in the brain, and the desiderative (*epithumētikon*), which Galen located in the liver. Where we feel love may not 'really' be the heart, but it is certain that we must 'love' our heart if we are to enjoy the quantity and quality of life that is the very object of this book.

Chapter 43
Respiratory* medicine and ENT

– it's all allergy and infection
– how to get rid of those blue and brown inhalers

I always wondered why the respiratory tract evolved so inefficiently for the purposes of acquiring oxygen. It would be far more efficient to have a one-way flow of air similar to the one-way flow of water over the gills of fish. The answer is because oxygen is potentially toxic and carbon dioxide retention is necessary for maintaining the correct acidity of the blood. This has clinical application because over-breathing, hyperventilation, causes deeply unpleasant symptoms because carbon dioxide is washed out of the lungs and bloodstream – in other words, carbon dioxide has not been retained in sufficient quantities. This may worsen asthma – indeed, during an acute attack most asthmatics

are hyperventilating; this is driven by adrenalin. A useful first aid treatment is to breathe and re-breathe into a paper bag (just cupped hands has a modest effect). Thus, some exhaled air is re-inhaled and so is higher in carbon dioxide. This reverses the symptoms of hyperventilation

Many of the problems of the lungs and upper airways arise because these areas are in direct contact with the outside world and so susceptible to infection. Air should be drawn in through the nose where the scroll bones or 'turbinates' of the nose create turbulence. This throws particulate matter, including microbes, against the lining of the respiratory tract where it is trapped by the sticky mucus lining. This lining sits over the hairs

***Historical note**: The path to human understanding of respiration is fascinating and reflects how we humans challenge received wisdom – the 'sapiens' bit that is often missing! Jean Fitting wrote a paper, 'From breathing to respiration'[1] in 2015 and its Abstract deserves full quotation:

'The purpose of breathing remained an enigma for a long time. The Hippocratic school described breathing patterns but did not associate breathing with the lungs. Empedocles and Plato postulated that breathing was linked to the passage of air through pores of the skin. This was refuted by Aristotle who believed that the role of breathing was to cool the heart. In Alexandria, breakthroughs were accomplished in the anatomy and physiology of the respiratory system. Later, Galen proposed an accurate description of the respiratory muscles and the mechanics of breathing. However, his heart-lung model was hampered by the traditional view of two non-communicating vascular systems – veins and arteries. After a period of stagnation in the Middle Ages, knowledge progressed with the discovery of the pulmonary circulation. The comprehension of the purpose of breathing progressed by steps thanks to Boyle and Mayow among others and culminated with the contribution of Priestley and the discovery of oxygen by Lavoisier. Only then was breathing recognized as fulfilling the purpose of respiration, or gas exchange. A century later, a controversy emerged concerning the active or passive transfer of oxygen from alveoli to the blood. August and Marie Krogh settled the dispute, showing that passive diffusion was sufficient to meet the oxygen needs.'

of cells which waft the mucus away, usually to be swallowed. The mucus-microbe gloop should drop into an acid bath of the stomach and this kills all invaders. Indeed, this is a major defence against disease.

If the immune system detects an invading microbe, then a first defence is a narrowing of the airways. This is called 'bronchospasm' and may result in noisy breathing with wheeze. This greatly increases turbulence and so filters out nasty invaders. Coughing and sneezing further help to expel unwanted microbes.

Acute and chronic infections of the airways

Such infections include: pharyngitis, tonsillitis, rhinitis, sinusitis, laryngitis, bronchitis, chest infections and bronchiectasis. Always treat these aggressively. Sweep the invaders off the beach at the first symptom of.[†]

Apply Groundhog Acute, especially iodine inhaled with a salt pipe. For children and babies, smear iodine oil (see Chapter 32: Iodine) around the nose and mouth; iodine is volatile and so when inhaled can do much good. Iodine oil in the ear is great for otitis externa and otitis media as the volatile iodine penetrates well and kills all on contact.

Also, vitamin C to bowel tolerance is a very good 'sweeper-off-er'.

Asthma and COPD

Asthma is a new disease. Children used to suffer

occasional wheezy bronchitis, which was a benign condition that resolved spontaneously. It has been replaced by asthma, a condition that apparently needs symptom-suppressing medication for life. This may be because the inhalers inhibit the very mechanisms that permit immune tolerance. Any allergy is not switched off. Bronchodilators like ventolin open up the airways so infection and pollutants can get in. Steroid inhalers suppress the immune response. Combine this with high-carb diets and there is an obvious recipe for infectious, allergic and toxic disaster. Asthma means much increased risk of COPD and barring from certain jobs, such as the armed forces. See this standing order from the RAF:

> *If you suffer from asthma or have done in the past, you cannot be considered for flying branches in the RAF. For ground branches and trades, individuals with a past history of asthma, wheezing or inhaler use may be eligible for service following review of the past medical history by medical staff. If you currently have asthma symptoms or a current prescription, or you use an inhaler for asthma or wheeze (regardless of cause), you are not eligible to apply for the Royal Air Force.*[3]

Treatment
Asthma and COPD have three common causes:
1. Infection – in chronic cases do not forget moulds and mycotoxins (see Chapter 16: Inflammation).
2. Allergy – dairy products are particularly

[†]**Linguistic note from Craig**: 'Of' is a preposition and one is taught never to end a sentence with a preposition. Sarah doesn't follow the rule book, and therein lies her charm. 'With' is also a preposition – prepositions show the relationship between the noun or pronoun and other words in a sentence. Anyway, the famous story goes that an editor had rearranged one of Churchill's sentences to avoid it ending in a preposition, so Churchill scribbled this note in reply: 'This is the sort of English up with which I will not put.'[2] Churchill was avoiding writing 'put up with' in order to lampoon his editor! *The Oxford Companion to the English Language* states that the original was in fact, 'This is the sort of bloody nonsense up with which I will not put.' So, Sarah and Churchill have this much in common, although she never lampoons me and is always very receptive to my editing.

catarrh-forming. Do the PK diet. Many cases of asthma are driven by allergy to gut flora so the PK diet should be combined with vitamin C to bowel tolerance.

3. Air pollution – avoid; consider using air filters (see Chapter 25: Reduce the toxic chemical burden).

Treatment

*   Groundhog Acute (page A2) and Chronic (page A3)
*   Inhaled magnesium (by nebuliser) or given intravenously is an excellent and safe bronchodilator which has effects over and above drug treatments. Sadly this is rarely used… follow the money.
*   Breathing exercises are of proven benefit. Buteyko breathing[4] works well, as does learning to sing and/or playing a wind instrument.

The aim is to put in place whatever you need so that the inhalers can be stopped. These are symptom suppressors with potential to accelerate the underlying pathology. Monitor progress using a peak flow meter. (This measures how well your lungs are able to expel air.) I now have three patients with bronchiectasis who have had no infections for a year as a result of the above interventions. One has been able to stop her blue and brown inhalers. In all cases, lung function has improved.

Chronic sinusitis

This is a greatly overlooked and under-rated problem. Sinuses are a comfortable site for any number of chronic infections. A typical sequence of events is dairy allergy which generates chronic catarrh followed by colonisation with yeast and/or bacteria. A further common sequel that I see is progression to a chronic fatigue syndrome. Indeed, Dr Joseph Brewer has shown that 90% of CFS/MEs will test positive for mycotoxins.[5]

Chronic middle ear infection, glue ear, nasal polyps and post-nasal drip

The surgeons love to dive in with sinus wash outs, grommets, sub-mucous resections and excisions of tonsils and adenoids. This may temporarily open up the airway but unless the underlying cause is treated, the problem will recur. Treat as for asthma, especially with the PK diet and iodine salt pipe.

Snoring

Snoring results from obstruction of the airway. It is an evolutionary disaster since this flags up to predators where you are hiding when at your most vulnerable. Partial obstruction may be due to an undershot jaw (see a good dentist or osteopath) or the oedema of allergy (usually dairy products) and/or hypothyroidism. Also see the causes of obstructive sleep apnoea in Chapter 8: Poisoning and deficiency clinical pictures.

Voice changes and loss of singing voice

These changes are due to a change of shape of the vocal cords. This may be due to a tumour, so get your chords looked at by an ENT surgeon. Otherwise, this is likely to be oedema from allergy and/or hypothyroidism.

Hyperventilation (over-breathing)

Hyperventilation is a stress response and driven by adrenalin. This is a totally appropriate response to our sabre-tooth tiger when we have to sprint, but in the modern world we either get adrenalin spikes in metabolic syndrome (as blood sugar falls) or from psychological or life stressors that do not demand a physical response. Problems arise when we breathe too much but do not match that with exercise.

Over-breathing means we wash carbon dioxide out of our blood. This has the effect of making oxygen stick more avidly to haemoglobin and so oxygen delivery to the tissues is reduced, with obvious consequences. Lowering carbon dioxide levels in the blood has other dire effects. It upsets the acidity of the blood and causes what is known in medical jargon as a respiratory alkalosis. This causes a mixture of symptoms from adrenalin (panic attacks, anxiety, tremor) to poor energy delivery (fatigue, foggy brain, feeling spaced out and dizzy).

If short-term relief of symptoms can be achieved by breathing into a paper bag (to re-inhale carbon dioxide and so correct the balance) that makes the diagnosis. Groundhog interventions cure. Much work has gone into breathing exercises, such as Buteyko, which are effective; I have tried them but find them so difficult that, for once, Groundhog is preferable – Yay!

Sarcoidosis

Sarcoidosis has long been a mystery disease. It is a nasty lung inflammation that bears many of the hallmarks of chronic infection, although no actual microbe has been clearly identified. However, this clinical and pathological picture demands Groundhog Chronic interventions. What is interesting is that sufferers are more likely to live in water-damaged buildings and good responses to antifungal therapy have been documented.[6,7,8] This raises the biologically plausible idea that mycotoxins are to blame (see Chapters 8, 15 and 34).

References

1. Fitting J. From breathing to respiration. *Respiration* 2015; 89: 82-87. www.karger.com/Article/FullText/369474

2. The American Heritage Book of English Usage: a practical and authoritative guide to contemporary English. Houghton Mifflin Harcourt 1996.

3. RAF recruitment guidelines: Medical conditions that preclude entry. December 2013. www.raf.mod.uk/recruitment/media/1652/medical-conditions-that-preclude-entry.pdf (accessed 5 December 2019)

4. Buteyko Breathing Association www.buteyko-breathing.org and Buteyko Works www.buteykoworks.com

5. Brewer JH, Thrasher JD, Straus DC, Madison RA, Hooper D. Detection of mycotoxins in patients with chronic fatigue syndrome. *Toxins* 2013; 5(4): 605-617. www.ncbi.nlm.nih.gov/pubmed/23580077

6. Tercelj M, Salobir B, Harlander M, Ryalnder R. Fungal exposure in homes of patients with sarcoidosis – an environmental exposure study. *Environ Health* 2011; 10(1): 8. www.ncbi.nlm.nih.gov/pubmed/21251285

7. Laney AS, Cragin LA, Blevins LZ, Sumner AD, et al. Sarcoidosis, asthma, and asthma-like symptoms among occupants of a historically water-damaged office building. *Indoor Air* 2009; 19(1): 83-90. www.ncbi.nlm.nih.gov/pubmed/19191928

8. Tercelj M, Salobir B, Zupancic M, Rylander R. Sarcoidosis Treatment with Antifungal Medication: A Follow-Up. *Pulmonary Medicine* 2014: Article ID 739673. www.hindawi.com/journals/pm/2014/739673/

Chapter 44
Gastroenterology

– diet and vitamin C done properly will do it all

We experience symptoms of any sort for a very good reason – they protect us from ourselves. How else can our intelligent guts tell us that we are eating the wrong foods other than by giving us symptoms? It seems that burping, posseting, vomiting babies are the new norm. They are literally screaming 'No' at us, but we continue to shovel down high-carbohydrate foods. The contents of breast milk simply reflect what is in Mother's blood, minus the blood cells. So, if Mother is eating carbs her blood sugars will be up and down like a yo-yo and babies will receive the regular adrenalin hit that results from such. No wonder they cry and can't sleep.

Adults are no different and doctors no better. Again, carbs are providing another cash-cow for Big Pharma. Drugs suppress symptoms (and are 'required' long term) and allow us to guzzle our way to an early grave.

Gut symptoms (and many others) arise largely for three reasons:
1. the upper fermenting gut
2. poor quality microbiome and
3. allergy.

To understand why we must first look at the what.

What constitutes normal gut function

The upper gut (mouth, oesophagus, stomach and small intestine) should be near sterile for the businesses of digesting meat and fat and absorbing minerals. Indeed, an acid stomach is also a vital part of defence against disease. Most attacking microbes enter the body through the mouth and nose. Those inhaled get stuck in the sticky mucus that lines the upper airways, which either drains directly into the stomach or is coughed up and swallowed. All these inhaled or ingested micro-organisms should fall into that acid bath and be killed.

By contrast, the lower gut (large bowel) is teeming with 'friendly' microbes that ferment fibre. Not only does this provide a fuel for the gut lining and the body, but there we see immune programming, synthesis of vitamins such as vitamins K and biotin and synthesis of neurotransmitters such as serotonin, cannabinoids and much more. Thousands of different species are involved, and their predator-prey inter-relationships are as complex as those of the animal kingdom. We disturb this at our peril. Indeed, longevity can be predicted by the diversity of the gut microbiome.

I struggle to find the necessary vocabulary

to describe this nourishing soup which is so essential for rude health and which is otherwise known as shit.* Perhaps this explains the complete contempt in which doctors seemingly hold the gut microbiome. They insist on starving it with Western diets and killing it with their drugs.

The upper fermenting gut

This is an inevitable part of high-carbohydrate Western diets. The upper gut may be able to cope temporarily with occasional carbohydrates which arrive during the autumn windfall, but the constant drip-feeding of meals, snacks and sweet drinks overwhelms its ability to do such. Microbes will move in wherever there is a free lunch, and the 'unfriendlies' love to ferment sugar and carbs. Yeasts were the first microbes recognised to do such, then the bacterium *Helicobacter pylori*, but we now know there are many others. This results in a multiplicity of symptoms and diseases.

So, what happens when we eat carbs…? Table 44.1 shows the effects.

Table 44.1: The effects of eating carbohydrates

Fermentation starts and so we get:	Mechanism	Resulting in
Microbial colonisation of the mouth:	Mouth colonised with *Streptococcus mutans*, yeasts and others – see below†	Dental plaque, coated tongue, gum disease, abscesses. Tooth brushing does not prevent rotting teeth Oral cancer
		These microbes spill over into the bloodstream and drive inflammation. This is a major risk factor for arterial disease in particular
		Dental interventions which are also dangerous – see Chapter 45
		Tooth loss so food cannot be chewed or enjoyed as much
Microbial colonisation of the stomach and small intestine with production of:	Carbs are fermented to produce gases such as carbon dioxide, hydrogen sulphide, hydrogen and methane	Burping, halitosis

*Note from Craig – Perhaps we should call it *divina misce* – divine mix!

†Dr Henry Butt, consultant gastroenterologist, commented that the microbes of the mouth are far nastier than those of the rectum, in response to which I asked, 'So should we greet others by kissing their bottoms?'

	Foods are fermented to produce toxins such as D lactate, ammonia and histamine	Foggy brain, liver toxicity, worsened allergy and much more
	Bacterial endotoxin and exotoxin Fungal mycotoxins	Directly toxic and implicated in many diseases such as organ failures (renal, hepatic, cardiac); they impair energy delivery mechanisms, cause immunosuppression, are carcinogenic and much more
	Low grade inflammation...	Inflammation drives cancer – there is increased risk of stomach cancer (and we know *H pylori* alone does this[1])
	... and so leaky gut	Leaky gut results in hypochlorhydria (low stomach acid) because hydrogen ions (protons) can no longer be concentrated in the lumen of the stomach – they leak out as fast as they are pumped in
	Bacterial translocation as microbes spill over into the bloodstream[2]	This drives inflammation at distal sites, so no part of the body is spared – see all subsequent chapters for details. This is a massive subject!
The hypochlorhydria of inflammation and leaky gut causes:	Failure of the pyloric sphincter plug hole to open normally, leading to...	...in babies, pyloric stenosis requiring surgery Pain and misery, bloating and feeling full
	...stomach contents bubbling up into the oesophagus causing inflammation	Reflux, heart burn and 'hiatus hernia' Inflammation drives Barratt's oesophagus (I now have three cases of Barratt's reversed with PK diet and vitamin C)
		Inflammation also drives oesophageal cancer, now on the rapid increase
	Malabsorption of protein	So it is fermented downstream by microbes – this may produce foul-smelling farts comprised of products that may be carcinogenic
	Malabsorption of minerals	Osteoporosis (and pretty much any pathology you care to mention)
	Upper gut unable to kill new invading microbes, ergo susceptibility to infection	Drives many pathologies – see our book *The Infection Game*

Treatment of the upper fermenting gut

As I get older, my medicine becomes more simple because I know the basic things done really well get you a long way. Starve the little wretches (the microbes) out with a PK diet (no carbs for them to ferment) and kill 'em with vitamin C to bowel-tolerance (see Chapter 31: Vitamin C). And that is it. For most.

Poor quality microbiome in the large intestine

The perfect microbiome results when the baby is inoculated at the point of birth with Mother's gut flora. Of course, this must be the gut flora of one on a PK diet... and her mother before her. These microbes must then be fed with the breast milk of Mother's PK diet. Baby must be weaned onto PK foods and continue with those for life. (Thank you, Michelle (see page 76.3), for really making me think about this.)

We know just a fraction of all there is to know about the microbiome. But what we do know is that the greater the diversity of microbes, the better is our health. My guess is that the microbiome is a microcosm of the animal and plant kingdom and an extension of the microbiome in soil. Every microbe has its preferred food, flourishes when that is available and switches into a dormant state when not, ready to spring up at the next windfall. I don't think we have to know every last detail of which microbe and which food. We simply have to follow the evolutionary principles that got us here in the first place, and that greatly simplifies treatment. More importantly, these are interventions that we can all put in place. So, let us follow Nature.

> natura nihil frustra facit.
> *Nature makes nothing useless.*
> *Politics A*, 1253.a8, by Aristotle (384 – 322 BC)

Treatment

Firstly, and yet again most importantly, eat a PK diet. This is rich in prebiotic, fermentable fibre. This should be varied as different foods come available in different seasons.

Secondly, garden. Just the business of digging, planting, weeding and harvesting means you will daily ingest and inhale soil bacteria, some of which will colonise any gaps in your gut microbiome. I wash my vegetables with the same grubby little paws that I garden with.

Thirdly, eat fermented foods. My favourites are sauerkrauts and fermented coconut milk (see our book *The PK Cookbook* for details).

And that is it. For most.

Allergy

At medical school we were taught that syphilis was the great mimic, producing any pathology. This has been replaced by allergy (and other chronic infections). One can be allergic to anything: foods, pollen, chemicals, bacteria and yeast, viruses, EM radiation, even sunshine, exercise and pressure (dermagraphism). But in the gut, the main issue is allergy to foods and gut flora.

Do not trust the allergy tests. So often I see patients who have tested negative for coeliac disease and been told it is safe to eat wheat. Indeed, I never ask for allergy tests – good detective work is the key. When I first started experimenting with elimination diets, the classic diet was lamb, pears and rice. I now know that was pretty hopeless since that would make a fermenting gut much worse. In fact, when I look back at those early attempts to treat irritable bowels I am embarrassed by my ignorance and humbled by my patients' forbearance and forgiveness. I now know that the starting point for treating allergy is the PK diet as part of Groundhog Basic, moving on to Groundhog Chronic. For most, that is all they have to do.

Table 44.2: Gut symptoms and diseases, and their treatment

Chronic symptoms and/or pathology	Treatment: Groundhog regimes, in particular...	Notes
Irritable bowel syndrome, reflux, hiatus hernia, indigestion, alternating diarrhoea and constipation. Ulcer disease.	Start with the PK diet Add in vitamin C to bowel tolerance	Any recent change in bowel habit should be investigated urgently with tests for faecal occult blood and faecal calprotectin
		Do not use acid blocking drugs which increase leaky gut and all complications of such, including oesophageal and stomach cancer and osteoporosis
Constipation, diverticular disease	Ditto	Constipation is a common symptom of hypothyroidism
Inflammatory bowel disease: Crohn's	Start with the PK diet Add in vitamin C to bowel tolerance	Consider treatment for the tuberculosis-like organism called *Mycobacterium avium subsp. paratuberculosis*
Inflammatory bowel disease: ulcerative colitis	Start with the PK diet Add in vitamin C to bowel tolerance	Faecal bacteriotherapy is of proven benefit and curative

With the above understanding, we can zip through the gut symptoms and pathologies, as shown in Table 44.2.

Gall bladder disease

The medical textbooks, undoubtedly written by men, will tell you this condition affects 'fair, fat, fertile females of forty'. Cheeky sods! The alliteration[‡] skills of these medical men clearly exceed their medical knowledge.

Gall bladder disease may afflict anyone eating a Western diet. I recently saw a teenager who had been diagnosed with gallstones. The problem is a low-fat diet. Bile contains cholesterol, which has a detergent-like effect to break large globules of fat in the small intestine into smaller 'micelles'

[‡]**Footnote:** Alliteration is a very old literary device. Here we have an English translation (by Seamus Heaney) of *Beowulf* which skilfully preserves the alliteration in the original text:

'He was four times a father, this fighter prince:
one by one they entered the world,
Heorogar, Hrothgar, the good Halga
and a daughter, I have heard, who was Onela's queen,
a balm in bed to the battle-scarred Swede.'

Seamus Heaney (13 April 1939 – 30 August 2013), Irish poet and playwright, was also a translator of significant note. *Beowulf* is an Old English epic poem consisting of 3182 alliterative lines. It was written between 975 and 1025. Given its reference to the daughter, this was probably written by men too!

so that the pancreatic enzymes can rapidly digest them. If cholesterol is too concentrated, it precipitates out as sludge or stones, and this occurs with high-carb, low-fat diets.

A logical treatment to dissolve stones and flush the gall bladder is, of course, a high fat diet combined with bile acids (called bile salts). The problem is that, in the short term, fat will make the gall bladder contract and if it does so onto a jagged gallstone then this is very painful. Patients are advised to eat a low-fat diet with short-term gain, long-term pain. This will generate more gallstones.

My advice would be for larger gallstones to be removed surgically. They act as a 'nidus' (that is, 'nest' in Latin) of infection and are a risk factor for gall bladder cancer. If they escape into the bile duct this causes an extremely painful colic. If they get stuck in the common bile duct you risk pancreatitis – a really nasty condition. Once removed, it is PK diet for life to prevent recurrence.

Smaller gallstones can be dissolved with bile acids (called bile acid factors) and, being small, if dislodged into the bile ducts should pass painlessly into the gut without the above complications. Roughly speaking, you can halve their size every six months of treatment. I would recommend the PK diet, bile salts 1 gram taken with all meals and vitamin C to bowel tolerance.

Pancreatitis

Pancreatitis too has much to do with Western diets. The three major causes are:

- gallstone (see above)
- alcoholism and
- poor antioxidant status.

It may also result from a poisoning, such as with organophosphate pesticides, or from toxic metals, such as nickel. All of these are preventable with Groundhog interventions. However, pay special attention to improving antioxidant status

(see Chapter 35), with selenium being particularly important. I would recommend 500 mcg daily for at least four months to restore levels.

Until the pancreas recovers, pancreatic enzymes are essential, otherwise raw materials for healing and repair are not available, or, worse, they are fermented by microbes and this adds to the body's toxic load.

Liver disease

The liver is truly remarkable considering what it has to deal with and put up with. Personified, it really is the best woman doctor! (Except Sarah – Craig) And the physician Galen saw it as one third part of the soul, as we have read (page 42.8). All the blood that circulates and absorbs nutrients from the gut ends up in the portal vein and thence to the liver. Of course, this contains those essential nutrients, but also a toxic soup of bacterial and fungal toxins, toxic plant products, such as lectins and alkaloids, as well as many fermentation products. If this soup passed directly into the systemic bloodstream, we would be poisoned within hours. The liver does a remarkable job in mopping up sugars with its glycogen sponge, detoxifying and further breaking down these nasties. It is so busy that at rest it consumes 27% of all the energy of the body – more than the brain and heart combined.

We all know alcohol causes fatty liver and cirrhosis. It still astonishes me how much alcohol has to be consumed in time and volume to cause this. That is testimony to the liver's amazing capacity to deal with toxic stress. It also makes me more comfortable with the joy of the occasional party when, yes, I drink too much! However, the real problem now is the epidemic of non-alcoholic fatty liver disease to which the doctors are responding with, 'Oh dear, poor you, what bad luck; we must monitor this carefully,' instead of 'Get on and do the effing PK diet'. Groundhog regimes reverse and cure.

Detoxification in the liver and Gilbert's syndrome

Broadly speaking, there are two stages to the liver's detoxification process. Stage one is an oxidation reaction to make molecules a bit more active in order that stage two can take place; stage 2 involves another molecule being stuck on. This tacking on of another molecule usually renders the toxin safer and more water soluble so that it can be excreted in urine. The tacking on could be of a sugar (glucuronidation), amino acid, glutathione or sulphate group.

People with Gilbert's syndrome do not have the ability to detox with the glucuronide pathway. They are slow detoxifiers. Symptomatic of this is bilirubin; this is slowly cleared away so levels in the blood run higher than expected. Gilbert's is a probability if the bilirubin is above 19 mcmol/l. Much higher and the patient becomes mildly jaundiced. Slow detox means they are at greater risk of any condition with a toxic cause (such as paracetamol poisoning); this includes chronic fatigue syndrome and, indeed, one study showed that 90% of patients with Gilbert's complained of fatigue. I like to see bilirubin running below 10 mcmol/l.

Most sufferers will be told that this is a benign biochemical abnormality that can be ignored. I treat Gilbert's with glutathione 250 mg for life. I also warn first-degree relatives since this is a genetic condition.

Conclusion

Now that we have sorted out the gut, let's make sure we still have teeth to eat with. Dentistry is next.

References

1. 'H pylori and cancer' at the Cancer Research UK website – www.cancerresearchuk.org/about-cancer/causes-of-cancer/infections-hpv-and-cancer/h-pylori-and-cancer
2. Berg RD. Bacterial translocation from the gastrointestinal tract. *Adv Exp Med Biol* 1999; 473: 11-30. www.ncbi.nlm.nih.gov/pubmed/10659341

Chapter 45
Dentists and their tools

– possibly even more dangerous than doctors

If we all followed Groundhog principles, dentists would soon be out of a job. Most dental disease is driven by infection as a result of the fermenting mouth. Carbohydrates in the diet are fermented by microbes that hide themselves away behind dental plaque (biofilm). Every time sugars or carbs are consumed, the numbers of bacteria increase rapidly. The tongue becomes coated – yes that surface crud that you scrape off is actually colonies of bacteria and fungi. Teeth are rotted, and gums invaded by infections (gingivitis). Gingivitis is the major cause of tooth loss. Brushing teeth is pretty ineffectual against microbial attack. Fed carbs, microbes double their numbers every 20 minutes.

Dentists wield a series of dangerous tools

Fluoride
Fluorid is in water, in toothpaste and painted on to the teeth, yet if fluoride was treated by the same standards as licensed drugs, it would be banned: the toxic dose is so close to the 'therapeutic' dose. Worse, there is little evidence that fluoride is effective in preventing dental decay – indeed, despite mass medication with fluoride, the commonest emergency operation for children is dental extraction of rotten teeth. Fluoride is toxic, driving cancer and probably osteoporosis. I see patients who are allergic to fluoride. Worse, there are negative effects on thyroid function.

We have referenced fully the effects of fluoridation in water in *The Infection Game*, but by way of example, in a 2005 study, it was found that 47% of children living in a New Delhi neighbourhood with an average water fluoride level of 4.37 ppm had evidence of clinical hypothyroidism attributable to fluoride. They found borderline low FT3 (free triiodothyronine – the active form of thyroid hormone) levels among all children exposed to fluoridated water.[1]

Dental metals
Metals are used in fillings, implants, bridges and braces. Dental amalgam includes mercury, silver, tin, cadmium, lead, antimony, copper and zinc. They cause problems because:
- Foreign bodies in the mouth encourage infections because microbes can hide away inside them; this is akin to providing homes for terrorists. We have a particular problem with root canal fillings – microbes from the fermenting mouth easily slip between the gum and the tooth and can become entrenched in the root. If numbers build up suddenly, an abscess may result. However, the more pernicious issue seems to be the chronic leak age of microbes into the

Table 45.1: Dental metals and the trouble they cause

Material	Toxic?	Immuno-toxic?	Harbours microbes?	Notes
Dental amalgam (includes mercury, silver, tin, cadmium, lead, antimony copper and zinc)	Yes	Yes	No – mercury kills microbes with the same efficiency that it kills human cells	Mercury is the most toxic element known to man apart from the radioactive elements. It leaks out of amalgam from the day it is inserted. No-one should be carrying any dental amalgam or, indeed, any metals in their mouth.
Root canals	No	Possibly	Yes	Ecomed doctors have seen many cases of CFS and arthritis and autoimmunity resolve when root canals are dealt with by a knowledgeable dentist
Braces, wires, mixed metals in the mouth	Probably. When two different metals are in contact in the wet environment of the mouth, there is a 'small battery' effect which increases the release of metals into the saliva	Indirectly	No	Metals in the mouth dissolve in saliva and are swallowed. Where these is a fermenting gut, hydrogen sulphide may be produced. This may convert an insoluble inorganic metal into a soluble organic metal which is much more easily absorbed and then bio-accumulates in the body – typically in the heart, brain bone marrow and kidneys
Other dental materials e.g. palladium, titanium, gold, platinum, cobalt, stainless steel, chromium, nickel	Yes	Some people become sensitised to metals – there is potential to be allergic to any dental metal	Some	Cripes – these dentists have much to answer for! As a child my teeth were trencher filled on the grounds that 'Darling, the fillings will be stronger than your teeth.' Perhaps – but I do not wish to be the corpse with the strongest teeth in the morgue. I have had all my mercury fillings removed and replaced.

bloodstream which have the potential to drive inflammation at distal sites, especially heart disease.

- Metals are toxic. Mercury-containing dental amalgam is the worst. Mercury is immuno-toxic – that is to say, it may switch on the immune system to drive allergy and auto-immunity.
- Mixed metals in the mouth generate a small battery effect which corrodes metals. This effect may generate an electrical field with potential to disrupt normal cell-cell communication. It is biologically plausible that there may be an electrical field generated between metals in the teeth and surgical implants elsewhere in the body – which cannot be good.

The problems related to each are summarised in Table 45.1.

Since toxic metals have such potential for harm, they should be considered in the aetiology of almost any disease. With symptoms of poor energy delivery, consider tests for measuring toxicity (urine elements with DMSA). With symptoms of inflammation, consider MELISA tests for immune activation against specific metals.

So what to do now?

- It is never too late to prevent dental decay. The PK diet instantly starves microbes out of the mouth.
- Get rid of the nasty metals – find a 'mercury-free dentist' who is aware.
- If you have an inflammation-related illness, then MELISA tests are essential, so you know which metals to avoid – see Chapter 15: Poisonings.
- If metals or equivalent are necessary, choose the least toxic material that you can afford. Titanium used to be the flavour of

the month, but titanium allergy is now common. Zirconium is the current choice but that may change. Ceramic is inert but technically difficult to work with.

- For established gum infections when microbes are deep rooted you may need antibiotics to get ahead of the game.
- For acute dental abscess, antibiotics are essential to save the tooth BUT see this as an early warning sign that the PK diet and Groundhog Chronic must be instigated at once.

Cavitations

Cavitations are holes in the jaw of dead bone (osteonecrosis) which will inevitably be colonised by bacteria. They may result from dental extraction and may indicate osteoporosis of the jaw. They act as a nidus of permanent chronic infection. Groundhog interventions may keep them at bay; you may need a good dentist to clean them out well and allow new bone to reform.

Personal experience

Craig: After a Kelmer test, as recommended by Sarah in 2004, which showed very high levels of mercury, I embarked on a series of six 1.5-hour dental appointments to have all my mercury dental amalgams replaced, again as recommended by Sarah. It is without doubt one of the most successful 'single' interventions I have done, in terms of a sudden and dramatic response. I was in a very bad way with my ME at that time, having been bedridden for long periods of time. I had to rest for three months (completely) before each dental appointment and afterwards I was totally exhausted for about six weeks. Cognitively I was changed almost over night after the first replacements and this just got better with each subsequent visit. There were times before the replacements when I could only just about count to 10; this was very emotionally distressing – I studied mathematics at university and it is very dear to me – in fact, my wife, Penny, calls maths my mistress! Soon after the replacements, I found that I could begin to write out solutions to complex maths problems again.

Never ever give up!

Sarah: I was reported to the General Medical Council (GMC) by the General Dental Council because, following a series of tests that showed mercury toxicity in a patient, I recommended the patient get rid of his dental amalgam. Unfortunately, his dentist chose to do this by extracting all his teeth. Thankfully, the patient received massive compensation to allow his dentition to be restored. I kicked the GMC and GDC into touch, so advancing my then cumulative score to Myhill 23, GMC nil. It currently stands at Myhill 30, GMC nil, with one result still pending at the time of going to press. So sang Brian when nailed to the cross:

> *Always look on the bright side of life.*
> *Life of Brian*, Monty Python

Reference

1. Susheela AK, Bhatnagar MV, Mondal NK. Excess fluoride ingestion and thyroid hormone derangements in children living in Delhi, India. *Fluoride* 2005; 38(2): 98-108. www.scopus.com/record/display.uri?eid=2-s2.0-21444459765&origin=inward&txGid=144d97676dc80ae8667ac6bd9ac848b9

Chapter 46
Nephrology and urology

– it is simple in principle, difficult in practice, but within everyone's grasp to cure

Isak Dinesen, in her *Seven Gothic Tales* has one of her characters speculate thus: 'What is man, when you come to think upon him, but a minutely set, ingenious machine for turning, with infinite artfulness, the red wine of Shiraz into urine?'*

In order to perform its infinite artfulness, the kidney is an organ that is greatly demanding of energy from minute to minute. If the blood pressure (and so circulation) drops for any length of time, the kidneys will fail.

Infections of the urinary tract (UTIs)

One imagines that urine is sterile. Not so. There are always some bacteria present. These come from the gut. The gut is slightly leaky, and some microbes get into the bloodstream (called bacterial translocation – see Chapter 11), pass through the kidneys and are excreted in the urine. The pathological definition of a UTI is triggered when microbes exceed 10,000 per ml of urine. So you may have 9999 microbes per ml and be told all is well.

With a PK high-fibre diet, we have fermentation of fibre in the large bowel and these friendly microbes which translocate cause no problem. Problems arise with high-carb diets and upper fermenting gut. There is potential for unfriendly microbes to translocate into the urinary tract and, if numbers build up to a critical level, the immune system senses a potentially dangerous invader and is switched on. This gives us the nasty symptoms of pain, frequency and burning micturition.

Kidney infections must always be taken seriously. Applying Groundhog Acute (page A2.1) with bowel-tolerance doses of vitamin C (10 grams every hour until diarrhoea – see Chapter 31) may do the trick. Antibiotics may be necessary, but antibiotics alone will not address the underlying causes, so the problem simply recurs. Indeed, by failing to apply Groundhog interventions one risks interstitial cystitis.

---

*__Footnote:__ Baroness Karen Christenze von Blixen-Finecke (born Dinesen; 17 April 1885 – 7 September 1962), Danish author who wrote under her pen names Isak Dinesen, in English-speaking countries, and Tania Blixen, in German-speaking countries. Her best known work is *Out of Africa*.

Interstitial cystitis (IC)

This clinical picture arises when there is inflammation of the urinary tract. Sufferers may have all the symptoms of cystitis, but urine tests do not show infection. This is because they have become sensitised to bacteria, so inflammation starts with levels of microbes far below the 10,000 microbes per ml needed to diagnose 'infection'. Standard treatment with long-term antibiotics will never cure the problem for all the reasons above. Sufferers are left with chronic pain and infection, with eventual incontinence and probably cancer.

Interstitial cystitis is an allergy problem. In order of likelihood think:

- Allergy to microbes from the fermenting gut (yeast and/or bacteria)
- Allergy to foods
- Allergy to chemicals – one of my patients had her IC triggered by photographic chemicals used in the dark room. Another was a pathologist with IC triggered by formaldehyde embalming fluids.

Treatment is Groundhog Chronic (page A3.1), especially the PK diet and vitamin C to bowel tolerance.

Prostate problems

Prostate problems too are an inevitable part of Western diets and lifestyles. The prostate may be:

- Inflamed – this is again driven by the above allergens (microbes, foods, chemicals) and/or chronic infection, including sexually transmitted diseases
- Enlarged – this is driven by growth promot-

ers, especially dairy products and insulin (a high-carb diet again).

The PSA is a useful test because this reflects the size of the prostate. It does not tell us if the enlargement is benign or malignant. In the interim, apply Groundhog Chronic (page A3.1). I have watched the PSAs of four men and when the PK diet is stuck to, the PSA level falls, but when the diet slips it rises.[†]

Some herbs are very helpful in treating prostate cancer – two of my patients have responded well to the Pfeifer protocol.[1]

Outflow obstruction

Outflow obstruction is characterised by symptoms of hesitancy, poor stream and terminal dribbling. Problems arise because:

- the bladder does not empty well, and stagnant urine gets infected
- back pressure on the kidneys can damage them because the prostate is so enlarged.

You will need a plumber (in the shape of a urologist) to deal with the obstruction, but Groundhog interventions should prevent complications.

Kidney stones

Kidney stones occur when solutes precipitate out in urine. Most stones are calcium oxalate. They may present with renal colic, which is very painful. With luck, the stone will pass – so pee through a sieve and hopefully collect the stone for analysis; then we can ask the question, why?

[†]**Note from Craig:** Craig's late father used to belong to a group of men, all aged over 65, called 'the Prostates'. Every Friday they would have a couple of drinks at a local pub and significantly more than a couple of visits to the toilet. They all accepted that this was part of the ageing process – do not accept it, it is not inevitable! One of the Prostates was Craig's old GP.

Table 46.1: Different types of kidney stone – frequency, causes and treatment

Composition	Colour	Frequency	Cause	Treatment to prevent stone formation
Calcium oxalate	Black or dark brown	Common	Oxalate in foods Oxalate is a mycotoxin and may be a fermenting gut product Too much calcium in the diet	PK diet (especially avoid dairy) Take magnesium 500 mg (this keeps calcium in solution) Vitamin C to bowel tolerance Urine test for mycotoxins
Calcium phosphate	Dirty white	Common	Too much calcium in the diet Too much phosphate	Vitamin C to bowel tolerance – calcium dissolves readily in mild acids
Uric acid	Yellow or reddish brown	5%	Uric acid is a mycotoxin	
Magnesium ammonium phosphate	Dirty white	10%	From recurrent urine infections	Dissolves well in vitamin C
Cystine		Rare	Appear in childhood – inborn error of metabolism	

Vitamin C has a reputation for causing stones, but this has no scientific basis nor is it biologically plausible. This myth appears to come from one single case history of a woman with stones who happened also to be taking vitamin C. The last thing Big Pharma wants is a safe, cheap, effective vitamin which multitasks – fake news has been a great money spinner for the industry – and it made sure every doctor heard this story.

Vitamin C in the urine binds calcium and decreases its free form. This means less chance of calcium separating out as calcium oxalate (stones). Also, the diuretic effect of vitamin C reduces the urine concentration of oxalate – fast moving rivers deposit little silt.

Oxalate is generated by many foods in the diet, including spinach (100-200 mg oxalate per ounce of spinach), rhubarb and beets. Tea and coffee are thought to be the largest source of oxalate in the diet of many people – up to 150-300 mg/day. This is considerably more than would likely be generated by an ascorbate dose of 1000 mg/day. However, the fungal fermenting gut and airways will generate oxalate – it is a mycotoxin.[2]

Chronic renal failure

Chronic renal failure is another disease on the increase. It is characterised by leaky kidneys (protein, salt and all minerals leak into the urine) and rising levels of creatinine in the blood. Recently it has been linked directly to glyphosate (the most commonly used pesticide) and contamination of food. At medical school renal disease was a nightmare to conquer because it was defined by immunological pathologies – all of which had nasty memory-defying names. However, the causes are the same as any other organ failure.

Table 46.2: Kidney problem – causes and how to treat

Problem	Cause	Treatment
The kidney needs a lot of energy to work...	Insufficient energy	Improve energy delivery mechanisms – see Chapter 30
...which makes it susceptible to toxins	Many drugs damage the kidneys Toxic metals bioaccumulate here Mycotoxins damage Pesticides damage	See Chapter 34
The kidney is a sieve so large immune complexes get stuck in it	These arise from allergy and autoimmunity	See Chapters 36 and 51
The kidney is a sieve so microbes get stuck in it	These come from the fermenting gut	See Chapter 44
The kidney becomes leaky...	...so all minerals and proteins are lost	Replace – see below

Creatinine

Creatinine is generated from muscles and protein consumed, then excreted by the kidneys. The creatinine level is taken as a measure of kidney function, but doctors forget the first part of the equation – i.e. that muscle and protein increase creatinine levels because creatinine is a breakdown product of protein. However, they do know that reducing protein intake will reduce creatinine levels – of course it will... because less creatinine is being generated. The poor patients are told that protein is damaging the kidneys – but this is not so. High creatinine is a symptom, not a cause, of renal damage. Protein is essential for healing and repair, so a low-protein diet is not desirable. There are obvious parallels with the cholesterol story (see Chapters 42 and 58).

Diuretics

Diuretics are another of my hated drugs. They work by mimicking chronic renal failure – they induce leaky kidney so not just sodium, but all minerals, leak out. The osmotic pressure created by such pulls out water and the patient pees like a racehorse. But this is dangerous medicine because that patient loses valuable raw materials. Worse, they are told by doctors not to eat salt.

Again, doctors have muddled cause and effect. Without salt and minerals, diuretics cannot work. So, the patient ends up on escalating doses of such, needing more and more to get the same result whilst becoming increasingly depleted of essentials. The correct advice to patients prescribed diuretics is to take more salt and minerals.

The best diuretic is vitamin C. This useful effect was published in a 1937 paper[3] and ignored. Why? Follow the money. All the conditions for which diuretics are used, such as high blood pressure, heart failure, fluid retention and lymphoedema, can be safely controlled with vitamin C until the true underlying cause has been dealt with using the Groundhog interventions.

Simpson's paradox

And finally as a warning to the wise of the potential pitfalls of blindly following bare statistics, there is a famous example concerning kidney stones. Charig et al (in 1986) authored a study comparing two different treatments and their conclusions can be summarised in Table 46.3.[4]

Table 46.3: Effectiveness of alternative treatments for kidney stone depending on the size of the stone being treated[4]

Stone size	Treatment A	Treatment B
Small stones	Group 1 93% (81/87)	Group 2 87% (234/270)
Large stones	Group 3 73% (192/263)	Group 4 69% (55/80)
Both	78% (273/350)	83% (289/350)

The reader will notice that:
- The better treatment, when looking at the entire population, is Treatment B with an overall success rate of 83%, compared with Treatment A's success rate of 78%.
- However, the better treatment for both small stones and large stones is Treatment A, with respective success rates of 93% (Treatment B, 87%) and 73% (Treatment B, 69%).

This is an example of a very common problem in statistical inference – that of Simpson's[‡] Paradox. In brief, this can be described as situations where a trend appears in several different groups of data but disappears or reverses when these groups are combined. So, in the case of the kidney stones study, if one only looked at the entire population and did not identify subgroups, then one would recommend the worse treatment method to everybody. This shows

[‡]**Historical note:** Edward Hugh Simpson CB (10 December 1922 – 5 February 2019) was a British code breaker, statistician and civil servant. He worked as a cryptanalyst at Bletchley Park from 1942 to 1945. In 2017, at the age of 95, Simpson contributed two chapters on the crypt-analytic process Banburismus developed by Alan Turing. Simpson 'appeared' in episodes of *The Simpsons* and *Numb3rs*.

the importance of looking beneath the figures, identifying any subgroups, and being the master of the figures rather than letting the figures be your master! Statistics are only as good as their initial design and of the person interpreting them. Sadly for patients, these inherent deficiencies in the application of statistics are often mis-used by Big Pharma to justify sub-optimal, and sometimes even useless, treatments.

References

1. Pfeifer Protocol. 20016. www.pfeifer-protocol.com (accessed 28 November 2019)
2. Orthomolecular.org. What really causes kidney stones. *Orthomolecular Medicine News Service* February 11, 2013. http://orthomolecular.org/resources/omns/v09n05.shtml [accessed 13 November 2019]
3. Abbasy MA. The diuretic action of vitamin C. *Biochemical Journal* 1937; 31(2): 339-342. doi: 10.1042/bj0310339
4. Charig CR, Webb DR, Wickham JE. Comparison of treatment of renal calculi by open surgery, percutaneous nephrolithotomy, and extracorporeal shockwave lithotripsy. *British Medical Journal (Clinical Research Edition)* 1986; 292(6524): 879-882. www.ncbi.nlm.nih.gov/pmc/articles/PMC1339981/

Chapter 47
Rheumatology and orthopaedics

– may be hard work to sort out but pain is highly motivating!

Just as 'The Prostates' (see Chapter 46) accepted ever more frequent visits to the toilet, we are given the clear impression by doctors that pain and degeneration are an inevitable part of ageing... 'Old age does not come alone'. So many of my patients have been told, 'What do you expect? It's your age'. Nonsense! These problems are not inevitable as evidenced by a look at the historical record. Here are the opening comments of a 1974 paper by Charles L Short in *Arthritis and Rheumatism*, the official journal of the American Rheumatism Association Section of The Arthritis Foundation:

The antiquity of rheumatoid arthritis, first clearly set off as an entity by Landre-Beauvais in 1800, is of more than historic interest. If the disease is actually of relatively recent origin, an environmental cause becomes likely. It is reasonably certain that it was identified by Sydenham in 1676. But studies in human palaeopathology, while revealing unmistakable examples of ankylosing spondylitis dating back to prehistoric times, have as yet failed to provide convincing evidence of the existence of rheumatoid arthritis prior to Sydenham's description.[1]

In addition, studies of 6000-year-old Native American skeletons found few signs of arthritis, despite the joint stress of their physically active lives.[2]

The body is excellent at healing and repair – I now have three patients whose hip or knee replacement surgery has been cancelled and they are drug free and pain free as a result of Groundhog interventions, viz: PK diet, nutritional supplements, physiotherapy and quality sleep. Given the freedom from inflammation, the energy and raw materials to heal and repair, the correct hormonal environment, stimuli and time, the body will heal. This gives us the principles of treatment for all.

Treatment of inflammatory or degenerative conditions

These conditions include:
- Bones and joints: osteoarthritis and inflammatory arthritis (rheumatoid, ankylosing spondylitis, psoriatic etc)
- 'Fibromyalgia and rheumatics'
- Connective tissue with:
  o bursitis (housemaid's knee, golfer's

elbow, jeep bottom)

o   tendonitis (tennis elbow, student's elbow, frozen shoulder)

o   blood vessel involvement (small and large vessel vasculitis, including temporal arteritis)

o   nerve problems – pain syndromes, post-herpetic neuralgia (page 48.3), trigeminal neuralgia (see page 6.4)

o   skin problems – premature ageing, systemic lupus erythematosus (SLE), systemic sclerosis or scleroderma.

In order of importance, the steps to follow are:

* Do not suppress symptoms with drugs
* Look for the cause of the inflammation
* Consume the raw materials for healing and repair
* Provide the energy to heal and repair
* Do the right sort of exercise
* Ensure the right hormonal environment.

Do not suppress symptoms with drugs

Pain is a vital symptom that tells us what is possible and allows us to safely use our bodies. Worse, many drugs used in rheumatology inhibit healing and repair and this accelerates the underlying pathology. Studies of patients receiving NSAIDs (non-steroidal anti-inflammatory drugs) for their hip arthritis showed that they needed surgery sooner than those who did not receive NSAIDs.[3] This paper in the *Journal of Prolotherapy* (2010) concluded: 'For those using NSAIDs compared to the patients who do not use them, joint replacements occur earlier and more quickly and frequently.'

Look for the cause of the inflammation (see Chapter 16)

Dr Honor Anthony, my friend, mentor and cancer researcher, suffered from arthritis. I recall her stating in 1985, 'All arthritis is allergy'. At the time I thought that could not be right. I now know she was spot on – if not allergy to foods then 'allergy'* to other incitants (substances that incite allergic responses). Dr John Mansfield described a patient with osteoarthritis of the hip due to house-dust mite allergy, cured with desensitising injections. Dairy products are a major cause of allergic muscles. I now know allergy, or an inflammatory process that I call allergy, drives much arthritis.

Such allergies may include:

* Allergy to microbes that spill over from the gut into the bloodstream. I suspect they get stuck in scar tissue (from historical damage – and we all have that) where they drive inflammation (as the immune system tries to get rid of them). Indeed, the Danish surgeon Hanne Albert sees success using antibiotics to treat osteoarthritic modic type 1 changes in the spine.[4] We know ankylosing spondylitis is driven by klebsiella bacteria and rheumatoid arthritis by proteus, both of which reside in the gut.[5, 6]
* Allergy to metals – consider this possibility if pain starts following surgery in which metals are used. This can be tested for using MELISA tests available through Biolab.

My view is the 'distinction' made between degenerative and inflammatory arthritis is almost irrelevant to intelligent treatment – good results are achieved with the same basic approach. We know arthritis is an inevitable part of metabolic syndrome, partly because sugar is

---

*__Footnote:__ I am using the word 'allergy' to describe a number of possible mechanisms, which include direct allergy to incitants, molecular mimicry which may extend to autoimmunity, low grade infection and probably other mechanisms yet to be discovered.

directly pro-inflammatory and partly because it encourages microbial overgrowth in the gut and body.

Consume the raw materials for healing and repair (see Chapter 35)

Take the basic package of supplements (page 79.1). If you have the time, make and drink bone broth. Bone-building supplements, such as glucosamine, silica and boron, are of proven benefit. Do not take high-dose calcium. Magnesium is just as important. Calcium and magnesium are absorbed by the same mechanism and so high doses of calcium inhibit magnesium absorption. Dairy products are a risk factor for osteoporosis. The key is vitamin D, which improves absorption of calcium and magnesium from the gut and ensures its deposition in bone.

Provide the energy to heal and repair (see Chapter 30)

I have seen cases of arthritis heal when hypothyroidism has been properly treated. Again, this illustrates the point that the immune system is responsible for healing and needs much energy to do so. I think this mechanism explains why niacinamide (vitamin B3) is of proven benefit – it improves mitochondrial function and therefore energy delivery. Quality sleep is also essential since this is when much repair goes on.

Do the right sort of exercise (see Chapter 23)

Healing and repair are directed by lines of force. A problem for astronauts is the lack of gravity – their bones and connective tissues literally melt away as the healing and repair grinds to a halt. This illustrates the point that the body is constantly building and breaking down, which makes perfect evolutionary sense – the body only allows sufficient energy for healing and repair as

to meet demand; anything more and precious resources are wasted. Use it, or lose it!

Ensure the right hormonal environment

The natural balance of building (anabolism) and breaking down (catabolism) is controlled by steroid hormones, one of which is vitamin D. As we age our adrenal function declines and with that our anabolic hormones. Taking adrenal glandulars and testicular glandulars (yes – even women can do this safely) may well help. Do not take HRT.

Polymyalgia rheumatica (PMR)

We are seeing epidemics of PMR. This condition is characterised by marked muscle stiffness, aching and pain which is much worse in the mornings and improves as the day goes on. Blood tests often show high inflammatory markers (erythrocyte sedimentation rate (ESR), C-reactive protein (CRP), or plasma viscosity), but these may be normal. PMR responds so quickly and reliably to steroids that if there is clinical suspicion, I think one is justified in using this diagnostically. The sufferer feels cured in a day or two! But then we have to work out the root cause and this has to be done in parallel with a slow reduction in the dose of steroids – not so fast as to allow the pro-inflammatory fire to blaze up again, but as quickly as possible to prevent steroid damage. We have to put the immune system in a straitjacket (see Chapter 36). The patient needs to be in charge of this process since symptoms determine the rate.

Allergic muscles and cramp

Both allergic muscles and cramp are extremely painful. Indeed, muscle pain is one of the most severe pains that one can experience. Labour pains[†] are, of course, muscle pains. Biliary colic and renal colic are also muscle pains – ask any sufferer how bad the pain is.

The diagnosis of allergic muscles and cramps is made more difficult because we often see delayed reactions, starting 24, or 48 hours, after allergen exposure and lasting for several days. Muscles can react in only one way, which is with contraction, and this can vary from a low-grade cramp to muscle tics or jumping, to acute lancinating pain so severe that the sufferer literally collapses. Typically, this just lasts a few seconds or minutes. One moment agony, the next moment fine. The sufferer appears to be a right old hypochondriac! I have never seen a rheumatologist diagnose allergic muscles because he never asks the question why. The mechanism is as above – tissue damage with bruising followed by sensitisation, commonly to dairy products. Pain is triggered by stretching the affected muscle. Initially, any stretch will cause it; then, as things settle down, only a sudden stretch will cause it. The sufferer protects him/herself from the pain by moving slowly. Other muscles in the vicinity of the allergic muscles may also go into spasm to protect against sudden inadvertent stretching and this causes a more generalised muscle spasm and stiffness.

Gentle regular exercise, such as walking, may be helpful and indeed some patients find that they have to exercise very intensely and very regularly to keep the problem at bay (if the allergen has not been recognised). Heat, a hot bath, and gentle massage help to relax the muscle in the short term, but the first movement after these interventions has to be done carefully or the spasm will be triggered. Diazepam affords some relief because, I suspect, it makes the irritable, allergic muscle less twitchy. I have two patients with 'stiff man syndrome' who have been much improved by identifying and desensitising to allergens (dairy products and metal allergy in their case).

Cramp, restless legs, jerking muscles, twitching muscles, tics

These may be part of the above allergic muscle problem. Alternatively, they may arise from dehydration. To hydrate the body needs not just water but also salt (to hold water within the cells), fat (to waterproof and provide a semi-permeable membrane) and heat (to power the fourth phase of water (see page 17.2)). Between layers of tissues I suspect magnesium is vital to enhance the friction-reducing effects of the fourth phase of water.[7]

Pinched nerves including sciatica, carpal tunnel syndrome, spondylosis, scoliosis

I suspect these conditions are too often ascribed to impingements of bone and wrongly treated as a result. Actually, the body is extremely good at reshaping bone, as I discovered myself.

[†]**Historical note:** The Romans had some interesting cures for labour pains: mothers to be were encouraged to partake of a drink, which had been powdered with sow's dung and fumes from hyena loin fat 'to bring forth an easy delivery'. Maybe this was more distraction technique than actual relief? (Sarah: This did not work for me. Nothing did!)

[‡]**Historical note:** Jacques Jean Lhermitte (20 January 1877 – 24 January 1959) was a French neurologist who studied spinal injuries during World War I, cementing his interest in neurology and leading to a later interest in neuropsychiatry. He has (at least) eight medically relevant eponyms bearing his name. Readers interested in eponymously named diseases are directed to https://en.wikipedia.org/wiki/List_of_eponymously_named_diseases. It is of note that only a few diseases are named after patients. Sometimes diseases or syndromes are named after fictional characters, such as 'Havisham syndrome', named after Miss Havisham, of Charlies Dickens's *Great Expectations* to describe a behavioural disorder usually observed in the elderly, characterised by gross self-neglect, and a lack of self-consciousness about personal habits.

I experienced what is known as 'Lhermitte's[‡] phenomenon' after the first occasion of breaking my neck, when I fractured all seven cervical vertebrae. If I flexed my neck, I felt a massive sensation of pins and needles down the whole of my body because of pinching of the spinal cord. I refused surgery and this symptom disappeared after four months.

Pinched nerves may result from allergic muscles or tissue swelling with oedema due to:

- Hypothyroidism – see Chapters 5, 13 and 30
- Inflammation from allergy or chronic infection – see above plus Chapter 16 and our book *The Infection Game*
- Mercury poisoning (perhaps any metal allergy). Mercury in particular accumulates in intervertebral discs. Scoliosis can be effectively treated with detox to get rid of toxic metals, combined with physiotherapy. (See the work of Rebecca ('Becky') Dutton who linked scoliosis in children to mercury in vaccinations.)
- Poor hydration – of course this depends on water, but also minerals, fat and warmth. Remember the fourth phase of water demands heat to hold water in its frictionless graphite configuration.
- Mechanical damage followed by poor quality healing and repair. See Chapter 35 for treatment, especially vitamin D 10,000 iu, niacinamide 1500 mg, boron 20 mg, organic silica 200 mg
- Poor posture – consult a physiotherapist or osteopath.

Craig was diagnosed with sciatica from his right buttock down his right leg. He experienced a recurring sharp shooting pain that had originally started when he had suddenly pulled the muscle, and after that it just seemed to keep on coming back... coming back, that is, until he became strict with the PK diet, since when he has had no reccurrences. The triggering allergen must have been a food type that he longer eats.

Osteoporosis

Osteoporosis is now accepted as an inevitable part of ageing but this is nonsense. It is entirely preventable and treatable (see Chapter 38). Dairy products increase the risk of osteoporosis because the proportion of calcium (Ca) to magnesium (Mg) is high[§] and this inhibits Mg absorption and its deposition in bone. One can solve this simply with adequate doses of vitamin D (at least 5000 iu daily) which improves absorption of calcium and magnesium from the diet and their natural assimilation in bone. The joke is that Ca and vitamin D are first-line NHS prescriptions for osteoporosis, and these make the problem worse for two reasons – they contain no Mg and the dose of vitamin D is far too low (800 iu) to have any significant effect. But this is good news for Big Pharma because the next line of management is their expensive bone builders – great work! Lifelong treatments make lots of money and lots of side effects,

However, an excellent treatment is strontium 250-500 mg daily. This is of proven value in reducing fracture rates and increasing bone density.[8, 9, 10, 11, 12, 13] Again, problems arise with prescribed strontium which uses an unnatural salt, namely the ranelate, and is made up with aspartame – which explains the risk of thromboembolism when Big Pharma strontium is used. Natural strontium chloride or citrate work well with no side effects.

Finally, monitor the response to treatment using heel ultrasound to measure bone density. This is accurate and involves no radiation.

[§]**Footnote:** The ratio of Ca to Mg in dairy products is 10:1, whereas our physiological requirements are for 2:1 – that is, two parts Ca to one part Mg.

Crystal arthropathies: gout, pseudogout and possibly others

Crystal arthropathies are extremely painful and result when crystals deposit out in the joints. Although gout can be prevented with drugs to reduce levels of uric acid in the blood, this really is symptom suppression. Uric acid is a useful antioxidant in the bloodstream. I subscribe to Costantini's theory that gout is a result of fungal infection, with the production of mycotoxins.[14]

One can diagnose a mycotoxin problem by measuring the level of such mycotoxins in urine.

Costantini points out that fungi produce uric acid and that most anti-gout drugs are also antifungal. We know metabolic syndrome is the major risk factor for gout because fungi can only ferment carbohydrates. The treatment of course is to get rid of the source of the fungal infections with Groundhog Acute interventions. Essentially, vitamin C to bowel tolerance is a good way of reducing fungi in the gut and the salt pipe with iodine is effective in clearing fungi from the upper and lower respiratory tract.

Fractures

Clearly professional help is needed in all cases, but the principles for treatment are RICE, which is to say:

- **REST** – immobilise and protect the fracture site by wrapping with a generous wad of cotton wool and then bandage firmly. This simple intervention greatly reduces pain.
- **ICE** – cooling the fracture site reduces bleeding and bruising.
- **COMPRESSION** – as above
- **ELEVATION** – again to reduce bruising.

Do not use painkillers because these inhibit healing and repair. The right amount of pain allows one to mobilise at the correct rate – that is, do what you can within pain limits since the lines of force generated in the process of such guide the laying down of new bone and connective tissue. These rules have allowed me to recover from fractures of the neck (on three occasion), and several other fractures: leg, collar bone, scapular, ribs, finger and possibly others. I have no residual pain.

Conclusion

- Do not suppress symptoms with drugs. Pain is painful in order to motivate one to make the difficult changes necessary to get rid of it.
- Use your brain to work out the cause and have the determination to see it through.

References

1. Short CL. The antiquity of rheumatoid arthritis. *Arthritis and Rheumatism* 1974; 17(3): 193-205.
2. [Smithsonian] What a 6,000-Year-Old Knee Can Teach Us About Arthritis. https://www.smithsonianmag.com/smart-news/knee-arthritis-old-problem-s-much-more-common-today-180964529/
3. Hauser RA. The Acceleration of Articular Cartilage Degeneration in Osteoarthritis by Nonsteroidal Anti-inflammatory Drugs. *Journal of Prolotherapy* 2010; (2)1: 305-322. http://journalofprolotherapy.com/the-acceleration-of-articular-cartilage-degeneration-in-osteoarthritis-by-nonsteroidal-anti-inflammatory-drugs/
4. Albert H, et al. Antibiotic treatment in patients with chronic low back pain and vertebral bone edema (Modic type 1 changes): a double-blind randomized clinical controlled trial of efficacy. *Eur Spine J* 2013; 22(4): 697–707. www.ncbi.nlm.nih.gov/pmc/articles/PMC3631045/
5. Rashid T, et al. The Link between Ankylosing Spondylitis, Crohn's Disease, Klebsiella, and Starch Consumption. *Clin Dev Immunol* 2013; 2013: 872632. www.ncbi.nlm.nih.gov/pmc/articles/PMC3678459/

6. Ebringer A, et al. Rheumatoid Arthritis is an Autoimmune Disease Triggered by Proteus. *Clin Dev Immunol* 2006; 13(1): 41–48. www.ncbi. nlm.nih.gov/pmc/articles/PMC2270745/

7. Pollack G. *Fourth Phase of Water: Beyond Solid, Liquid & Vapor.* www.amazon.co.uk/ Fourth-Phase-Water-Beyond-Liquid/ dp/0962689548

8. McCaslin FE Jr, Janes JM. The effect of strontium lactate in the treatment of osteoporosis. *Proc Staff Meetings Mayo Clin* 1959; 34: 329-334.

9. Marie PJ, Hott M. Short term effects of fluoride and strontium on bone formation and resorption in the mouse. *Metabolism* 1986; 35: 547-551.

10. Gaby AR. *Preventing and reversing osteoporosis.* Prima Publishing, Rocklin, CA, 1994.

11. Marie PJ, Skoryna SC, Pivon RJ, Chabot G, Glorieux FH, Stara JF. Histomorphometry of bone changes in stable strontium therapy. In: Hrmphill [spelling?] DD (Ed). *Trace substances in environmental health XIX</ital>).* University of Missouri, Columbia, Missouri, 1985, 193-208.

12. Meunier PJ, Slosman DO, Delmas PD, Sebert JL, et al. Strontium ranelate: dose-dependent effects in establishing postmenopausal vertebral osteoporosis – a 2-year randomized placebo con-trolled trial. *J Clin Endocrinol Metab* 2002; 87(5): 2060-2066.

13. Meunier PJ, Roux C, Seeman E, Ortolani S, et al. The effects of strontium ranelate on the risk of vertebral fracture in women with postmeno-pausal osteoporosis. *N Engl J Med* 2004; 350(5): 459-468.

14. Costantini AV. Fungal bionics – a new concept of the aetiology of gout and hyperuricaemia. *Pediatric Research* 1988; 24: 15. www.nature. com/articles/pr1988417

Chapter 48
Dermatology

Dermatology has been described as the art of finding a Latin name and then prescribing an antibiotic steroid cream. Again, patients are reassured that they have a 'diagnosis' when of course eczema, dermatitis, psoriasis, lichen planus, ichthyosis and acne are clinical pictures, not diagnoses. Eczema is further broken down into discoid, atopic, dyshidrotic, nummular, seborrhoeic, stasis, venous and other such. Again, this is astrology, not astronomy. The real crime is the unthinking use of steroid creams and ointments. We know these make psoriasis worse. They inhibit the healing and repair of the immune system and so the skin thins and ages prematurely.

I now know that very many skin lesions are driven by allergy and infection. As you will have now realised, there is a continuum, with overt infection on the left, allergy on the right and a mix in the middle which I describe as allergy to microbes. So, for example, impetigo is a pure staphylococcal driven skin infection, while some eczemas clear completely with the elimination of dairy products (pure allergy), but many are a halfway house of allergy to microbes with, staphlococci and fungi being the commonest offenders. This is why Groundhog interventions are so effective in treating so many skin conditions. Acne is a disease of Westerners – it does not exist in primitive societies. (See our book *The Infection Game* and below for more on this point.)

Cuts, grazes, wounds, burns, spots, active eczema and other skin breaches

Clean any breaches of the skin as best you can, ideally with copious amounts of Lugol's iodine (approximately 10 ml of Lugol's 15% in 500 ml of water) to physically washout any dirt or other such contaminants. If you are caught out in the wild, then peeing over and scrubbing the wound works well too – urine is near sterile. If there is any hint of foreign bodies, such as splinters, gravel or ingrained dirt, then surgical treatment may be necessary – wounds never heal if there are foreign bodies present.

Allow the wound to dry. Once dry, smother it with iodine oil (see Chapter 32 for the recipe); you can see the yellow stain of iodine – keep it yellow!

Keep the wound dressed until the skin heals over to prevent further contamination.

Superficial pathology

Use iodine oil to treat all skin conditions and superficial pathology such as:
- Bacterial infection: infected spots, boils and abscesses, including styes (eyelash infection), paronychia (nailbed infection), im-

petigo, erysipelas, folliculitis (hair follicles), pilonidal sinus, ischiorectal (bum) abscess and other nasty inflamed lumps. Also nail infections, ear infections.

- Viral infections: chicken pox, cold sores, genital herpes, orf, warts, verrucas, molluscom contagiosum (sounds like another Harry Potter spell – but in this case the magic cure is iodine).
- Fungal infections: cradlecap, skin fungal infections: tinea, ringworm, athlete's foot, dhobi itch, jock rot, gym itch, scrot rot, pityriasis.
- If you are not sure what the lesion is, you can do no harm with iodine.

At the first sign of any abscess or boil, apply Groundhog Acute together with topical iodine oil ad lib or, even better, pure Lugol's iodine 15%. This alone may get rid of the problem.

If the infection is around your eyes or nose, then take this very seriously – there is potential for the infection to spread back into the brain and cause a cavernous sinus thrombosis. Antibiotics are essential protection against this nasty possibility.

However, once a boil is maturing avoid antibiotics. If they are effective, then the boil will stop growing and you will be left with a permanent lump, an 'antibiotic-oma' which may cause problems in the future. Instead, poultice or hot-bathe the boil to draw it to a head and discharge. There is nothing more satisfying than to see the gungy contents expelled, with instant relief.

Cellulitis

Cellulitis is a potentially lethal extension of the above. If a local infection has not been adequately dealt with, then a red line will be seen streaking up to the local lymph node, which will swell to a painful hot lump as it fights the infection. This is a prelude to septicaemia and must always be taken seriously. In addition to applying all the above and Groundhog Acute, systemic antibiotics are essential, possibly even intravenous. Urgent and professional attention is necessary.

Acne

Acne is a miserable affliction that scars the life of sufferers when they are at their most vulnerable. It afflicts up to 95% of adolescents in Western societies.[1] By contrast, in a study of 1200 Kitavan* subjects examined (including 300 aged 15-25 years), no case of acne (grade 1 with multiple comedones or grades 2-4) was observed. Of 115 Aché subjects examined (including 15 aged 15-25 years) over 843 days, no case of active acne (grades 1-4) was observed.

This tells us that Western diets and lifestyles are to blame and explains why the PK diet is highly effective. From my experience I know there are at least two causes of acne – carbohydrates (probably mediated by the fermenting gut) and allergy to dairy products. Groundhog Basic is highly effective at curing acne. Of course, I am applying this to that age of patient least willing to take advice from an old crone like me. I

*Footnote: Kitava is one of the four major islands in the Trobriand Islands archipelago group of the Solomon Sea, located in Milne Bay Province of south eastern Papua New Guinea. The Kitavan diet is uninfluenced by modern Western diet and comprises an abundance of foods that have a low glycaemic index rating. There is also practically no diabetes, cardiovascular disease leading to stroke or congestive heart failure, dementia or high blood pressure among native Kitavans. The Aché are an indigenous people of Paraguay; they are hunter-gatherers.

have a rule of thumb that I can do very little to help those between the age of 14 and 24 because they already know all there is to know about Life.

> *I am not young enough to know everything.*
> *The Admirable Crichton*, JM Barrie, and Oscar Wilde – attribution uncertain (JM Barrie: 9 May 1860 – 19 June 1937; Oscar Wilde: 16 October 1854 – 30 November 1900)

However, vanity is a powerful motivating influence and I have a few notable successes in persuasion. Most importantly, do not use RoAccutane (isotretinoin). It is a major risk factor for suicide. I have one patient who has suffered constant severe headaches since taking a short course in 1999 (see Chapter 58).

Body odour (BO)

Sweat has almost no smell. It is simply blood but without the large bits like cells and proteins. It does contain sugar, and the higher the blood sugar the more sugar there is in sweat. This provides a free lunch for microbes on the skin. They love moist conditions and so thrive in armpits, tits and other naughty bits.

If your microbes ferment this sugar to something that smells nasty, then you too will smell nasty. BO is part of the metabolic syndrome of Westerners eating carbohydrate-based diets. Treatment of course is Groundhog Basic, perhaps combined with topical iodine.

To illustrate the above point, there have been interesting experiments done to change the offending microbes. The sufferer has plastered his smelly areas with antiseptics to kill the indigenous flora. He has then received a sweaty donation, ideally from a non-stinking family member, and thereby recolonised offending departments. The problem has been greatly relieved. The prospect

of this procedure has provided useful clinical leverage for those reluctant to fully embrace Groundhog…

If you need to be further persuaded, consider this. The conventional treatment is to use deodorant. This works because it contains aluminium, which kills all microbes. Unfortunately, it also kills humans – aluminium is well absorbed through the skin and causes Alzheimer's. It may contribute to the development of breast cancer and may explain why cancers are more common in the upper outer quadrant of the breast.[2]

Shingles (varicella zoster virus, human herpes virus 3 or HHV3) (see Chapter 49: Neurology)

Shingles is not really a skin infection but an infection of the nerves which manifest with a nasty rash. It is caused by the chicken pox virus. One has to have had prior infection with chicken pox. This explains why you can catch chicken pox from someone with shingles, but not the other way around. The virus then lives in the spinal cord and comes to life if the body's defences go down. Indeed, when I see shingles in any person I wonder why – is there an underlying nasty, such as a tumour?

Not only is shingles very painful, but there is also a risk of a long-standing post-herpetic neuralgia (I think of this as viral allergy). Post-herpetic neuralgia affects nerve fibres and the skin, causing burning pain that lasts long after the rash and blisters of shingles have disappeared. Shingles must be treated aggressively. In order of priority:

- Groundhog Acute (page A2.1)
- Smother with iodine oil (see Chapter 32) ad lib so the area is constantly stained yellow, and
- Take anti-virals such as acyclovir 800 mg x 5 daily until the rash has healed. This may mean a few weeks of treatment. But this

is important in order to reduce the risk of post-herpetic neuralgia.

Varicose (or venous) ulcers

Typically, these present in older people, initially with thin and discoloured skin, sometimes associated with varicose veins and thread veins, over the shin and ankle. The skin breaks down and refuses to heal. I think there are at least three strands to the treatment of venous ulcers.

1. Pooling of blood in the legs. When the primitive ape stood up this made him a better hunter. He could run down his prey and have arms available to hurl stones and spears. But, after years of being vertical, it brought certain disadvantages – poor drainage of the sinus cavities, a tendency to groin hernias, a tendency to incontinence and a high-pressure system in the lower half of the body with potential to cause piles and varicose veins. This high-pressure system is partly responsible for varicose ulcers. Venous blood pools and toxins are not cleared. Venous return can be massively improved by graduated pressure tights – the idea here is that the compression must be greatest in the toe and foot and least at the top of the leg. With any exercise, the venous blood is massaged away, and this prevents stagnation. The fit of the stocking must be perfect; obviously if it is tighter at the top than the bottom the situation will be made worse. Get yourself a pair of tights from daylong.co.uk. If you are sitting down, then your legs must be up (ideally at the level of the heart so the venous pressure in the legs is almost zero – a recliner chair is a great start). If you are not sitting down, then wear tights and move.

2. Allergy to microbes from the fermenting gut. Before the skin breaks down the pre-ulcer skin shows all the hallmarks of inflammation.

3. Chronic infection. As soon as skin is breached, the microbes move in and make themselves at home. They find a warm free lunch of sugar and moisture.

Once the mechanism of damage is clear, treatment follows logically. In order of priority:

- Groundhog (for the fermenting gut)
- Graduated pressure stockings, recliner chair and exercise.
- Treat open ulcers as above for all skin breaches – topical iodine for starters. Antibiotics may be needed to get ahead of the game.
- Continue with Groundhog for life – otherwise the problem will simply recur for the same reasons that it arose in the first place.

Finally, be mindful that if the ulcer is not healing despite doing all the above, then it should be biopsied – sometimes there is malignant change.

Multi-resistant *Staphylococcus aureus* (MRSA)

This microbe is a particular problem in hospitals where there are open wounds. Hospitals create a perfect storm where none of the Groundhog imperatives are in place and antibiotics are heavily used. This is an ideal habitat for growing antibiotic-resistant strains of microbe. Sick patients are fed junk food diets, high in sugar and refined carbohydrate. Vitamin supplements are often forbidden. Relatives are encouraged to bring in fruit, though fruit is a bag of sugar and feeds microbes. These disastrous conditions occur just when the need for a healthy diet and lifestyle is greatest. Hospitals are dangerous places to be.

In hospital, emphasis is on prevention. If you

find yourself stuck in hospital, do not permit anyone to touch your wound without first seeing them either wash their hands or don surgical gloves. Do your best to apply Groundhog. After I broke my neck and was stuck in a neurosurgical unit, I was saved from starvation (the hospital 'food' was inedible) by my lovely daughter who appeared with good food, supplements and water.

Lichen planus, lichen sclerosus, lichen striatus, lichen aureus, lichen nitidus

'Lichen' simply means thickening of the skin, which may occur due to friction. But these conditions are very often driven by fungal infection and Groundhog interventions combined with iodine work really well.

Morgellon's syndrome

This syndrome is a lovely example of how doctors blame patients when they do not know the cause of a condition. For years patients were accused of 'dermatological hypochondriasis with delusional behaviour'. There is good evidence that the ghastly itching of Morgellon's is similar to lice – it is an insect infestation. It should be treated as such. There are no easy answers here but some have been cured with ivermectin. I would combine this with topical iodine oil and possibly antibiotics because it is highly likely there will be secondary infection with bacteria.

Skin cancer

The relatively benign and common basal cell carcinoma (rodent ulcer) and the squamous type

Both basal cell carcinoma and squamous type are driven by inflammation which may be from skin burnt by sunshine or chronic infection. Diagnosed and treated early they never kill. An excellent and effective herbal treatment accessible to all is curaderm. Its developer, Dr Cham, points out that the membranes of cancer cells differ from those of normal cells and this makes them susceptible to attack from solacidine glycosides in eggplant (aubergine) extract. The idea is that solacidine gets into the malignant cells and dissolves the membranes of its lysosomes, which rupture to release digestive enzymes which digest and dissolve the lump. Normal cells are unaffected. This makes it a joy to use because one cannot go wrong. Even if the diagnosis is wrong, no damage ensues.

However, be mindful that 100% cures never happen and if you have a recurrence or a non-responder you must consult about surgical removal.

The uncommon and dangerous malignant melanoma

Contrary to popular belief, malignant melanoma is not caused by sunshine. If it were it would have the same distribution as the common cancers of the skin. It does not. Melanomas can appear anywhere on the body. We need a high index of suspicion to ensure early and effective medical and surgical treatment. Look for any change in size, shape, colour, consistency or thickness. Look for irregularity of shape or colour. With any associated symptoms, such as itch, bleed, redness or inflammation, you must act. Treated early gives a 99% cure; late gives a less than 10% cure.

Conclusion

Throughout time, the skin has been seen as a potent symbol of beauty. The English playwright and poet, Christopher Marlowe (baptised 26

February 1564 – died 30 May 1593) wrote of Helen of Troy's face that:

> *Was this the face that launch'd a thousand ships,*
> *And burnt the topless towers of Ilium?*
> *Sweet Helen, make me immortal with a kiss.*
> *Her lips suck forth my soul: see where it flies!*
> *Come, Helen, come, give me my soul again.*
> *Here will I dwell, for heaven is in these lips.*

Hopefully, this chapter has shown that the face, and the skin, are not just things of beauty but also that infections can gain entry to the body here and that disease lurks there too and that one must be alert to one's δέρμα (derma, or skin), and treat any problems accordingly.

References

1. Cordain L, Lindeberg S, Hurtado M, Hill K, Eaton SB, Brand-Miller J. Acne vulgaris: a disease of Western civilization. *Arch Dermatol* 2002; 138(12): 1584-1590. www.ncbi.nlm.nih.gov/pubmed/12472346
2. Darbre PD. Aluminium, antiperspirants and breast cancer. *J Inorg Biochem* 2005; 99(9): 1912-1919. www.ncbi.nlm.nih.gov/pubmed/16045991

Chapter 49
Neurology*

Remember that ATP (see page 5.1) multitasks. It is not just the energy molecule, but is also a neurotransmitter in its own right. To be precise, it is a co-transmitter – neurotransmitters such as dopamine, GABA, serotonin and acetylcholine do not work unless ATP is present. These neurotransmitters are needed for good neurological function. Improving energy delivery mechanisms is the starting point to treat all neurological, psychiatric and psychological disease.

Table 49.1: Neurological symptoms, mechanisms and treatments

Symptom or clinical picture	Mechanism – ALWAYS poor energy delivery	Treatment – Groundhog Chronic, especially energy delivery mechanisms (Chapter 30) and especially the paleo-ketogenic (PK) diet
Migraine and chronic headaches (see below)	Allergy to foods, to chemicals Poor energy delivery	PK diet
Any psychological or psychiatric symptom Autism, behavioural disorders	See Chapter 50 – one cannot separate neurology from psychiatry; I suspect the mechanisms are age sensitive	Psychiatry – see Chapter 50 Autism – see Chapter 56: Paediatrics
	Poor energy delivery	PK diet

*Linguistic note: 'Neuron' (and thereby 'neurology') is directly from the Greek νεῦρον (neûron, 'nerve'), originally meaning 'sinew, tendon, cord, or bowstring'. It is interesting how sometimes the original meanings of words 'show themselves' in how we use them in their modern context. For example, in terms of 'nervous disorders', we often refer to a person as being 'highly strung', harking back to the original 'bowstring' meaning of neuron, and we talk of people feeling 'tense', just as a bowstring might be tense.

Symptom or clinical picture	Mechanism – ALWAYS poor energy delivery	Treatment – Groundhog Chronic, especially energy delivery mechanisms (Chapter 30) and especially the paleo-ketogenic (PK) diet
Foggy brain, poor short-term memory, slow cognitive skills eventually progressing to... Dementia (see below)	Poor energy delivery mechanisms	Improve energy delivery – see Chapter 30, especially PK diet and hypothyroidism
	...including small strokes and TIAs that may go unnoticed	See below
	Inflammation due to infection (e.g. syphilis, Lyme), allergy, autoimmunity	See Chapters 16 and 36
	Poisoning due to addiction, toxic metals, pesticides, VOCs Deficiencies of vitamins	Chapters 8 for symptoms of toxicity and deficiency Chapter 25 for how to reduce the toxic burden Chapter 34 for tools for detoxing
	Prions	See prion disease below
		AND see dementia below
Epilepsy and fits	Head injury and other post traumatic injuries with scarring	See epilepsy and fits below PK diet Magnesium
	All the above	
Tourette's[†] – this bridges psychiatry and neurology with symptoms in both camps. I see this as a form of epilepsy	Ditto	Ditto See epilepsy below
Strokes and TIAs	Thrombosis of the arterial wall Embolus Bleeds	See stroke and TIAs below
Alzheimer's,[†] Parkinson's,[†1] motor neurone disease, multisystem atrophy, Huntington's chorea*	Prion disorders	See Chapter 18 and below

Multiple sclerosis	Prion disorder driven by fungi and mycotoxins Often poor antioxidant status	Groundhog Chronic Urine test for mycotoxins See Chapter 36
Pain syndromes e.g. Tic doloreaux, post-herpetic neuralgia, 'allergic nerves'	Allergy to microbes	See below – Chronic pain syndromes Topical iodine oil ad lib – see Chapter 32: Iodine Vitamin C to bowel tolerance
Movement disorders e.g. Tourette's		
Brain tumours	Vaccination Electromagnetic radiation (mobile phones)	See Chapter 53: Oncology PK diet Vitamin C to bowel tolerance

Migraine

There are several threads to migraine:

- Allergy – We know food can cause migraine and this is usually clinically obvious. I suspect part of the mechanism is allergic muscles in the scalp which would explain why migraine affects one side of the head at a time.
- Poor blood supply to the brain – Indeed, this may be so impaired as to cause neurological deficit such as hemiplegia. A patent foramen ovale (a hole in the heart that fails to close naturally during fetal development) is a recognised trigger of hemiplegic migraine. Constricted allergic blood vessels may also impair the blood supply to the brain. Vasoactive amines also narrow the arteries; these may be present in red wine and aged cheeses. More reason to go PK!
- Poor energy delivery – Many factors to do with energy delivery may trigger a migraine,

†**Footnote**: Tourette's syndrome, Alzheimer's disease, Parkinson's disease and Huntington's‡ chorea are all further examples of eponymous diseases, named after physicians – see Chapter 47. James Parkinson (11 April 1755 – 21 December 1824), like many of his time, was a polymath, having interests not only in surgery but also in apothecary, geology, palaeontology and political activism. He was also adept at shorthand and insisted that all surgeons should learn it well so that they could take full medical histories quickly. In addition to the eponymous disease, his name is remembered in several fossil organisms, for example the ammonite *Parkinsonia parkinsoni*, the crinoid *Apiocrinus parkinsoni*, the snail *Rostellaria parkinsoni*, and the tree *Nipadites parkinsoni*.

‡**Footnote**: Returning to eponymous diseases, before we move onto psychiatry there is room enough to remember one of the other physicians after whom a disease is named – Huntington's disease, or Huntington's chorea. George Huntington (9 April 1850 – 3 March 1916) was an American physician and his father and grandfather were also physicians in the same family practice; their combined longitudinal observations described the hereditary disease bearing his name across multiple generations of a family in East Hampton on Long Island. Sir William Osler said of the paper in which Huntington described the illness that: 'In the history of medicine, there are few instances in which a disease has been more accurately, more graphically or more briefly described.'[9] You can decide for yourself – the paper is reproduced on Wikisource and in the *Journal of Neuropsychiatry and Clinical Neurosciences* as a 'Classic Article'.[9]

such as low blood sugar (in the non-keto-adapted), missing sleep or exhaustion. Migraines may occur as part of a stress response (the symptom the brain gives us when it knows it does not have the energy to deal with demand)

- Poisoning – Mycotoxins are a known cause of migraine – see Chapter 8.

Intravenous magnesium instantly relieves the pain of migraine, and associated symptoms, in all cases. It multitasks as a vasodilator, muscle re-laxant and improves energy delivery through its effect on mitochondria.[1] Indeed, when I worked in general practice intravenous magnesium was my favourite emergency drug for treating acute chest pain, acute asthma attacks, thrombotic strokes and, of course, migraine (see Chapter 58).

I suspect Mark Twain suffered from migraine and his were severe:

> *Do not undervalue the headache. While it is as its sharpest it seems a bad investment; but when relief begins, the unexpired remainder is worth four dollars a minute.*

Dementia

Many use the words 'dementia' and 'Alzheimer's' interchangeably to mean the same thing. This is muddled thinking, again. Dementia is the symptom, Alzheimer's a pathological diagnosis indicating a prion disorder. See below for the treatment of prion disorders.

Dementia responds fantastically well to Groundhog Chronic. We know this from the work of consultant neurologist Dale Bredesen who reverses dementia with such a regime. As noted before, in Chapter 21, Dr Dale Bredesen has published twice in this area to show what can be achieved.[2, 3] In practice, this rarely happens because Groundhog is so difficult, and carers do not want to withhold the patient's 'only pleasure'

– that is, their addiction. Even highly intelligent people, exhibiting the early stages of dementia as a symptom, find fantastically complex rationali-sations for their addiction with the most recent I heard being:

> *I was five in 1940 when food rationing started and 19 when the last items, meat and bacon, came off ration. During most of that time it would have been impossible to satisfy an appetite largely on protein. Indeed, it would have been downright anti-social to try. To this day my immediate reaction to egg and bacon would be to reach for bread to fill up. As my daughter would say, 'You can take a boy out of the 1940s, but you can't take the 1940s out of the man.'*

Ayn Rand, Russian-American writer and philosopher (2 February 1905 – 6 March 1982) summed up this thought process as: 'Rationalization is a process of not perceiving reality, but of attempting to make reality fit one's emotions.' (From *Philosophy: Who Needs It?*)

Strokes and TIAs (transient ischaemic attacks)

Strokes and TIAs result from the same mechanisms; the only difference is the outcome, with strokes causing permanent neurological damage. If anything should be a wake-up call to do Groundhog interventions, then it is surely this. You are just a brain, and a stroke is as serious as a personality change or amputation. Do not be reassured by doctors telling you that a few pills will prevent a future catastrophic fatal stroke.

It is vital to diagnose the mechanism early through urgent high-tech scans because early ef-fective treatment is life changing. Altogether 85% of strokes result from blood clots, which may be:

- local thrombosis of an artery

- distal thrombosis of an artery (for example, triggered by an atherosclerotic plaque in the arteries of the neck)
- embolus from a clot having formed in the heart (typically in atrial fibrillation)
- embolus from a leg vein which has slipped through a patent foramen ovale (hole in the heart – actually this is common) so bypassing the lungs.

Alternatively, a stroke may be the result of a bleed into the brain. This may result from:
- subarachnoid haemorrhage (which is extremely painful – it feels like a hammer blow to the back of the head)
- bleeding from an arterio-venous malformation
- over-treatment with blood thinners (warfarin, heparin, aspirin and NSAIDs, anticoagulants, apixaban and other 'abans')

Where there has been a clot, treatment should be with clot busters such as injected altiprase. The sooner this is given the better; after 4.5 hours it is too late. One could also use bolus magnesium sulphate: 4-10ml of 50% magnesium sulphate injected slowly over 2-3 minutes. Dr Sam Browne, an NHS GP, detailed how this would reverse symptoms of a stroke within minutes.[4]

(I recall a long conversation with a dear friend who was fearful of an end of life as a hemiplegic. Because we both knew that the chances of timely clot-busting therapy in practical reality was virtually zero, she decided that in the event of a stroke she would wish for intravenous magnesium. That would mean either the stroke would reverse, or she would rapidly die. I too would make that choice.)

If there is a bleeding stroke, then vitamin K should be injected, and the patient referred urgently to a neurosurgeon.

In both cases, hyperbaric oxygen (oxygen under pressure) is essential, but in practice rarely available. Only oxygen under pressure will increase the oxygen-carrying capacity of the blood, which helps to reduce the volume of tissue that is damaged.

Epilepsy and fits

I think of these as electrical storms of the brain. They are always dangerous and 'sudden unexplained adult death in epilepsy' (SUDEP) a risk. I suspect SUDEP is similar to 'sudden adult death' (SAD) syndrome. Almost certainly both result from cardiac arrest, but why?

Calcium is needed for heart muscle to contract and pump blood into the arteries, magnesium for it to relax and refill. SUDEP and SAD are both associated with extra energy expenditure – SUDEP as the body is convulsing, SAD with intense exercise. For example, the Great Northern Run of 2005 saw four participants die of SAD within 55 minutes. Conditions were especially hot. Intensive exercise is demanding of magnesium as well as inducing magnesium loss (in sweat and urine). Acute magnesium deficiency would mean the heart would be unable to relax to fill with blood and it would stop beating. Within minutes of death, magnesium would leak out of cells and so a magnesium deficiency would not be apparent at post mortem. The true diagnosis is then not made.

Magnesium is a great treatment for epilepsy. This is well established in the treatment of pre-eclampsia where oral magnesium prevents fits and intravenous magnesium cures an acute attack (see Chapter 55). It is also a great treatment for status epilepticus and works when all drug therapy has failed. For more see 'The Role of Magnesium in Neurological Disorders' by Kirkland et al for a discussion of magnesium and its efficacy for epilepsy and other neurological conditions, and also the World Health Organization's 'Recommendations for Prevention and Treatment of Pre-Eclampsia and Eclampsia'[5, 6]

Before drugs were available, the ketogenic diet was *the* treatment for epilepsy. It remains the best treatment. The mechanism by which a ketogenic diet works has several strands. It improves energy delivery to the brain, it reduces brain damage from oxygen free radicals and increases GABA – gamma aminobutyric acid, one of the 'happy' neurotransmitters. Because the diet is difficult, and as we know doctors do not like to ask patients to do difficult things (probably because they are worse addicts and cannot do them themselves), it has gone out of fashion. Worse than that, doctors actively discourage the ketogenic diet. One mother's battle to cure her epileptic son became the subject of a film, *First do no harm* starring Meryl Streep (my favourite actress).

An important source on this is Kim and Rho's 2008 paper, 'The ketogenic diet and epilepsy', which concluded that: 'While the mechanisms underlying the broad clinical efficacy of the ketogenic diet remain unclear, there is growing evidence that the ketogenic diet alters the fundamental biochemistry of neurons in a manner that not only inhibits neuronal hyperexcitability but also induces a protective effect. Thus, the ketogenic diet may ultimately be useful in the treatment of a variety of neurological disorders.'[7] See also the paper 'Ketogenic diet for treatment of epilepsy' by Rogovik and Goldman, 2010.[8]

Doctors forget to remind patients that the anti-epileptic drugs have nasty side effects – for example, they are highly damaging to the unborn baby. They have so many side effects that they have to be remembered by a mnemonic that goes from the A of ataxia to the H of hepatitis… and more.

Shingles (varicella zoster virus, human herpes virus 3 or HHV3)

This is dealt with in Chapter 48: Dermatology (page 48.1).

Chronic pain syndrome

This is one of the laughable 'diagnoses' dreamt up by doctors who do not think causation. It is as risible a diagnosis as chronic fatigue syndrome. Craig and I look forward to hearing about the 'chronic feeling ill syndrome'! We may not know the cause of pain for sure but at least let's come up with a biologically plausible mechanism that can be put to the test by the intelligent and determined patient. Pain is highly motivating. Simply the fact that it usually starts with an acute pain gives us a clue to causation. Much is microbe driven inflammation so in addition to Groundhog Chronic go back to Chapter 36 for the tools for damping down inflammation and reprogramming the immune system.

Prion disorders

As detailed in Chapter 18, there are well-recognised toxic and infectious associates – go through the check list in Table 49.1 and consider:

- tests for toxicity (see Chapter 15: Toxic metals, pesticides, VOCs and mycotoxins), and
- tests for chronic infection (see Appendix 5 from *The Infection Game*).

Table 49.2: Neurological diseases, their associated prions and causes

Disease	Which prion	Associated with:
Alzheimer's disease	Amyloid beta protein	Aluminium toxicity (as, for example, in dialysis dementia) See link below
		Mercury toxicity e.g. the Mad Hatter in *Alice in Wonderland*
		Borrelia (Lyme disease), toxoplasmosis, herpes virus 1 (cold sores), herpes virus 2 (genital herpes), cytomegalovirus, cryptococcus, cystercercosis, mycoplasma, syphilis, HIV. Creutzfeld-Jacob disease (CJD) (the infectious particle is uncertain), possibly *Helicobacter pylori* and *Chlamydia pneumoniae*, fungal infection
Parkinson's disease	Alpha synuclein	Manganese poisoning (miners in South Africa)
		Organophosphate pesticides
		Helicobacter pylori, borrelia, mycoplasma, Erhlichia, anaplasma
Motor neurone disease	SOD1 (copper-zinc superoxide dismutase – antioxidant enzyme)	Manganese poisoning
		...and cycad (a natural toxin from beans); 10% of the deaths on the island of Guam were due to MND from cycad
		Poliovirus, retrovirus, mycoplasma, borrelia, HHV6
Multisystem atrophy	A variant of alpha synuclein	Pesticide exposure, especially organophosphates (remember glyphosate, the most used pesticide today, is also an organophosphate)
Creutzfeld-Jacob disease (CJD)	PrPSc (scrapie isoform of the prion protein)	Organophosphate pesticides
		Manganese poisoning
	Innoculation with PrPSc	Blood transfusion or surgery Theoretically through vaccination
Familial fatal insomnia	PRNP (prion protein)	Genetic mutation that runs in families. Thankfully very rare

Having done your best to diagnose what is going on, we then have to deal with the loss of tissues. In the future, stem cell therapy will be the way forward. In any event, should you have any symptoms or other pathology, put in place Groundhog Chronic. At the very least I would expect this to slow disease progression until stem cell therapy becomes available.

References

1. Demirkaya S, Vural O, Dora B, Topcuoglu MA. Efficacy of IV magnesium in acute migraine attacks. *Headache* 2001; 4(2): 171-177. www.ncbi.nlm.nih.gov/pubmed/11251702

2. Bredesen DE.Reversal of cognitive decline: A novel therapeutic program. *Aging (Albany NY)* 2014; 6(9): 707–717. www.ncbi.nlm.nih.gov/pmc/articles/PMC4221920/ and

3. Bredesen DE. Reversal of cognitive decline in Alzheimer's disease. *Aging (Albany NY)* 2016; 8(6): 1250–1258. www.ncbi.nlm.nih.gov/pmc/articles/PMC4931830/

4. The Case for Intravenous Magnesium Treatment of Arterial Disease in General Practice: Review of 34 Years of Experience' *Journal of Nutritional Medicine* (1994) 4, 169-177 http://www.mgwater.com/browne01.shtml

5. Kirkland AE, Sarlo GL, Holton KF. The Role of Magnesium in Neurological Disorders. *Nutrients* 2018; 10(6): 730. doi: 10.3390/nu10060730 www.ncbi.nlm.nih.gov/pmc/articles/PMC6024559/#B114-nutrients-10-00730

6. Chapter 4: Evidence and recommendations (Section 31: Magnesium). In: WHO Recommendations for Prevention and Treatment of Pre-Eclampsia and Eclampsia. World Health Organization, Geneva, 2011. www.ncbi.nlm.nih.gov/books/NBK140560/#_ch4_s31_

7. Kim DY, Rho JM. The ketogenic diet and epilepsy. *Curr Opin Clin Nutr Metab Care* 2008; 11(2): 113-120. doi: 10.1097/MCO.0b013e3282f44c06. www.ncbi.nlm.nih.gov/pubmed/18301085

8. Rogovik AL, Goldman RD. Ketogenic diet for treatment of epilepsy. *Can Fam Physician* 2010; 56(6): 540–542. www.ncbi.nlm.nih.gov/pmc/articles/PMC2902940/

9. Huntington G. On chorea. *The Medical and Surgical Reporter* 1872; 26(15); 317-321. https://en.wikisource.org/wiki/On_Chorea and https://neuro.psychiatryonline.org/doi/full/10.1176/jnp.15.1.109

Chapter 50
Psychiatry

Only once or twice has Craig thought of a good riposte 'at the time', rather than some five or six hours later, as is the way for most of us. One such time was when he was being assessed for a course of psychiatric treatment for his ME, back in 1994. He was rejected for the trials (phew!) and perhaps this conversation goes some way to explain that rejection:

Psychiatrist: So, do you have any interests?

Craig: Yes, I quite like unexplained events, the X-Files, Forteana and so on.

Psychiatrist: Hmmmm… interesting… A man who likes unexplained events and who suffers from an unexplained illness…

Craig: Hmmmm… interesting… A psychiatrist with delusional thought patterns….

The brain is like a computer – it is comprised of software and hardware. Psychotherapy *may* be very skilful at dealing with the former, but the psychiatrists, who should know better, ignore the latter. There are several elephants in the room detailed below, but let us first linger on how modern psychiatry is practised so you can see that it has no logic and no scientific basis.

How modern psychiatry is practised

Psychiatrists make 'diagnoses' based on lists of symptoms. They join them together randomly and as a result, the psychiatrists' bible, *The Diagnostic and Statistical Manual of Mental Disorders IV*, lists 297 possible 'diagnoses' made up of different groups of symptoms. This is akin to the ancients looking at the night sky and making shapes like the Great Bear or Orion. All those symptom stars give us lots of lovely constellations but this cannot be described as science. And guess what? Big Pharma has ensured that every star sign has a drug with which one can treat that picture. This is Astrology. Should one of my patients develop a psychiatric condition, then I want them treated by Astronomy – in other words, a proper science-based approach. 'Ho, ho!' I can hear these astrologists cry, 'We are working with a scientific model – it is all about neurotransmitters. The depressed patients need more of the happy ones and we can do that with drugs.' But there is not a scrap, let me repeat, not one scrap of evidence to support this notion.

The interested reader should, by way of example, see the paper by Lacasse and Leo, 'Serotonin and depression: A disconnect between the advertisements and the scientific literature',[1] which states that: 'With direct proof of serotonin deficiency in any mental disorder lacking...' And this paper is by no means the most hard-hitting of those disputing the 'psychiatric model'.

I am no expert in psychiatry, but I can at least postulate biologically plausible mechanisms for symptoms which result in treatment regimens that are completely safe and, as importantly, put the patient in control of their symptoms. Once they understand the physical mechanisms that are resulting in such mental pain, they are well motivated to do the regimes. With the new-found energy that results, they are better able to be helped by psychologists who can detail techniques to reprogram the software.

With the full understanding and co-operation of willing patients, together with close monitoring, I know these regimes are highly effective. (Sigh... by making these heretical statements I can feel another attack from the General Medical Council coming on.) So, what are the important mechanisms which underpin much of psychiatry?

The mechanisms underpinning psychiatric disease

In order of importance, these mechanisms are:
1. Addiction and symptom suppression
2. The fermenting brain
3. Poor energy delivery mechanisms
4. The raw materials for the brain to function
5. Chronic infection
6. Toxicity
7. Immunotoxicity
8. Prion disorders.

1. Addiction and symptom suppression

In the short term, addiction masks symptoms. We all use them all the time. Coffee and tea to wake up and get going; alcohol to chill out. Used occasionally in modest doses they are good servants. Psychiatric disease results when these servants become masters. As detailed, addiction gives us the false impression of endless energy. That is why cocaine is such a great party animal. Endless energy is reflected in our face which becomes lit up and sexually attractive. We have the energy to dance all night, the jokes are funnier, our conversation is quick witted and hilarious as the ideas flow. Sometimes the energy expenditure is so excessive that disaster results. When a drug death is reported, I never hear the mechanism of such. But I suspect the imbiber has unknowingly and unsuspectingly slipped into energy deficit and suddenly the body does not have the energy for life, and so death ensues.

The psychiatric patient exhibits all the symptoms of addiction withdrawal (and others – see below) – namely, lethargy and low mood expressed with a dull, miserable, 'unattractive'* face. Eye contact is lost. Behaviour becomes anti-social, confidence melts away and hypochondria, avoidance of exercise and introversion result. The depressed, anxious patient is the 'party pooper' to continue with the analogy above.

It never fails to amaze me how psychiatrists have picked up on some chapters of the addiction story but are oblivious to others. Any young person attending casualty with an acute psychosis will, as a routine, be tested for drugs with the commonest offenders being cannabis, amphetamine, cocaine, LSD, alcohol and ecstasy. On the

*Footnote: Once again, I am using the adjectives 'attractive' and 'unattractive' as described in Chapter 5. 'Party pooper' may seem 'glib' words to describe anxiety and depression, but remember that 'pooped out' is an expression that most likely derives from 19th century sailors to indicate how they felt, and what happened, when they were caught unawares on the poop or aft deck of a ship when a wave crashed down and washed over them. These sailors were overwhelmed and often lost at sea.

few visits I have made to psychiatric wards, the patients are constantly self-medicating with addictions. Commonly these are sweet drinks, biscuits, chocolate, caffeine and, if the opportunity presents, nicotine. Any escapees are characterised by an excursion to the off-licence. These patients are not weak-willed because they know not what they do – they are suffering terribly and going for the temporary relief they reliably achieve. Whilst the obvious links to 'illegal highs' have been made, the greatest addiction of all has yet to be fully recognised. Sugar (and carbs that are rapidly digested to sugar) is cheap, socially acceptable, widely available (indeed, difficult to avoid) and horribly convenient. Some of the worst addicts are fruitaholics, and fructose, metabolically speaking, is worse than the white stuff.

There are some glimmers of hope in the scientific literature – for example, see the paper by Avena et al, 'Evidence for sugar addiction: Behavioral and neurochemical effects of intermittent, excessive sugar intake'[2] which concludes that: 'The evidence supports the hypothesis that under certain circumstances rats can become sugar dependent. This may translate to some human conditions as suggested by the literature on eating disorders and obesity.'

Most psychiatric treatments are of the addictive symptom-suppression type, which simply increase the addictive load with a (perhaps slightly less toxic) drug dependency. All have potential nasty side effects. Although marketed as not being habit forming, SSRIs are addictive. They also cause acute suicidal ideation. Benzodiazepines slow reaction times, which makes for accidents;

major tranquillisers induce metabolic syndrome and premature death. But perhaps the most pernicious aspect of psychiatric prescriptions is that patients are misled into believing that the root cause of their disease is being treated. When it becomes apparent that they are addicted to the prescription drug, they understandably conclude that they are mad and are no longer in control and cannot help themselves. Dependency on others and loss of confidence and personality follow – what has come to be known as 'gaslighting'.[†]

2. The fermenting brain

We know that microbes easily get from the gut into the bloodstream to drive pathology at distal sites and these include the brain. Work by Nishihara[3] suggests that where there is a fermenting gut there may also be a fermenting brain. There is potential, and this is biologically plausible, that neurotransmitters in the brain may be fermented into LSD-, amphetamine– and cocaine-like molecules. This may explain why the ketogenic diet has such a great record of success in treating psychosis. Any such benefits may be further enhanced by attention to the fermenting gut.

3. Poor energy delivery mechanisms

AGAIN, remember that ATP (see page 5.1) multitasks. It is not just the energy molecule; it is also a neurotransmitter in its own right. To be precise, it is a co-transmitter – neurotransmitters such as dopamine, GABA, serotonin and acetylcholine do not work unless ATP is present.

[†]**Linguistic note**: The term 'gaslighting' is used to describe the psychological manipulation of someone into doubting their own sanity, and the use of these prescription drugs is a clear example of this. The term derives from the film *Gaslight*, a 1944 American film, adapted from Patrick Hamilton's 1938 play *Gas Light*, about a woman whose husband manipulates her into believing that she is going insane. Patrick Hamilton (17 March 1904 – 23 September 1962) was an English playwright and novelist. A gifted man, Hamilton succumbed to addictions himself – he started to consume alcohol excessively whilst a young man and as a result of this life-long addiction, he died of cirrhosis of the liver and kidney failure.

Improving energy delivery is also the starting point for all neurological and psychological disease.

Drs Carl Pfeifer and Abram Hoffer pioneered the nutritional treatment of psychosis with ketogenic diets and high doses of vitamin C. This of course addresses both the above issues of carbohydrates as an addiction and the fermenting gut-brain link – carbs and sugars are removed from the diet and vitamin C kills the bugs causing the fermentation. A further effective tool was the use of high-dose niacinamide (vitamin B3, 3 to 10 grams daily, the dose being individually titrated). I was interested to hear this because this is the commonest deficiency I see in my chronic fatigue patients where there is poor mitochondrial function. It would make perfect sense that improving energy delivery mechanisms to the brain would benefit a range of symptoms characterised by poor energy. Similarly, a great treatment for depression is high-dose vitamin B12 by injection – for example, 5 mg (that is, 5000 mcg) daily. Indeed, this treatment is so effective that any patient with bipolar mood disorder (i.e. a tendency to go 'high') must be warned to stop using B12 injections at the first hint of their mood going up.[4]

Thyroid disease may present with psychiatric illness, but this is rarely recognised by the psychiatrists who ignore the hardware and invariably look to a symptom suppressing software approach. Hyperthyroidism may present with psychosis, hypothyroidism with myxoedema madness. If energy delivery to the brain is slow, then this manifests at first with foggy brain but progresses eventually to dementia. Dr Richard Asher[‡] was able to discharge many patients from psychiatric hospitals simply by starting them on thyroid hormones.[5]

4. The raw materials for the brain to function

These obviously come from the diet but also the microbiome. Indeed, all neurotransmitters can be found in the gut, many being the product of fermentation by friendly bacteria in the large bowel. For example, we know that *E coli* can ferment tryptophan (an amino acid present in meat) to serotonin. Tryptophan 8 to 12 grams daily is of proven effectiveness in the treatment of depression. Of course, this is far too cheap and safe for Big Pharma which has effectively sidelined this natural antidepressant (see The Prozac story, page 58.5).

5. Chronic infection

The best known infectious cause of psychiatric disease is syphilis. Tertiary syphilis progresses to 'general paralysis of the insane' (GPI). I remember reading a wonderful case history of an 80-year-old woman who suddenly started to behave without the normal social inhibitions, dressing wildly and flirting outrageously. She was diagnosed with tertiary syphilis but refused treatment because she was enjoying herself too much. I made the terrible mistake of telling my daughters that a sign of secondary syphilis was a saddle-shaped nose as the nasal bones collapsed. The trouble was every time we met a new person the girls would sidle round for a profile view to see if they could diagnose!

We are currently seeing epidemics of a different treponemal infection – namely, Lyme disease. This too may present with psychiatric symptoms or dementia. Many microbes can access the brain and an infectious cause should always be considered (see Appendix 5 in our book *The Infection Game*).

[‡]**Historical note**: Dr Richard Asher (3 April 1912 – 25 April 1969) married Margaret Augusta Eliot and his father-in-law gave him a complete set of the *Oxford English Dictionary* as a wedding gift. This gift was allegedly the reason for Asher's reputation as a medical etymologist.

6. Toxicity

See Chapters 15 and 34 for the what, why and how to get rid of pesticides, volatile organic compounds (VOCs), toxic metals and mycotoxins. Organophosphate pesticides induce acute suicidal ideation. The Countess of Mar described how she found herself wanting to drive her Landrover off the side of a hill following sheep dipping.

7. Immunotoxicity

We are seeing epidemics of young people and children who are not living up to their full intellectual genetic potential. Clinical pictures include autism, Asperger's, attention deficit disorder, dyslexia, dyspraxia, hyperactivity and other such. This will be multifactorial, but vaccination is a big player; see Chapter 51 for the why and Chapter 56: Paediatrics.

8. Prion disorders

Prion disoders may also present with psychiatric symptoms – see Chapter 49: Neurology.

Treatment

The important point to grasp here is that psychiatric disease has a physical (hardware) dimension that is almost invariably overlooked. Thankfully the tools of the trade to deal with this are within the grasp of us all. It really does not matter what the clinical picture is – depression, psychosis, bipolar, anxiety – the approach to treatment is the same and in order of priority is set out in Table 50.1.

Treatments for specific psychiatric diagnoses

Depression

Do all the above. Tryptophan 10 grams daily is a great treatment for depression as it is fermented into serotonin by friendly *E coli* in the gut. See Chapter 58 for why this is not routine practice.

Vitamin B12 by injection – see Chapter 33.

Post-traumatic stress disorder (PTSD)

Life is inevitably stressful, and we all have skeletons in the cupboard. During sleep we relive the events of the day and remember the important things and rationalise the damaging memories. But if sleep is disturbed by adrenalin, then those memories are relived in a hormonally stressful environment, thereby reinforcing them. This is an obvious vicious cycle. The treatment is obvious too – stop adrenalin release at night with the PK diet, thereby blocking any damaging memories that may be lurking. In addition, this can be done with a beta blocker, such as propranolol (take care with asthmatics). Indeed, this intervention is of proven benefit.

Sadly, I hear that 13% of children currently suffer from PTSD. I suspect this has become so much more common because of high-carb diets with adrenalin spiking at night that compounds any psychological distress.

Table 50.1: The tools of the trade for reversing psychiatric illness

Groundhog Chronic	To improve energy delivery mechanisms: supply the raw materials for normal brain function special attention to the thyroid and to sleep and to mitochondrial function
Abolish all addictions	With time you may be able to do a 'deal with the devil'. Make addictions your servant, not your master. I use caffeine and alcohol in this way
Treat the fermenting brain	By treating the fermenting gut – PK diet and vitamin C to bowel tolerance
Look for toxic causes	Pesticides Volatile organic compounds (glue sniffers) Toxic metals (the Mad Hatter from *Alice in Wonderland*) Porphyria (the madness of King George III) Mycotoxins – see Chapter 8. Easily diagnosed with a urine test – see Chapter 15
Identify chronic infections which may need specific antimicrobials to deal with them	Psychosis has been long associated with acute infection. The microbes known to cause psychiatric disease include syphilis (general paralysis of the insane), Lyme disease, HIV and other retro viruses, Epstein-Barr virus (EBV – with exposure under the age of 4 years), herpes simplex and genital herpes. Herpes viruses, including EBV, may have a role. I can see no biologically plausible reason why many other microbes may not be implicated. If all the above interventions did not result in resolution then I would wish to do the full gamut of tests for infectious disease – see Appendix 5 and *The Infection Game*
Look for mycotoxins	Moulds contaminating foods ferment to produce LSD (bread baking). Moulds from other sources may contribute to the total toxic load

Conclusion

Not only is the practice of psychiatry mediaeval in its diagnosis, it is similarly primitive in many of its treatments. The symptom-supressing chemical straitjacket is the norm. Barbaric treatments have included insulin coma therapy, metrazole-induced seizures, lobotomies and ECT (electro-convulsive shock therapy). The logic and biological plausibility of these treatments continue to elude me.

References

1. Lacasse JR, Leo J. Serotonin and depression: A disconnect between the advertisements and the scientific literature. *PLoS Med* 2005; 2(12): e392. www.ncbi.nlm.nih.gov/pmc/articles/PMC1277931/
2. Avena N, et al. Evidence for sugar addiction: Behavioral and neurochemical effects of intermittent, excessive sugar intake. *Neurosci Biobehav Rev* 2008; 32(1): 20–39. www.ncbi.nlm.nih.gov/pmc/articles/PMC2235907/
3. Nishihara K. Disclosure of the major causes of mental illness—mitochondrial deterioration in brain neurons via opportunistic infection. www.drmyhill.co.uk/drmyhill/images/d/dc/NISHIHARA.pdf
4. Hoffer A. Psychosis cured with vitamin therapy: Nutrition protocols and case histories of Dr A Hoffer. www.doctoryourself.com/hoffer_psychosis.html
5. Asher R. Myxoedematous madness. *Br Med J* 1949; 2(4627): 555–562. www.ncbi.nlm.nih.gov/pmc/articles/PMC2051123/

Chapter 51
Immunology

– allergy and autoimmunity
– the problems of vaccination

One in 20 Westerners now has an autoimmune condition (which amounts to a self-destructive civil war). In fact in the USA, this figure rises to one in 15.[1] Benaroya Research conclude that 5 million American men and 18 million American women have autoimmune disease.

Allergy UK estimates that 44% of British adults have at least one allergy (when the immune system attacks the benign and harmless outsider). Both autoimmunity and allergy present with symptoms of inflammation (Chapter 7).[2]

Principles of treatment for allergy and autoimmunity

Having one allergy and/or an autoimmune condition greatly increases the risk of others. Furthermore, both these conditions run in families. Since the commonest triggers for both are acute infection, vaccination and silicone, you must avoid these. Allergy and autoimmunity are much easier to switch on than to switch off, and so awareness and prevention are vital.

So, the overall strategy is:
- Groundhog Chronic (Appendix 3)
- Groundhog Acute (Appendix 2) at the first sign of any infection. (Stock your first aid box now and include a copy of our book *The Infection Game*)
- Live in as unpolluted an environment as possible, avoiding moulds and chemicals
- Be wary of any dental, surgical or cosmetic interventions that require metals or silicones – these are good at switching on the immune system. (This syndrome is called ASIA – autoimmune syndrome induced by adjuvants)
- Choose your holidays wisely to avoid vaccination and do not be blackmailed into the flu vaccination.

Table 51.1: Specific autoimmune diseases and their treatments

Common autoimmune conditions	Probable triggers	The tools of the trade for treatment are detailed in Chapter 36, but especially vital are:
Thyroid problems: Hashimoto's Hypothyroidism Graves' disease Hyperthyroidism	Viral infection Vaccination, especially hepatitis B Metals, especially lead, aluminium, mercury	See Chapter 41: Endocrinology
Rheumatoid arthritis	Allergy to gut microbes	PK diet and vitamin C to bowel tolerance
Systemic lupus erythematosus ('lupus')	Probably viral – EBV	PK diet and vitamin C to bowel tolerance
Ulcerative colitis	Allergy to foods Major gut dysbiosis	PK diet and vitamin C to bowel tolerance Consider faecal bacteriotherapy
Crohn's disease	Allergy to food Chronic infection with *Mycobacterium avium paratuberculosis*	PK diet and vitamin C to bowel tolerance Long-term antibiotics
Multiple sclerosis (MS)	Viral infection (EBV) Toxic metals, especially mercury Moulds and mycotoxins Poor antioxidant status	PK diet and vitamin C to bowel tolerance Measure and get rid Measure and get rid Quench the inflammatory fire (see Chapter 36) High dose vitamin B12 by injection, e.g. 5 mg daily often helpful
Type 1 diabetes mellitus	The main risk factors are vaccination, vitamin D deficiency and consumption of dairy products	PK diet (see our book *Prevent and Cure Diabetes*) Insulin
Autoimmune Addison's disease (adrenal atrophy)	Viral infection Vaccination	See Chapter 41: Endocrinology

Since there are about 200 cell types in the body and 20 types of cell organelle, there is potential for 220 different autoimmune diseases. But the principles of management are the same.

What do immunologists do?

I think immunologists rate amongst the most dangerous of doctors because they wield tools with so much potential for harm. These tools are:

Immunosuppressives

Vaccinations

Immunosuppressives

In suppressing the immune system, we know not what we do. The immune system and the brain are functionally indistinguishable. Both are sensitive and responsive, process information in a way that involves memory and intelligent decision-making, and then react appropriately. The immune system too has a hardware component which constitutes the body's army. White cells make up the officers and foot soldiers. Both wield weapons such as antibodies and cytokines. There is an elaborate 'software' system of communication involving hormones, prostaglandins, interferons, leucotrienes, eicosanoids, cytokines, chemokines and much more. Like the brain, all functions are intricate, delicate and complicated. Drug suppression of the immune system inevitably leads to early death and disease by degeneration or cancer. Immune suppression is like treating the inflamed brain with a club – yes, you knock it out but cause terrible damage in the process.

Immunologists try to classify autoimmune and allergic diseases by mechanism. We have the unimaginative titles of 'type I, 2, 3 and 4 allergy' or 'hypersensitivity reactions'. These are irrelevant to clinical practice other than to select a drug to fit. These drugs include steroids, methotrexate (and other anticancer drugs), gold, hydroxychloroquine, azothiaprine, NSAIDs, rituximab and other 'imabs', cyclosporin and mycophenylate (which are both mycotoxins). This completely misses the important intellectual point of causation. This drug approach crushes the messenger. Again, we are smothering the flames but not extinguishing the fire. When the drugs are stopped, disease flares (that is, if the immune system has the energy to do such).

Vaccinations

It is a fact, little short of astonishing, that the effectiveness of vaccination is unproven. When vaccinations were introduced, rates of infectious disease were already falling thanks to Victorian engineers, better nutrition, warmer homes and good hygiene. Vaccines had no impact on this rate of decline. Indeed, recent studies have shown that vaccines increase death rates in children. Furthermore, febrile illnesses (illnesses that include fever) of childhood protect against later disease, including brain tumours and autoimmunity. Fevers in childhood represent an essential part of programming the immune software. I think of this as training the army to tolerate the local rebels and renegades. We can use good nursing care (warmth, rest, love, hydrating fluids) together with vitamin C and iodine to ensure that the renegades never prevail – that is to say, we can safely allow our children to experience the normal infections of childhood without risk of serious complications. Bring back the chicken pox parties!

> *All truth passes through three stages.*
> *First, it is ridiculed. Second, it is violently*
> *opposed. Third, it is accepted as being self-*
> *evident.*
>
> Arthur Schopenhauer, German
> philosopher (1788 – 1860)

Thankfully, with vaccination we are, at last, on the cusp of stage three. We know that this is biologically plausible for the following reasons:

1. Vaccinationals are immunotoxic
2. Adjuvants used are toxic in their own right
3. Most vaccinations are administered by injection
4. Viral vaccines must be 'grown' on animal tissue
5. Preservatives in vaccines are directly toxic

1. Vaccinations are immunotoxic

The immune system is intelligent. It will, quite rightly too, ignore an injection of dead microbes.

Vaccinations only elicit an immune reaction if what is called an 'immune adjuvant' is included. Essentially, this is a wake-up call to the immune system to put it on red alert. The intention of vaccination is for the immune system to react solely to the viral or bacterial antigens contained within the vaccination and so stimulate immunity. But adjuvants may wake up the immune system inappropriately, with the potential to switch on allergies and/or auto-immunity. Indeed, we know that MMR, hepatitis B vaccination, influenza, DPT, typhoid and others all switch on allergic reactions, such as reactive arthritis, erythema nodosum, urticaria and vasculitis, as well as autoimmune disease, such as rheumatoid arthritis, systemic lupus erythematosus (SLE) and type 1 diabetes. For example, a paper by JF Maillefert et al concluded that in a sample size of 22 patients: 'The observed disorders were as follows: rheumatoid arthritis for six patients; exacerbation of a previously non-diagnosed systemic lupus erythematosus for two; post-vaccinal arthritis for five; polyarthralgia–myalgia for four; suspected or biopsy-proved vasculitis for three; miscellaneous for two.'[3]

2. The adjuvants used are toxic in their own right

Mercury as thiomerosal has been widely used. Lyn Redwood – a remarkable woman who has done much to bring light to bear on this issue – determined that her son had been exposed, through vaccination, to 125 times the Environmental Protection Agency safety limits for mercury. He developed severe pervasive neurodevelopmental disorder.[4]

Aluminium is increasingly used instead of mercury, but is no less toxic. It too is a known neurotoxin and is associated with Alzheimer's disease and autism.

Formaldehyde, another known neurotoxin (and indeed a pesticide), may be used. For a useful summary regarding formaldehyde and its neurodegenerative effects, please see the paper by which concludes that: 'This aldehyde is a well-established neurotoxin that affects memory, learning, and behavior. In addition, in several pathological conditions, including Alzheimer's disease, an increase in the expression of formaldehyde-generating enzymes and elevated levels of formaldehyde in brain have been reported.'[5]

The hydrocarbon squalene may switch on autoimmunity. Increasingly, a delivery mechanism known as a 'virosome' is used; these allow viruses to fuse with target cells. This further bypasses the body's natural defences against viral attack.

3. Most vaccinations are administered by injection

Altogether, 90% of the immune system is associated with the gut. Injections bypass the body's natural defences and allow viruses and bacteria access to otherwise protected tissues, such as the central intelligence agency processing departments of the immune system and, of course, the brain. This is a computer hackers' dream. Our normal firewalls are bypassed giving direct access to our intelligence systems, so that they can be reprogrammed to work for the hacker's virus. This is a biologically plausible explanation for the many neurodegenerative clinical pictures that we see that follow vaccination and, of course, immune disruption. As recently as January 2017, Douglas Leslie et al of Yale University School of Medicine concluded that: 'Subjects with newly diagnosed AN* were more likely than controls to have had any vaccination in the previous 3 months [hazard ratio (HR) 1.80, 95% confidence interval 1.21-2.68]. Influenza vaccinations during the prior 3, 6, and 12 months were also associated with incident diagnoses of AN, OCD, and an anxiety disorder. Several other associations were also significant with HRs greater than 1.40 (hepatitis A with OCD and AN; hepatitis B with AN; and meningitis with AN and chronic tic disorder).'[6]

4. Viral vaccines must be 'grown' on animal tissues

Viral vaccines must be grown on animal tissues, such as mice or monkey cells, because they need the host machinery of these animal cells to replicate. There is potential for viruses or prions already contained within those animal tissues to also be cultured and get into the vaccine. A major concern, well hidden at the time, was that during the BSE epidemic many vaccines were grown on bovine material with huge potential to spread new variant CJD.

The research scientist Judy Mikovits[†] discovered that at least 30% of vaccines were contaminated with gamma-retroviruses (such as XMRV (xenotrophic murine leukaemia virus)). These viruses are associated with autism, CFS, Alzheimer's, Parkinson's and motor neurone disease. Indeed, the FDA confirms that vaccines may be contaminated with foreign proteins and viruses which are 'tumourigenic'.[7]

Meanwhile, HPV vaccines are: 'Not only unproven to protect against cervical cancer, but Dangerous and Unnecessary,' according to Sarah Kalell in response to a request by the Cancer Association of South Africa (CANSA) to substantiate the claim that HPV vaccines cause death, disability and chronic health problems.[8]

5. Preservatives in vaccines are also directly toxic

The preservatives in vaccines include cetyltrimethylammonium bromide, monosodium glutamate, 2-phenoxyethanol and polysorbate-80. To choose just one of these preservatives, the study by Musshoff et al on the effects of 2-phenoxyethanol concludes that: '2-phenoxyethanol (ethylene glycol monophenyl ether) caused a considerable reduction of NMDA-induced membrane currents... The results indicate a neurotoxic potential for 2-phenoxyethanol.'[9]

Allergic disease

For a general approach, see Chapter 36. For the approach to specific diseases, see Table 51.2.

---

*Footnote: AN stands for 'anorexia nervosa'.

†Historical note: Judy A Mikovits, PhD, is an ME/CFS researcher and was previously the research director at the Whittemore Peterson Institute (now the Nevada Center for Biomedical Research). Dr Mikovits led the team that published a paper suggesting a connection between the XMRV retrovirus and ME/CFS. As a result of this paper, Mikovits felt the full force of scientific prejudices regarding ME/CFS, and eventually she was fired from the WPI in 2011. After her sacking, there was a legal dispute with the WPI – Dr Mikovits was actually arrested and imprisoned at this time. All charges, including criminal charges of theft, brought by the WPI against Dr Mikovits, were eventually dropped. This book is not the place for a full recounting of the circumstances surrounding these events but, for example, at one time, Dr Mikovits was banned from even setting foot on the NCI (National Cancer Institute) campus, a prohibition which would be enforced by security. The full story is told in the excellent book, *Plague: One Scientist's Intrepid Search for the Truth About Human Retroviruses and Chronic Fatigue Syndrome (ME/CFS), Autism, and Other Diseases*, written by Kent Heckenlively (a former attorney) and Judy Mikovits.

Table 51.2: Common allergic conditions – triggering allergens and treatments

Common allergic conditions	The common allergens	The tools of the trade for treatment are detailed in Chapter 36, but especially vital are:
Asthma and rhinitis Seasonal hayfever	Dairy products	PK diet
	Pollen, HDM, animal/bird dander	Plus avoid, desensitise (see Chapter 36)
	Viral infections Bacterial infections Fungal infections producing mycotoxins Microbes from the fermenting gut	Plus Groundhog Acute and Chronic Iodine salt pipe Vitamin C to bowel tolerance Antimicrobials (antibiotics and antifungals) – you will need a doctor to prescribe
Eczema	Dairy, grains, yeast eggs Chronic infection of the skin with staphylococci or fungi Microbes from the fermenting gut	PK diet Iodine oil (iodine with coconut oil – see Chapter 32) Vitamin C to bowel tolerance
Dermatitis (eczema due to contact allergens)	Household cleaners and washing powders Metals e.g. jewellery, piercings	Avoid
Urticaria and angio-oedema	Microbes from the fermenting gut Metals	PK diet Vitamin C to bowel tolerance
Anaphylaxis	Foods: nuts, dairy, shellfish, eggs, fish, fruits Wasp and bee stings Chemicals, NSAIDs e.g. aspirin, latex, general anasthetics Exercise induced	See below
Migraine and headaches	Food Chemicals (especially smelly ones like perfume, air fresheners)	See Chapter 49: Neurology
The allergic brain – hyperactivity, foggy brain	Many foods... and other factors	See Chapter 56: Paediatrics
Irritable bowel syndrome	Dairy, grains, yeast	PK diet

	Microbes from the fermenting gut	Vitamin C to bowel tolerance
Arthritis and connective tissue pain, polymyalgia rheumatica, temporal arteritis, vasculitis	Food Microbes from the fermenting gut Toxic metals	See Chapter 47: Rheumatology
The allergic perineum (interstitial cystitis, vaginitis, prostatitis, epididymitis etc)	Foods, often yeast Microbes from the fermenting gut Toxic metals Latex Rarely, semen	See Chapter 46: Urology
The allergic heart e.g. rheumatic heart disease	Streptococci	Allergic reactions may also manifest with pulse changes. The Dr Arthur Coca pulse test means an allergy is likely if the pulse changes by more than 10 beats per minute after exposure. This test is not definitive but may be a useful clinical guide. You can access the full 110-page *The Pulse Test* free of charge here: https://soiland-health.org/wp-content/ ---uplo ads/02/0201hyglibcat/020108. coca.pdf
Any part of the body may react allergically	Any or all of the above	

Anaphylaxis

Anaphylaxis[†] is a major allergic reaction with the potential to kill. Common triggers are detailed above. How do you know you are pre-anaphylactic? Firstly, if you suffer from type I allergy (the immediate, classical type, with asthma, urticaria, angio-oedema). Secondly, if you have ever had a previous anaphylactic

---

[†]**Historical note**: As has been seen, allergies and autoimmunity can have devastating effects on the health (and even death) of people, but they can also change the course of history. The son of the Roman emperor Claudius (10-13 BC to 54 AD), Britannicus, is recorded as having suffered from an allergy to horse dander, with contemporary reporters noting that when so exposed, his eyes would swell up and he would develop a severe rash. Britannicus was heir apparent, but due to his allergies, he was seen as 'weak' and he was severely hampered from many ceremonial and other duties that required close contact with horses. When Britannicus's mother died, Claudius remarried, this time Agrippina the Younger. She had a son named Nero, and Claudius adopted him. Nero soon won the favour of the public, and he was named emperor in 54 AD instead of the 'weak' Britannicus. So, an allergy to horse dander gave the world Nero as emperor of Rome. (I think I would be shot by my Latin teacher for making such leaps, just in the name of a good story! Craig)

reaction or near miss. This is important because with time, and lack of Groundhog treatments or desensitisation, anaphylactic reactions become more serious and more life threatening.

Early symptoms include itchy skin, flushed skin, blotchy skin, a raised red itchy rash, swelling of the mouth, tickling, tingling or itching of the throat, mouth and lips. and stomach ache.

Firstly, take a dose of antihistamines – any type will do. Crunch it up in the mouth and swallow. Apply cold water or ice packs to the affected area – sometimes this is sufficient to stop the reaction.

If the above symptoms progress, or if there is any hint of further reactions, do not waste time. Use injected adrenaline or an EpiPen.

Later symptoms include marked swelling of the lips or tongue, difficulty in swallowing, wheeze or difficulty in breathing, change in voice or inability to speak, drowsiness, blue lips, feeling faint, loss of consciousness. The pulse may be going fast, or conversely might be going very slowly. Blood pressure may fall.

If in doubt whether or not to use an EpiPen or adrenaline by injection, use it. No-one has ever died following an intramuscular injection of adrenaline given early in an anaphylactic attack. The injection needs to be into the muscle.

Some people need a second injection of EpiPen, so make sure you always have two to hand. Should you ever require an EpiPen injection, then you need to be seen and assessed by a doctor as soon as reasonably possible. If you need the EpiPen, also take prednisolone 30 mg (6 tablets) or hydrocortisone 100 mg. These take up to six hours to work but they help prevent a second attack.

How to use an EpiPen/adrenalin
This is what you need to do:
- Pull off the grey safety cap.
- Place the black tip onto the side of the thigh at right angles to the leg.
- Press hard into the thigh until you hear the pen click (the injection can be given through clothing).
- Hold in place for 10 seconds.
- Remove EpiPen; note what time it is.

There is a very useful website called www.epipen.co.uk with useful resources if you are in the UK:

They can send you an EpiPen dummy trainer pen

There is a demonstration video of how to use your EpiPen

There is an EpiPen expiry service

Adrenalin has a short lifespan, so do check the dates on your ampoules and EpiPen regularly. I like all my patients to have three EpiPens – one for the house, one for the car and one for the handbag (or manbag).

References

1. Benaroya Research Institute. Autoimmune diseases. www.benaroyaresearch.org/what-is-bri/disease-information/autoimmune-diseases (accessed 28 November 2019).
2. Allergy UK. Allergy prevalence: useful facts and figures. www.allergyuk.org/assets/000/001/369/Stats_for_Website_original.pdf?1505209830 (accessed 28 November 2019)
3. Maillefert JF, Sibilia J, Toussirot E, Vignon E, et al. Rheumatic disorders developed after hepatitis B vaccination. *Rheumatology* 1999; 38(10): 978-983. doi.org/10.1093/rheumatology/38.10.978 https://academic.oup.com/rheumatology/article/38/10/978/1783598/Rheumatic-disorders-developed-after-hepatitis-B
4. www.wikidoc.org/index.php/Lyn_Redwood (Brief introduction to Lyn Redwood and her work)
5. Tuulpule K, Dringen R. Formaldehyde in brain: an overlooked player in neurodegeneration? *Journal of Neurochemistry* 2013; 127(1): 7-21. Doi: org/10.1111/jnc.12356 http://onlinelibrary.wiley.com/doi/10.1111/jnc.12356/abstract

6. Leslie D, Kobre RA, Richmand BJ, Guloksuz SA, Leckman JF. Temporal association of certain neuropsychiatric disorders following vaccination of children and adolescents: a pilot case-control study. *Front Psychiatry* 2017; 8: 3. doi: 10.3389/fpsyt.2017.00003. www.ncbi.nlm.nih.gov/pubmed/28154539

7. Khan AS. Investigating viruses in cells used to make vaccines; and evaluating the potential threat posed by transmission of viruses to humans. US Food and Drug Administration. 02/01/2018 www.fda.gov/BiologicsBloodVaccines/ScienceResearch/BiologicsResearchAreas/ucm127327.htm

8. Sarah Kalell. The Cancer Association of South Africa (CANSA) HPV Vaccines cause death, disability and chronic health problems. September 2015. http://sanevax.org/wp-content/uploads/2015/10/CANSA-Reply-September-2015-HPV-Vaccine.pdf (accessed 28 November 2019)

9. Musshoff U, Madeja M, Binding N, Witting U, Speckmann EJ. Effects of 2-phenoxyethanol on N-methyl-D-aspartate (NMDA) receptor-mediated ion currents. *Arch Toxicol* 1999; 73(1): 55-59. www.ncbi.nlm.nih.gov/pubmed/10207615

Chapter 52
New killers of the 21st century

– environmental pollution
– immunotoxicity by chemicals, metals and silicones
– electro-magnetic pollution
– wind turbine syndrome
– doubtless more to come...

We Do Not Inherit the Earth from Our Ancestors; We Borrow It from Our Children.
Of unknown and disputed origin[1]

These new killers include:
- Poisoning by chemicals: sick building syndrome, Gulf War syndrome, sheep dip flu, aerotoxic syndrome, 9/11 syndrome, fluoride, dental amalgam, cosmetics (especially hair dyes and deodorants)
- Immunotoxicity by chemicals, metals and silicones
- Electro-magnetic pollution by wifi, mobile phones, cordless phone, electric vehicles
- Wind turbine syndrome
- and doubtless more to come.

These are the diseases of Westerners arising as a direct result of pollution of the environment. Most go unrecognised by the Establishment for at least three reasons:
- The underlying cause is an industry essential. Follow the money.
- The compensation and benefits for disease would be financially unaffordable.

- Lack of effective treatment.

The symptoms of the above problems include: Establishment denial that such a syndrome exists (that might include Government Inquiries – I know, I have given evidence; they listen carefully, document thoroughly then ignore in the final report).

The disease is described as psychosomatic – it's all in the mind
- Patients organise themselves into self-help groups
- Doctors who support such patients are vilified and targeted by Big-Pharma-sponsored actions (I know, I am one such)
- Individual legal actions for compensation for damage. With successful actions, gagging clauses are included.

For the specific details of such a case – that of chronic fatigue syndrome/myalgic encephalitis (CFS/ME), see Chapter 1 of our book *Diagnosis and Treatment of Chronic Fatigue Syndrome and Myalgic Encephaltis – it's mitochondria, not hypochondria*.

There is no space here to detail the decades

of stories of my battles and campaigns over the above issues. That is another book. For me, this started with coal miners in Nottinghamshire with pneumoconiosis from inhaling coal dust. Even the radiologists dared not diagnose this correctly in fear of retribution. The best one could hope for was a report stating, 'mottling of the lungs consistent with a diagnosis of pneumoconiosis'. I then moved on to sick building syndrome in the 1980s when we saw people poisoned by the formaldehyde of cavity wall insulation – now banned. On moving to the Welsh borders, I recognised farmers poisoned by organophosphate chemicals used in sheep dip, cattle pour-ons, fly control in the dairy and crop sprays. I used to do a double act with the amazing Mark Purdey who described the link between BSE and organophosphates in a series of compelling papers and scientific experiments. This wonderful research was stymied by MAFF who banned all research into BSE except by government controlled (whoops, I mean licensed) laboratories.[2]

From here it was not difficult to diagnose Gulf War syndrome – resulting from a toxic cocktail of organophosphates, multiple vaccinations and biological warfare. The many cases of autism could be explained by vaccination and other toxic exposures. I have seen over 250 women with chronic disease following silicone breast implants. I have one young man patient forced to live in the middle of freezing nowhere in order to avoid the electromagnetic pollution that results in a mental and physical pole-axing. I see increasing numbers of patients rendered sick by the infrasound of wind turbines who can only be relieved of symptoms by moving house.

Sadly, there will be many other new syndromes that will fit the above paradigm, I have no doubt.

Symptoms of 21st-century killers

In addition to the section that follows, see Chapter 8 for symptoms of poisonings and deficiencies.

Clinical pictures induced by 21st-century killers

Just as we have Koch's postulates*[3] to describe an infectious disease, we have a characteristic clinical picture that describes toxicity-induced disease.

---

*Historical note: 'Koch's postulates' were set out in 1890 by the German physician and bacteriologist Heinrich Hermann Robert Koch (11 December 1843 – 27 May 1910) as criteria for judging whether a given bacterium is the cause of a given disease. His postulates are as follows:

The bacterium must be present in every case of the disease.

The bacterium must be isolated from the host with the disease and grown in pure culture.

The specific disease must be reproduced when a pure culture of the bacterium is inoculated into a healthy susceptible host.

The bacterium must be recoverable from the experimentally infected host.

These postulates are not perfect – for example, leprosy cannot be 'grown in pure culture' in the laboratory – but they did represent a massive step forward. (Koch received the Nobel Prize in Physiology or Medicine in 1905 for his research into tuberculosis.)

Table 52.1

Clinical picture	Mechanism
There is an initial over-whelming exposure which triggers local symptoms with local inflammation and pain (such as rhinitis, asthma, vomiting, diarrhoea, acute confusion, collapse)	Acute poisoning
If the exposure is unremitting, the inflammation becomes more general, with malaise, headache, muscle pain, joint pain and chronic fatigue.	Chronic poisoning
With subsequent exposures, the immune system starts to react to much lower concentrations of toxin. This is allergy. It has been dubbed TILT (toxicant-induced loss of tolerance). The commonest offending chemicals are perfumes, air fresheners and cleaning agents. One experiences the same symptoms as above, but at much lower exposures of chemical. Sufferers develop an exquisite sense of smell and may be able to detect chemicals that others cannot. This sensitisation may switch on chronic inflammation with increasing disability.	Sensitisation to single toxins
Sufferers start to react to other chemicals by which they have been poisoned. This is called the spreading phenomenon. A combination of TILT and the spreading phenomenon makes 21st-century life almost impossible for some since these chemicals are ubiquitously present in the modern polluted world and nigh on impossible to avoid completely. If exposure is unavoidable, then we see premature ageing, accelerated pathology and death.	Sensitisation to multiple toxins

Like infection, we start with an exposure which initially triggers local symptoms but progresses to a more general picture. Like infection, immune learning, experience and memory mean that we react sooner and at lower levels of exposure and with increasingly serious disease. In the short term, there is acute inflammation; in the medium term, chronic inflammation and increasing disability; in the long term, premature ageing, accelerated pathology and death.

Treatment of 21st-century killers

Treating these relatively new killers is easy in principle but difficult in practice. The principal actions are:

- Groundhog Chronic – see Appendix 3
  Avoid the incitant – see Chapter 25: Reduce the toxic chemical burden
- Get rid of poisons stuck in the body – see Chapter 34: Tools for detoxing
- Put in place interventions to improve en-

ergy delivery mechanisms – see Chapter 30: Tools to improve energy delivery

- Put in place interventions to reduce the inflammation that has been switched on – see Chapter 36: Tools to switch off chronic inflammation

References

1. Quote Investigator. We do not inherit the earth from our ancestors; we borrow it from our children. 22 January 2013. https://quoteinvestigator.com/2013/01/22/borrow-earth/ (accessed 29 November 2019)
2. Wikipedia. Mark Purdey. https://en.wikipedia.org/wiki/Mark_Purdey (accessed 29 November 2019)
3. Sheil WC Jr. Medical definition of Koch's postulates. MedicineNet. medicinenet.com/script/main/art/asp? articlekey=7105 (accessed 24 March 2020)

Chapter 53
Oncology

– you need all the tools to kill cancer

I do not pretend to be a cancer expert, but I know of some fundamental principles which apply across the board and are relevant to the prevention and treatment of virtually all cancers.

Once a diagnosis of cancer has been given, there will be trillions of cancer cells already established. For a tumour to be visible on a scan, there must be between a thousand million and a million million cells present. Anything that can be done to reduce this total load is going to be helpful. Standard conventional approaches to cancer – surgery, radiotherapy and chemotherapy – all have their place. The problem is targeting treatment so that as much of the tumour is killed as possible while normal cells are spared. In practice, this is a very difficult balancing act. However, there are other things that can be done, over and above, which not only make these treatments more effective, but greatly reduce the side effects from such therapies. In my experience, and evidence from a large body of medical literature, these interventions improve the chances of survival. They are set out in Table 53.1.

Table 53.1: The fundamental principles behind extra anti-cancer therapies

What	Why	How
Starve the cancerous growth	Cancers can only grow on sugar and refined carbohydrates The British Society of Integrated Oncologists recommends a ketogenic diet for all cancer patients and numerous studies support this[1]	Paleo ketogenic (PK) diet

What	Why	How
Kill the cancer with vitamin C	It is biologically plausible that this is effective because as cancer cells are starved of sugar, they increase their mechanisms for uptake of sugar. Because vitamin C chemically 'looks' like sugar, the cancer cells grab vitamin C instead. This is not a fuel and so cancer cells are killed as they are starved out of existence. Intravenous vitamin C works even better but it is difficult to find a doctor who can supply it	Vitamin C to bowel tolerance Vitamin C intravenously is of proven benefit. Indeed, it is on the cusp of becoming a standard part of the chemotherapy of all cancers. High quality medical studies have traditionally been thin on the ground in this area – follow the money – vitamin C cannot be patented. But, as one example, in 2019 a well-designed study for Breast Cancer concluded favourably.[*2] As more studies like this are published, we will see IV Vit C be incorporated into the 'standard' chemotherapy treatments of all cancers.
Identify growth promoters: female sex hormones, dairy, insulin	Cancers grow faster in the presence of growth promotors Obesity is associated with higher insulin levels	PK diet Aim to lose weight to a normal BMI Avoid the Pill and HRT Identify oestrogen mimics (e.g. soya) and get rid of these
Ensure excellent nutritional status with vitamins and minerals	This allows healing and repair	Basic package as per Groundhog
Look for an infectious associate...	...that may be susceptible to treatment Many cancers are driven by infection – see *The Infection Game*	
Improve antioxidant status	To mop up free radicals created by the cancer treatments and limit side effects	See Chapter 36: Tools to switch off chronic inflammation
Sleep well	Sleep is when healing and repair take place	See Chapter 22: Sleep

*Footnote: A recent study by Lee et al (2019) concluded that 'Combining high-dose vitamin C with conventional anti-cancer drugs can have therapeutic advantages against breast cancer cells.' Indeed, even on its own intravenous vitamin C 'significantly decreased cell viability of all breast cancer cell lines, particularly of MCF-7 cells.'[2]

Identify cancer triggers	To prevent more cancers developing Look for toxins – tests are essential: DNA adducts is ideal but if not available, measure toxic metals, VOCs and pesticides (see Chapter 25)	Do a good detox regime (to get rid of exogenous tumour initiators and growth promoters) See Chapter 34: Detoxing
Exercise	Within your limits	Exercise inhibits cancer
Improve energy delivery mechanisms	To ensure the immune system has the energy to fight	
Use natural anticancer substances	To enhance the effects of all else. I see this as a small 'bolt-on extra', not the answer in itself. So many use these hoping that herbals alone will do the trick but…	…they rarely do – do it all!
Consider heating regimes	Cancer cells cannot tolerate heat as well as normal cells	Heating regimes are of proven benefit in many cancers[†]
Monitor the effects of treatment with tumour markers	To assess progress. Some tumours have a unique marker. A cheap-to-measure tumour marker is lactate dehydrogenase, which is part of routine liver function tests and a marker of cell damage	If you are not winning, then you must work harder at the regimes!

Starve out the cancer cells

Cancers are evolutionarily primitive cells and can only survive on glucose. In this respect they are very much like yeast and rely entirely on anaerobic metabolism. Glucose is fermented in the absence of oxygen to produce energy. This is very inefficient and produces lactic acid. Indeed, this inefficient burning of glucose probably explains the cancer 'cachexia' (weight loss) seen in advanced cases.

Normally animal and, of course, human cells get the vast majority of their energy from the processes carried out in the mitochondria. This is extremely efficient; mitochondria can use not just glucose, but also fat and protein as sources of energy. All these uses require oxygen. The reason it is important to understand this is because mitochondria control cell division. If mitochondria are switched off, this control is lost, and the cell turns into a cancerous cell. Indeed, this may well be part of the mechanism by which cancer begins.

[†]**Footnote:** Once again, the availability of good research data is limited – 'heat' cannot be patented. But also once again, some good studies are now being done. For example, Skitzki et al (2009)[3] state: 'The use of hyperthermia as an adjunct to cancer immunotherapy is supported by an increasing number of research data. Both preclinical and clinical data results have demonstrated improved antitumor immune responses with the addition of mild hyperthermia.'

The difference between a cancer cell and a normal cell, therefore, is how it gets its energy. By substantially reducing sugar supply, one starves out the cancer cell. In this event, cancer cells up-grade the mechanism by which they absorb sugar, which is the same mechanism by which they absorb vitamin C, and vitamin C is extremely toxic to cancer cells.

So, the first two key interventions are:

- The ketogenic diet
- High-dose vitamin C – take to bowel tolerance. The cheapest source is ascorbic acid, but if this is not tolerated then magnesium ascorbate can be used instead. Because vitamin C has such a short half-life in the blood, it needs to be given in lots of small doses throughout the day. If available, consider intravenous vitamins C, but there is no point trying this until you are up to bowel tolerance oral doses because that may be all that is necessary.

In this approach, we mimic human warfare – we starve the enemy (with the ketogenic diet), and we kill the enemy (with vitamin C).

References

1. Ketogenic Diet Resource. Ketogenic Medical Research. www.ketogenic-diet-resource.com/medical-research.html#cancer (accessed 29 November 2019)
2. Lee SJ, Jeong JH, Lee IH, Lee J, et al. Effect of High-dose Vitamin C Combined With Anticancer Treatment on Breast Cancer Cells. *Anticancer Res* 2019; 39(2): 751-758. www.ncbi.nlm.nih.gov/pubmed/30711954
3. Skitzki JJ, Rapesky EA, Evans SS. Hyperthermia as an immunotherapy strategy for cancer. *Current Opinion in Investigational Drugs* 2009; 10(6): 550-558.

Chapter 54
Women's health

– men are from Mars, women are from Venus

Men and women differ because they have very different evolutionary strategies to promote the survival of their genes. The Man's best strategy is to make himself as appealing to as many women as he can and father as many children as possible. The one-night stand for him is the most efficient ploy, then shimmy off and woo another. Conversely the Woman's best chance of survival of her genes is to invest all her energy into a safe environment for raising a child; this needs long-term planning, a proper secure nest and infrastructure of help from relatives and friends. These strategies mean men and women have very different drives, loyalties and game plans. It is indeed the case that, to quote the title of the 1991 book by American author and relationship counsellor, John Gray: *Men are from Mars, Women are from Venus.**

Having said that, there are other evolutionary ploys, as detailed by Sandy Toksvig: 'Some species propagate their genes by having millions of offspring, investing no effort in their maturation in the hope that a few would survive. Others have a few offspring but nurture them carefully. My mother used a unique strategy – she had one child, did nothing and hoped for the best.'

These behavioural differences result from sex hormones. Testosterone drives attention-grabbing, risk-taking behaviour. Look at those red stags who invest huge amounts of nutritional resources into growing antlers every year. During the rut, they stop eating and fight other males endlessly to impress those watching hinds. A quick bonk and the stags are back fighting again for the privilege. (Having said that, it has been observed that when the mature stags are fighting, a younger pricket – a male fallow deer in its second year, having straight, unbranched antlers – may

---

***Roman mythological note**: Venus is the name of a Roman goddess. Her domain encompassed love, beauty, desire, sex, fertility, prosperity and victory. Her name is indistinguishable from the Latin noun *venus* ('sexual love' and 'sexual desire'). Julius Caesar claimed Venus as an ancestor. Mars was the god of war and also an agricultural guardian; he represented military power as a way to secure peace. Venus was betrothed to Vulcan, god of Fire, but she found him boring, so she and Mars had a passionate affair. Vulcan suspected what was going on and, being a blacksmith, made a fine metallic mesh and secreted it on a couch whereupon Venus and Mars were ensnared and humiliated in front of the other gods on Mount Olympus. With Mars, Venus gave birth to Timor (Phobos), representing fear in battle; his twin Metus (Deimos) who was the personification of terror; Concordia, the goddess of harmony; and the Cupids who represent the different aspects of love. Concordia is the good news here: she denotes agreement in marriage and like-mindedness – an example of what can happen when men and women combine to their best. (The astronomically minded will have noted that Phobos and Deimos are both moons of Mars.)

seize the opportunity to nip in and cover a female (the scientific term for this is a 'sneaky fucker').) But stags can literally starve and fight themselves to death. This activity takes place in the autumn and many males enter winter in an exhausted state and do not survive. Testosterone is there for the genes, to the detriment of the individual.

Female sex hormones too exist for the benefit of our selfish genes and to the detriment of women. They are not essential for life – children and post-menopausal women live very well without them. They are only necessary for the business of reproduction and that is a very dangerous matter. Why so?

- Sexual intercourse is a high-risk activity which carries the potential for acquisition of serious infections
- We do stupid things in the pursuit of orgasm. Female sex hormones induce the sorts of desires and madnesses that are an immediate prerequisite for sex
- To create and grow babies we need growth promoters. Cancer is just one step away from such and *all* female sex hormones are growth promoting
- To prevent Mother rejecting baby as a foreigner (the baby is, of course, genetically different) female sex hormones suppress the immune system; this too is potentially dangerous
- To prevent Mother bleeding to death with childbirth, her blood becomes stickier. This is a risk for thromboembolic disease: heart attacks and venous thrombosis with pulmonary embolism
- To store food for breast feeding, female sex hormones induce metabolic syndrome with associated cravings, weight gain and hypertension
- Female sex hormones, including oxytocin, make us love our children so much. Human children are completely dependent on their mothers for years, so a high degree of anxiety and hypervigilance in Mother is

essential to keep children safe.

With this understanding of female sex hormones, we can make sense of the clinical problems that arise.

The Pill and HRT are dangerous medicines

The Pill and HRT are dangerous medicines for all the reasons given above: they increase the risk of cancer, heart disease, arterial disease, thrombosis and stroke. The risk of developing these diseases is increased by the immune suppressant effects. They encourage a toxic cocktail of infection with carcinogenic viruses (HPV and HHV 2), immune suppression so that these viruses proliferate to initiate cancer, then the growth promotion that further drives cancer. No wonder we are seeing epidemics of cervical cancer in young women, and this has been made worse by HPV vaccinations (see below). Female sex hormones can make us psychologically unstable sometimes to the point of madness. Indeed, the term hysteria comes from the Greek word for uterus, *hystera* (ὑστέρα). In ancient, Greece a wandering and discontented uterus was blamed for that dreaded female ailment of excessive emotion.

In the short term, I suspect female sex hormones mask the symptom of fatigue (the business of procreation and child-rearing is very hard work) and this makes them addictive.

Premenstural tension (PMT)

Evolution never intended any woman to ever see a period. Either she was too young, or too old, or pregnant, breastfeeding or starving. Symptoms associated with the menstrual cycle were never meant to be! Indeed, I suspect most symptoms associated with such are actually symptoms of poor energy delivery and can be effectively treated by Groundhog interventions and improving energy delivery mechanisms, in particular by tackling hypothyroidism (see Chapter 30: Tools to improve energy delivery).

Menstrual irregularities

A regular menstrual cycle results from the regular production of an egg. Eggs are produced when the brain considers it safe to do so. This needs good energy delivery mechanisms, freedom from inflammation, a safe physical and psychological environment and a good state of nutrition. Female athletes often lose their menstrual cycle as they become super fit simply because they do not have the reserves of fat to allow pregnancy and breastfeeding. This is not a problem and reverses reliably well.

A regular vaginal bleed can immediately be established by prescribing the Pill, but this is symptom-suppressing, dangerous medicine. Indeed, it can result in an early menopause. I saw a young woman patient who went into menopause aged 24 with amenorrhoea and menopausal levels of the two female hormones follicle stimulating hormone (FSH) and luteinising hormone (LH) after being prescribed the Pill.

Endometriosis

Endometriosis results when a piece of the lining of the uterus (womb) ends up elsewhere in the body. This displaced tissue is sensitive to hormones and so swells and bleeds with each and every hormone cycle. This results in pain, which typically starts before a period and stops after. There is a clear association with yeast, but I am not sure what the mechanism is. However, treatment with Groundhog Chronic is very helpful, especially attention to tools for treating the fermenting gut (see Chapter 29).

Menopausal problems

The miserable hot flushes of the menopause result from a desperate last-ditch attempt by our selfish genes to produce another pregnancy. I suspect it is the high levels of FSH and LH, which are frantically kicking the ovaries to squeeze out that last egg, that are responsible for these. FSH and LH are released from the pituitary gland in bursts and the spike in levels of such has profound vasodilatory effects. However, evolution does not care that the temporary caretaker of genes cannot sleep. Evolution is solely interested in new babies and their survival.

Of course, HRT will abolish hot flushes instantly, but that is a high-risk strategy. There are no simple answers, but Groundhog interventions greatly help, especially sorting out thyroid and adrenal issues and using testicular glandulars, 1-2 grams daily.

Vulvitis, vaginitis, vulvodyndia and lichen planus

I suspect all these conditions are driven by microbes; this may be allergy to microbes from the fermenting gut and/or low grade microbial presence. Groundhog Chronic together with topical iodine oil are effective treatments.

HPV vaccination

Before human papilloma virus (HPV) vaccination was introduced, the incidence and death rates from cervical cancer were falling. Now they are rising in the very age groups that have received the vaccine. Why should that be? There are over 200 strains of HPV, of which 12 are carcinogenic. Not all strains are represented in the vaccine. If this vaccine is given to a woman who is already infected with a strain of HPV, then this seems to kick-start the process of carcinogenesis. Even virgin girls may be already infected with HPV since the virus passes vertically from mother to daughter. It is shocking to think that a vaccine designed to prevent cancer is actually encouraging it.

Women who have received the vaccine arrive at the false conclusion that they are protected from cancer. This may encourage risk taking, such as unprotected sex, use of the Pill and failure to attend screening clinics for cervical cancer. Post-marketing studies and observations show that HPV vaccination causes many problems, including:

- Chronic fatigue syndrome (I know this all too well from my many patients) – HPV seems particularly effective at switching on inflammation
- Arthritis and pain syndromes, autoimmunity (ASIA syndromes) – see Chapter 51: Immunology
- Impaired fertility subsequently (in rats HPV reduced fertility by 25%)
- Death (which, in true Big Pharma underwhelming style, is listed as an 'adverse effect').

The bottom line is that vaccination for HPV is bad news and must be avoided.

Conclusion

Lest I have given too bleak a view of what it is to be a woman (or man), let us finish with some wisdom. First, Oscar Wilde (16 October 1854 – 30 November 1900) on women from his play *The Ideal Husband*:

> *Women are never disarmed by compliments. Men always are.*

And then Virginia Woolf (25 January 1882 – 28 March 1942) on gender in *A Room of One's Own*:

> *I would venture to guess that Anon, who wrote so many poems without signing them, was often a woman.*

Ultimately, however, we must remember that the selfish gene is at play with us all and this is perhaps summed up best by Mark Twain (30 November 1835 – 21 April 1910):

> *What would men be without women? Scarce, sir... mighty scarce.*

Chapter 55
Preconception, pregnancy and paleo breast-feeding

– you must 'get your shit together' for the sake of your kids

If there is any one moment in your life to do Groundhog it should be during this window of time when you are going to have a baby. Feel free to mess your own life up, but do not impose that on the next generation. The business of building and programming our lovely children is far more complex than normal adult biology and biochemistry. Interference with this process means malign effects may persist for life and even affect subsequent generations. This was established in the 1930s by Franz Pottenger, who experimented with cats by feeding them cooked-meat diets. Of course, Goundhog for cats is raw meat and raw milk. The cooked-diet cats developed degenerative diseases. When they bred, by the third generation they lost fertility and of those that did manage to conceive, no kittens survived.[1]

A further example of this is the stilboestrol story. This hormone was prescribed to 1000 New Zealand women at risk of miscarriage. Many of the girls born developed vaginal cancer as teenagers, with some new cases appearing in their sixth decade. Grandsons were born with genital abnormalities.[2]

We start life as a single cell type which then has to divide into at least 200 different tissues, and 20 different cell organelles, all of which must grow in the correct three-dimensional space, and then interact perfectly. This continues right through childhood. Words fail me in my attempt to describe this miraculous process. Exposure to toxins like metals, pesticides, volatile organic compounds (VOCs) and mycotoxins (from fungi) is like throwing a handful of sand into a finely tuned engine. Disaster. But get the regimes right and you will set up your children for good physical, mental and immunological health for life – the best birthday present of all.

What follows is a counsel of perfection, and this is **the** time for a virtuoso Groundhog performance. Given that young Groundhogs are called chucklings, maybe we should call this 'Groundhog Chuckling'?

The Groundhog CHUCKLING of preconceptual care

Table 55.1: What to do preconception to ensure optimal health for baby

What to do	Especially	Why
Get Groundhog Basic well established	The PK diet	The perfect fuel for foetal growth, especially brain development, is fat and ketones.
	Micronutrients (see Appendix 1 and Appendix 2)	In the doses recommended these are completely safe, indeed desirable during pregnancy
	Avoid vaccinations...	...because of toxicity and immunotoxicity (see Chapter 51)
Tests to exclude sexually transmitted disease	Should be done if either you or your partner are not virgins	Many STDs are associated with pregnancy problems and birth defects, especially HIV, syphilis, cytomegalo virus (CMV), gonorrhoea, chlamydia, bacterial vaginosis, herpes, streptococci and other such
		You may need prescription drugs to get rid of these – see Chapter 39 and also our book *The Infection Game*
Test for rubella antibodies	If you need rubella vaccine then make sure this is given well before pregnancy	It is a complete nonsense that rubella antibody tests are not normally done until 12 weeks of pregnancy; by this time it is too late as the damage of new rubella infection occurs during the first 12 weeks
Test for blood groups	If you are rhesus negative, you will need anti-D globulin injected during pregnancy to avoid haemolytic disease of the newborn (HDN)	BUT this contains thimerosal 30 mcg/ml. Thimerosal is about 50% ethyl mercury by weight. Hence, a patient who had received a dose of RhoGAM (0.7 ml on average) would have received 10.5 mcg of ethyl mercury. Bad news, but better than risking HDN
		See below for how to mitigate the toxicity of vaccination
Routine bloods to check for anaemia, liver or kidney disease	If any history of problems	

Routine blood for thyroid levels	If any problems with fatigue, or family history or other thyroid symptoms (see Chapters 5 and 13)	The IQ of the baby is inversely proportionate to the thyroid stimulating hormone (TSH) level. My view is if the TSH is above 1.5, consider treatment with thyroid hormones. The need for thyroid hormones increases by 50% during pregnancy and hypothyroidism can develop rapidly and at a stage of foetal development when they are most vital. Re-check blood ever 12 weeks and again post-partum
Test for toxic metals (urine elements with DMSA)	I recommend this as a routine since toxic metal problems are almost impossible to avoid and it is impossible to predict what abnormalities they may cause	Mercury, lead, arsenic, cadmium and nickel are all mutagens. Aluminium probably is. Platinum and palladium may be mutagens. The lower the total body load, the better for reasons of cocktail and biochemical bottlenecks (see Chapter 15: Poisonings)
Genova toxic effects CORE test[3]	If there is any history of exposure to toxic chemicals	This test is done on a urine sample. It is a bit pricey but vital in order to prevent foetal damage. Heating regimes remove toxic chemicals reliably well (see Chapter 35: Tools for healing and repair)
		See Chapter 25: Reduce the chemical burden, to review possible toxins
		Tests of toxicity are vital if you are planning to breast feed. Breast milk is a fatty liquid and fat-soluble pesticides, VOCs and toxic metals will be excreted in breast milk. Indeed, it is estimated that one third of Mother's body burden of chemicals will be dumped into her baby. There is a global distillation of organochlorine pesticides with bioaccumulation in the food chain from plankton upwards. Inuit Indian mothers can no longer safely breast feed – they risk seriously poisoning their babies*
		Allow time for all the above to become established so you will not expose the baby to detox, diet and die-off reactions (see Chapter 28)

*Footnote: See the paper by Dewailly et al[4] which concludes: 'The Inuit mothers exhibit the greatest body burden known to occur from exposure to organochlorine residues present in the environment by virtue of their location at the highest trophic level of the Arctic food web.'

Vaccinations for the mother

If you have to receive a vaccination, and the only one I recommend is the one to avoid haemolytic disease of the newborn (see above), then do all possible to mitigate the toxic effects of the adjuvants mercury and aluminium. Only have the vaccine on a day when you feel 100% well (so often serious vaccine reactions happen when they are given to someone already ill).

Take DMSA 15 mg per kg of bodyweight 30 minutes before the vaccine is given. This will grab hold of aluminium or mercury that leaks away from the injection site. This is a very safe intervention and considerably safer than exposure to toxic metals.[5]

Take a clay such as Toxaprevent 3 grams at night for two weeks in order to grab toxic metals as they are excreted in bile. Also, take all the supplements as detailed in Chapter 34: Tools for detoxing, and carry on for at least one month

To find out what is in individual vaccines, take a look at the US's Centers for Disease Control and Prevention (CDC) document, 'Vaccine Excipient and Media Summary Excipients Included in U.S. Vaccines, by Vaccine'.[6]

Infertility

Infertility is a fast-growing problem, so much so that one in 10 couples looking to procreate now attends a fertility clinic.[†] Very little analysis goes into the mechanism of infertility, but it is really very straightforward.

[†]**Story from Craig:** Penny and I had some trouble conceiving. The process to determine what the 'issue' was involved me (Craig) attending a clinic to have my 'wedding tackle' checked out. This started well, with a single (female) doctor crouching in front of me, measuring testicular size using an orchidometer[‡]. Results were fairly normal, though with one a little bigger than the other. But then the doctor asked whether a few students could come in and do the same examination. I agreed, only to be greeted by a line of approximately 30 (all female, except the very last one – a 'Rugby-playing type') trainee doctors and nurses, who, each in turn, crouched and confirmed the size readings... I looked out of the window and counted the leaves on a nearby oak tree! It was all worth it – Georgina Claire was born on 11 May 1992 at 5.28 am. (Sarah – I have no idea what this examination could achieve other than a funny story!)

[‡]**Medical note–** The orchidometer was introduced in 1966 by Swiss paediatric endocrinologist Professor Andrea Prader of the University of Zurich. It consists of a string of 12 numbered wooden or plastic beads of increasing size from about 1 to 25 ml in volume. Doctors sometimes informally refer to them as 'Prader's balls' or the 'medical worry beads'. Prader (23 December 1919 – 3 June 2001) has the eponymous disease Prader-Willi syndrome named after him – sufferers develop a constant hunger, leading to issues such as obesity and type 2 diabetes.

Table 55.2: Possible causes of infertility and what to do about them

The problem	Why	What do to in addition to Groundhog Basic
Low sperm count or too many malformed sperm	Poisoning	See Chapters 8, 15, 25 and 34 for symptoms, mechanisms, sources of and how to detox
	Chronic infection	Get tested at a sexually transmitted disease clinic See *The Infection Game*
	Poor energy delivery mechanisms	Improve energy delivery mechanisms See Chapter 30; hypothyroidism is a greatly overlooked cause (and further results in low testosterone)
	Micronutrient deficiency	Groundhog Basic addresses most deficiences but consider nutritional tests at Biolab
Mother not producing an egg (often indicated by no or irregular periods)	Ditto above	A useful test to look at how many eggs she has left is of anti-mullerian hormone[§]
Fallopian tubes blocked so the egg cannot get to the womb	Usually blocked due to chronic infection	Yes, you will need the surgeons to help you here
Unfavourable environment in the womb	Chronic infection	Get tested at a sexually transmitted disease clinic See *The Infection Game*

It is important to analyse possible underlying causes and treat them properly because if they are not addressed, the risk of miscarriages and birth defects increases, for the same reason that there is infertility. Nature is not stupid – we know that if the system is 'forced' against its will by hormone injections, this greatly increases such complications. Again, symptom suppression is dangerous. Indeed, I have several patients whose CFS was triggered by fertility treatments. I have

§**Footnote:** Women are born with their lifetime supply of eggs, and these gradually decrease in both quality and quantity with age. Anti-mullerian hormone (AMH) is a hormone secreted by cells in developing egg sacs (follicles). The level of AMH in a woman's blood is generally a good indicator of her ovarian reserve.

Table 55.3: Interventions during pregnancy and childbirth

What to do	Especially if...	Why
Continue Groundhog Basic	The high levels of female sex hormones promote metabolic syndrome with the risk of type 2 diabetes, hypertension and eclampsia, thrombosis with sticky blood and growth promotion with the risk of cancer	The paleo-ketogenic (PK) diet mitigates all these effects
	Nutritional supplements Take extra magnesium 300 mg daily	Good levels of vitamin D and magnesium protect against pre-eclampsia[8]
Stay fit	Labour is called labour for good reasons – it is hard work	Keep exercising
Stock up your First Aid box as in Appendix 2: Groundhog Acute	Mother is relatively immunosuppressed and so at increased risk of infection – all infections are potentially damaging to babies	'By failing to prepare, you are preparing to fail' to quote Benjamin Franklin (17 January 1706 – 17 April 1790), Founding Father of the United States of America, and polymath, known as the 'First American'
Do your best to avoid unnecessary exposure to infection	Toxoplasmosis if acquired in pregnancy carries the risks of miscarriage and birth defects	Now is not the time to get a cat. If you do have one, avoid its turds – that is a Daddy job!
Work especially hard to avoid toxic exposures		See Chapter 25: Reduce the toxic chemical burden
Childbirth – plan for a hospital delivery	We have the technology – let's use it! 'Home deliveries are for pizzas, not babies': Dr Adam Kaye, obstetrician	Childbirth is a dangerous business for Mother and Baby. At any moment Mother risks a major bleed. Obstructed labours are common... and there are other obstetric disasters and unforeseen neonatal complications
Breast feeding		Carry on
Improve energy delivery mechanisms with the PK diet, sleep Check for hypothyroidism	Post-partum depression	Poor energy delivery can result in low mood The keto-adapted baby does not suffer hypoglycaemia; its brain works best running on fat. These babies sleep well so their mothers do also. See the case history 'Green Mother' in Chapter 76

even more whose infertility has been successfully treated by the above interventions. The pioneer of this treatment was Nim Barnes who developed the Foresight regimes: 'Between 2002 and 2009 1578 couples completed the full Foresight programme. Altogether, 1417 babies were born. There was a 89.8% success rate. There were 52 pairs of twins and three sets of triplets. There were 42 miscarriages. Only two single births were premature, no birth defect and no low birth weight babies.'[7]

Pregnancy sickness

The mother's sickness during early pregnancy is a vital part of foetal protection. As detailed above, babies are exquisitely sensitive to toxic stress. All plant food is toxic; if you look at life from the point of view of a plant it does not want to be eaten and so it renders itself as toxic as possible with lectins, alkaloids, glycosides and other such. We humans have a wonderful liver that detoxes to render such plant material less toxic, but even a low level of toxicity is enough to poison the developing foetus. So, Nature – and isn't she so clever to do this (how does she know?) – makes Mother vomit up the nasty foods causing the problem.|

Of course, animals, birds and fish have different defences. They do not need to be toxic because they can escape. This is further reason to eat these foods during early pregnancy and further explains the success of Dr Brewer's work… see next.

Pregnancy anaemia

The mother's haemoglobin level is expected to drop during pregnancy as her blood volume increases. This is normal. The trouble is, many doctors treat 'blind' by prescribing iron supplements. This is sloppy medicine. Iron blocks zinc absorption and one ends up with zinc-deficient babies. Iron should not be prescribed in pregnancy without first checking ferritin levels. If these are low, then use an iron supplement, but take this away from other minerals (or it will block their absorption) and with vitamin C (to enhance absorption). Re-test after three months to make sure levels have corrected.

Pre-eclampsia and eclampsia (high blood pressure, oedema, convulsions and death)

Interestingly this problem is much more common in developing countries and is directly related to poor nutrition. We got a clue from the work of Dr Tom Brewer, an obstetrician working in the poorer states of America in the 1950s, who abolished pre-eclampsia (and premature babies) in 750 patients by feeding them a highly nutritious diet. By contrast the 'control' group of mothers eating 'normal' diets suffered 59 cases of pre-eclampsia, five cases of eclampsia and 37 premature births.[8]

The MAGPIE study, published in the *Lancet* further demonstrated the importance of magnesium. The Royal College of Obstetricians and Gynaecologists concluded: 'Magnesium sulphate

|Footnote: In researching the best foods for pregnancy, I stumbled over the American Pregnancy Association's advice to eat, in the event of nausea and sickness, 'flavoured popsicles' whose ingredients include, amongst others, sugar, corn syrup, gum and aspartame. Dear, oh dear – the antithesis of Groundhog. Indeed, *Groundhog negativus*!

is the therapy of choice to control seizures. A loading dose of 4 g should be given by infusion pump over 5–10 minutes, followed by a further infusion of 1 g/hour maintained for 24 hours after the last seizure. Recurrent seizures should be treated with either a further bolus of 2 g magnesium sulphate or an increase in the infusion rate to 1.5 g or 2.0 g/hour.[9]

Groundhog interventions address all the above issues and should prevent all risk of such complications.

Post-partum depression and psychosis

As you have read in Chapter 50: Psychiatry, so much mental disease arises from poor energy delivery mechanisms. If Mother* believes she does not have the energetic mental, physical and emotional reserves to deal with Baby's needs, then the brain will produce energy-sparing symptoms like depression and fatigue. A baby who is fed a high-carb diet (either because Mother herself eats a high-carb diet and is breast feeding or because all formula milks are full of sugar) cannot sleep for any length of time, so Mother's symptoms are compounded by chronic lack of sleep. Indeed, I know of no better way to induce chronic fatigue than to prevent sleep. Those babies fed a PK diet should sleep 10-12 hours a night – see below.

Breast feeding

Breast milk is best for physical, mental and immune development, for the contented happy baby who sleeps well and for the avoidance of infection – breast milk is full of antibodies which protect baby. But mother needs to eat a PK diet for the best results.

Mother's PK diet is essential

Food that mother consumes is digested in her gut, but small food and fat particles pass directly into her bloodstream and/or lymphatics and straight into the breast milk. If mother is eating a Western diet high in carbohydrates and containing dairy products, this may cause problems for the baby for exactly the same reasons they cause problems for adults, vis:

- Allergy. 'Three-month colic' is common and clearly an allergy issue. Indeed, this was my introduction to allergy. My firstborn, Ruth, had terrible colic. I was up most nights trying to comfort her. My then husband Nick's only comment was, 'You're the effing doctor – you sort it out.' Cutting out the dairy products was a eureka moment – within 24 hours Ruth stopped howling and slept for longer than two-hour stretches.

- Metabolic syndrome – If mother is eating a carbohydrate-based diet, a video of her blood sugar levels would look like the Rocky Mountains. This would be paralleled by sugar levels in her breast milk. As her baby's blood sugar spikes, insulin will be produced and her baby will get too fat. Insulin brings blood sugar down rapidly, the brain panics thinking it is about to run out of fuel, and adrenalin levels shoot up. Baby wakes crying, irritable and fretful, perhaps

---

*Social note: Modern parenting and families do not fit a stereotype. I shall work with the hypothesis that 'Mother' still bears the brunt of the work – I hope the dear reader will both forgive this sweeping generalisation and understand that one has to make such in order to make progress with the intellectual argument. If breast feeding (as one should), then it must be Mother who gets up to do the night-time feeds. But evidence for the bias towards 'Mother' doing the lion's (lioness's?) share of work abounds. For example, a recent study found that 'Fathers relaxed for 47 per cent of the time that their partners were looking after the child, while mothers did the same for only 16 per cent of the time that their partners were performing childcare duties.'[10, 11]

with jerky limb movements.

- Sleep. Adrenalin wakes the sleeping baby. By contrast, the adrenalin free, non-stressed, ketogenic baby sleeps 10-12 hours at night and more in the day. This makes perfect evolutionary sense – a screaming baby at night is an open invitation to predators. Mother needs to forage for food in the day to maintain the supply of breast milk. Not working is not an option.
- Oral thrush. Fill a baby's mouth with sweet milk and it will ferment. The commonest organism to cause this is candida.
- Fermenting upper gut. Fill a baby's upper gut with sweet milk and it will ferment. This results in wind (the need to be 'burped'), posseting and vomiting.
- Fermenting skin. High blood sugar means sugars seep onto the skin and are colonised, usually by fungi. Cradle cap is a fungal infection of the scalp. Most nappy rashes are fungal infections of the groin.
- Abnormal fermenting microbes and so offensive nappies. The nappies of PK breast-fed babies are almost odourless.

All this makes perfect evolutionary sense. The restless, irritable, sleepless, screaming, smelly baby will alert predators to the possibility of an easy meal.

Breast milk is full of antibodies which protect babies from infection. All vitamins that mother consumes will pass into her breast milk. Great. Importantly, vitamin C passes through and protects her baby at this vulnerable age. This gives us all the more reason not to vaccinate since the baby is perfectly protected by mother's breast milk. Should any snuffle develop, this is effectively and safely treated as below.

Protection from allergies

The baby's immune system learns to accept that which it is exposed to (see 'Reprogramming the immune system' in Chapter 16). Mothers have been told not to wean babies with nuts on the grounds this may trigger allergy. Actually, the reverse is true. Babies raised in Israel are fed a peanut-based rusk ('Bamba') and peanut allergy there is rare. Du Toit et al, in their study looking at this phenomenon concluded that: 'The early introduction of peanuts significantly decreased the frequency of the development of peanut allergy among children at high risk for this allergy and modulated immune responses to peanuts.'[12]

Babies receiving PK breast milk can be safely weaned onto PK foods at 4 months, because their immune system has already been exposed to these. As detailed in Chapter 16, mother chews her PK food to ensure it is soft, free from bones, mixed with her saliva and easily swallowed. Kissing is a useful evolutionary tool to transfer the food into the baby's mouth. Indeed, this is why (as I say in the earlier chapter) kissing, and breasts are so attractive to men – they need to know their partners can feed their offspring well. (As previously noted also, 'smart is sexy' too; perhaps this is because intelligent partners will look after both the offspring and the man? – Craig)

Good for mother. Breast feeding causes nipple stimulation with release of the love hormone oxytocin. Mothers need to be in love with their babies because without such they would not care and without that no baby will thrive.

Remember the breast-fed baby may not gain weight as fast as the bottle-fed. This is usually cause for midwives to bully vulnerable mothers. The infant weight charts are set for breast-fed babies. When I was working in the NHS, it was my experience that the midwives were not happy until the baby's cheeks met in front of its nose. But fat babies make for fat adults and that shortens life. The rough rule-of-thumb is that babies should have doubled their birth weight at six months and tripled it at one year.

Do not vaccinate

Chapter 51 explains why not. We do not need to vaccinate because we have far safer methods of dealing with infection. Indeed, childhood febrile (feverish) illness is an essential part of immune programming that stands us in good stead for life. Breast feeding is highly protective against infection.

Weaning

This can be easy. When baby shows an interest, which may be at 4 months, feed a PK diet, as above. From an immune perspective, the weaning diet is then the same as breast[†] milk. I would recommend continuing with breast feeding for as long as socially and comfortably possible – ideally at least one year.

Cot death

The Richardson Report into cot death elegantly explains all the facts of the cot death epidemic. This is something all parents with babies need to know about. The idea is biologically plausible: all mattresses are impregnated with fire retardants, antimony and phosphorus, often with arsenic as a contaminant. When a baby lies on a mattress, inevitably secretions fall into the mattress through posseting, saliva, nasal secretions or vomit. This allows the growth of the fungus, *Scopulariopsis brevicaulis*. This fungus feeds on human secretions and is normally present in all bedding materials which are rich in such. However, this fungus attacks fire retardants in such a way as to release poisonous gases – namely, phosphine, stibine and arsine. These gases are heavier than air, so they concentrate in the mattress. Babies may be much more susceptible to these poisons than adults. The early symptoms of poisoning are headache and irritability. They may cause death, possibly through respiratory depression or heart failure, because they act as cholinesterase inhibitors, in the same way as organophoshates. These are the same chemicals as those used in germ warfare and in pesticides (their effects are probably similar to nerve gases used in chemical warfare).

This hypothesis explains the facts of cot death:

- Cot death is unknown in Japan where boron is used as a fire retardant. However, when the Japanese come to live in the West and use our bedding materials, they experience the same incidence of cot death.
- It occurs more often during a mild illness when a baby has a temperature. An increase in a baby's body temperature from 37 degrees (normal) to 42 degrees causes a 20-fold increase in poison gas production.
- It occurs more in winter when parents overwrap their babies and turn the central heating on. Many deaths occur in the early morning when the central heating turns on automatically. Indeed, the incidence of cot deaths exactly parallels heating bills.
- It is more common in boys because their metabolic rate is 15% higher than girls so they are more likely to overheat.
- It is uncommon in first-born babies on new mattresses because the fungus has not had time to establish itself in the mattress.

[†]**Linguistic note:** Depending on where you look, there are well in excess of 100 words in the English language to describe the female breast. *Cosmopolitan* magazine lists 101 here: www.cosmopolitan.com/uk/body/a47859/101-different-names-boobs/ *The Oxford Dictionaries* online list the archaic form 'embonpoint' from the French meaning 'in good condition'. A British term is 'bristols'; one theory is that this is rhyming Cockney slang with the English League football team, 'Bristol City' and that Bristol was 'chosen' rather than, say Leicester City, for the added benefit of alliteration. I could go on, but I won't! Craig.

Subsequent children are less likely to have a new mattress and second-hand mattresses will already be inoculated with the fungus. Deaths in babies under one month have always been on mattresses previously used by other children. There is a high incidence of cot death in Armed Service families who are provided with mattresses (which will already have been infected with *Scopulariopsis brevicaulis*) in their houses.

- Babies who lie on their tummies inhale gases directly from the mattress. Cot death is less common in babies over 5 months because by this time they are strong enough to lift their heads off the mattress or rollover and avoid inhaling the poison gases.
- Babies dying of cot death have abnormally high levels of antimony in their blood (from stibine gas).
- The high incidence of cot death in Aborigine babies is due to their use of sheepskins for babies to sleep on. There are high levels of arsenic in sheep wool (arsenic levels are high in the soil and it is excreted in the wool); this is broken down by the fungus to produce arsine gas which kills the babies.
- Cot death is more common in low birth weight or otherwise disadvantaged babies, probably because they are more susceptible to poisoning.

Prevention of cot death

As a result of this report, specific recommendations have been made:

- All mattresses should be covered with polythene to prevent release of poisonous gases. They should be washed regularly or replaced. (My personal advice would be also to use a folded cotton sheet which could be washed regularly to clear out secretions and get rid of the fungus. Best of all would be a Japanese futon/mattress that uses boron

as a fire retardant.) 'Vented mattresses' are particularly bad because they allow large accumulations of posset, vomit, nasal secretions, saliva etc to accumulate in them and encourage heavy growth of the fungus.
- Babies should not be overwrapped (I recommend in particular the head should never be covered as this is a vital cooling device.) A window should be left open in the bedroom and central heating set at a minimum level.
- Babies should be laid on their backs, not on their tummies. This advice of course explains the success of the 'Back to Sleep' campaign. It has been estimated that this advice alone has saved the lives of 15,000 babies between 1991 and 2014.

I now hear (to be confirmed) that phosporus, arsenic and antimony compounds are no longer used as fire retardants in mattresses. However, it is likely they have been replaced by poly-brominated biphenyls (PBBs). These are also toxic compounds, which may or may not contribute to cot death but are extremely toxic in their own right and no baby should be exposed to them. One should also be aware that sheepskins may come from sheep that have been dipped and those dipping chemicals, which may include organophosphates, may still be present in the wool. I think the above advice for mattress for babies holds good – that is, choose a natural, organic material that can be regularly washed, such as organic cotton or organic wool for all the baby's bedclothes.

References

1. McKay P. Review of *Pottenger's Cats A Study in Nutrition, 1939* 2008. https://pdfs.semanticscholar.org/adc0/34665300a4919735a60ee534d43971bdfd21.pdf (accessed 28 November 2019)
2. Paul C, Harrison-Woolrych M. Stilboestrol gone

but not forgotten. *MedSafe: Prescriber Update* 2006; 27(1): 9-11. https://medsafe.govt.nz/profs/PUarticles/DES2006.htm (accessed 28 November 2019)

3. Genova Diagnostics. Toxic Effects CORE. www.gdx.net/product/toxic-effects-core-test-urine-blood (accessed 28 November 2019)

4. Dewailly E, Ayotte P, Bruneau S, Laliberte C, Muir DC, Norstrum RJ. Inuit exposure to organochlorines through the aquatic food chain in arctic Québec. *Environ Health Perspect* 1993; 101(7): 618–620. www.ncbi.nlm.nih.gov/pmc/articles/PMC1519892/

5. Bridges C. Effect of DMPS and DMSA on the placental and fetal deposition of methylmercury. *Placenta* 2009; 30(9): 800–805. doi: 10.1289/ehp.93101618 www.ncbi.nlm.nih.gov/pmc/articles/PMC2739879/

6. CDC. Vaccine Excipient Summary: Excipients included in US Vaccines, by Vaccine. January 2019. www.cdc.gov/vaccines/pubs/pinkbook/downloads/appendices/B/excipient-table-2.pdf (accessed 28 November 2019)

7. Barnes N. *How to Conceive Healthy Babies – the natural way.* New Generation Publishing, 2014.

8. Jones J. The Dr Brewer Pregnancy Diet: Pre-eclampsia. www.drbrewerpregnancydiet.com/id36.html (accessed 28 November 2019)

9. The Magpie Trial Collaborative Group. Do women with pre-eclampsia, and their babies, benefit from magnesium sulphate? The Magpie Trial – a random placebo-controlled trial. *Lancet* 2002; 359(9321): 1877-1890. doi: https://doi.org/10.1016/S0140-6736(02)08778-0 www.thelancet.com/journals/lancet/article/PIIS0140-6736(02)08778-0/fulltext

10. www.medicalnewstoday.com/articles/319687.php

11. Parker K. Despite progress, women still bear heavier load than men in balancing work and family. Pew Research Center, 10 March 2015. www.pewresearch.org/fact-tank/2015/03/10/women-still-bear-heavier-load-than-men-balancing-work-family/ (accessed 28 November 2019)

12. Du Toit G, Roberts G, Sayre PH, Bahnson HT, et al. Randomized Trial of Peanut Consumption in Infants at Risk for Peanut Allergy. *N Engl J Med* 2015; 372: 803-813. doi: 10.1056/NEJMoa1414850 www.nejm.org/doi/full/10.1056/NEJMoa1414850?query=featured_home#t=article

Chapter 56
Paediatrics

> *Those who educate children well are more to be honoured than they who produce them; for these only gave them life, those the art of living well.*
> Aristotle, Greek philosopher,
> 384 BC – 322 BC

Apply all that has gone before in this book (and see Chapter 38 on how to slow the ageing process for an overview). Remember that one has to be as principled with children as with adults. Perhaps more so since a healthy childhood makes for a healthy adult. In raising children on carbohydrate diets, we are simply imposing our addictions on them and setting them up for an addictive tendency for life. They cope with the stresses of adolescence through addiction, which may manifest with eating disorders, binge drinking, smoking or vaping, or other such legal and/or illegal highs. This is bad education.

I am very fortunate that my mother was a good cook and strict in matters of food. Snacking was a cardinal sin. We always sat down to a fry-up for breakfast and a proper cooked lunch or supper based on meat and vegetables. Otherwise, it was leftovers. Of course, we enjoyed the occasional carbohydrate bonanza. I rarely recall being hungry or even thinking much about food. I was as happy spending pocket money on *The Beano** as on a bull's eye gobstopper. The point here is that children raised on PK diets do not feel deprived – they simply accept such as the norm. This is proper education.

The vaccination question

Do not vaccinate your children for two good reasons:
* Vaccination does not prevent disease and we have excellent Groundhog tools of proven benefit which are completely safe.
* Vaccination has serious side effects which may persist for life. For details of the why see Chapter 51: Immunology.

---

*Literary note: *The Beano* is the longest-running British children's comic magazine, first appearing on 30th July 1938. Dennis the Menace only made his first appearance in issue number 452. During the Second World War, paper shortages meant the comic was reduced to 12 pages every two weeks.

Table 56.1: Common problems in children not raised according to Groundhog principles

Problem	Why	Reason to do Groundhog especially
Tooth decay	Fermenting mouth	PK diet Toothbrushing does little to prevent tooth decay See Chapter 45: Dentists
Colic, eczema, rhinitis, asthma, croup	Allergy, most often to dairy	PK diet Also see Chapter 51: Immunology
	May also be triggered by infection	Groundhog Acute
Coughs, colds and ear infections (kids are 'expected' to have eight episodes a year[1]) Gastroenteritis	Poor immunity. Any such infection should be minor and pass within 24 hours	Groundhog Acute
Gut symptoms – tummy ache, burping, bloating	Allergy, fermenting gut	PK diet Vitamin C
Acute febrile illnesses	A vital part of immune programming	Groundhog Acute Do not suppress symptoms Good nursing care: rest, warmth, fluids, love Vitamin C Iodine salt pipe for respiratory symptoms Topical iodine oil for mumps, chicken pox lesions, swollen lymph nodes
Joint pain	Allergy to foods Allergy to microbes from the fermenting gut	PK diet Vitamin C to bowel tolerance
Anxiety disorders, depression, and attention deficit hyperactivity disorder, eating disorders and anorexia/bulimia	See Chapter 50: Psychiatry Carbohydrate addiction Immunotoxicity Toxicity Fermenting brain Poor energy delivery mechanisms	Easy to treat with the PK diet Do not vaccinate (see Chapter 51) Detox regimes (see Chapters 8, 15, 25 and 34) Treat as for fermenting gut – PK diet, vitamin C to bowel tolerance Improve energy delivery (see Chapters 5, 11, 12, 13, 14, 30)
Autism, atypical autism, Asperger's, Rett's, childhood disintegrative disorder	These are not diagnoses but psychiatric clinical pictures (see Chapter 50 and below)	Good results achieved with all the above and Groundhog Chronic (see Appendix 3) Especially consider immunotoxicity from vaccinations (see Chapter 51) and toxicity

Graham Worrall[1] states that:

'On average, adults get 4 to 6 colds per year, while children get 6 to 8 of them.'

> Boyhood, like measles, is one of those complaints which a man should catch young and have done with, for when it comes in middle life it is apt to be serious.
> P.G Wodehouse, English author and humourist, 15 October 1881 – 14 February 1975

Acute febrile illness in children

Children are no longer allowed to be ill. Parents are encouraged to suppress symptoms at the first sign of any. But the immune system needs educating, just as the brain does. Depriving the child's immune system of exposure to the soil in our organic gardens, the friendly lick of our beloved pets and the contact of grubby pals is like depriving our brains of sight, hearing, touch and smell. Just as the brain must experience all to survive, so must the immune system.

Allow children to be exposed to the infections that have been with us for thousands of years. An educated immune system protects us from future nasties, including cancer. With Groundhog interventions we can reduce the threat of a terrifying book to an Enid Blyton jolly, but both teach us to read. (My particular love was *The Secret Island*.)

> Provided no mischief can be done either by physician or nurse, it is the most safe and slight of all diseases.
> Sir Thomas Sydenham on smallpox[†]

Autism, atypical autism, Asperger's, Rett's, childhood disintegrative disorder

We have an epidemic of special needs ('special educational needs and disability' or SEND) children, with these problems affecting an estimated one in seven.[2] It has been predicted that by 2025 50% of US kids will be autistic. There have to be ecological reasons for this epidemic; there are many biologically plausible players, with an obvious cocktail effect. The sooner one can treat these children, the better the results. And results are often very good.

[†]**Footnote:** Thomas Sydenham (10 September 1624 – 29 December 1689) was an English physician and the author of *Observationes Medicae*. This text survived as a standard medical reference book for over 200 years and led to Sydenham being known as the 'English Hippocrates'.

Table 56.2: Causes of SENDs in children and what to do about them

Trigger	Mechanism	Treatment
Vaccination	Direct poisoning by aluminium, mercury or other such (see Chapter 51)	Get rid of toxic metals (see Chapter 34)
	Immune toxicity	Reduce inflammation (see Chapter 36)
	Chronic infection	Groundhog Chronic (Appendix 3)
Western diets	Addiction Adrenalin of metabolic syndrome Allergy	PK diet
Abnormal gut microbiome	Associated with fermenting brain. Dr Andrew Wakefield found live measles virus in the bowel wall of autistic kids... as did many other doctors!	PK diet Vitamin C to bowel tolerance See Chapter 44: Gastroenterology
Pesticide exposure		Get rid of VOCs etc (see Chapter 25: Reduce the toxic chemical burden)
Mycotoxins		See Chapter 51: Immunology

If you have any doubts about the veracity of the vaccination-autism link, see the film *Vaxxed*. This details a whistle-blower within the American CDC (Centers for Disease Control and Prevention), Dr William Thompson, who released unpublished CDC research data clearly showing a link between vaccination and autism. This was particularly strong in African American boys. Had Thompson published the data, then he would have been arrested under the Official Secrets Act. Meanwhile, Robert F Kennedy Jr and the Children's Health Defense were recently able to obtain CDC records through a FOIA request for the unvaccinated study done back in 1999. The results were damning against vaccines but were not made public.[4] The film invited Congress to investigate the claim so that unpublished data could be properly analysed and to protect Thompson from a jail sentence. Congress has yet to rise to this challenge. Why? Autism is the most expensive disease ever – sufferers need care for life. Should a link be proven, compensation cases would follow that would bankrupt the country. As ever, follow the money.

Having said that, several courts have accepted the link between vaccination and autism and have settled for large amounts. The Hannah Poling case was followed by 70 others. In Italy, the courts awarded Ryan Mojabi and his family a multi-million-dollar settlement for autism as the result of an injury from the measles-mumps-rubella (MMR) vaccine.

Genetic diseases

There is a tendency to ascribe problems to the genes so that 'nothing more can be done'. Nonsense. Dr Henry Turkel greatly improved the health of children with Down's syndrome through attention to diet, supplements and hypothyroidism. Any genetic disease may be tackled using all the principles in this book. For a quick review of Turkel's work in this area please see www.doctoryourself.com/turkel.html – *Down Syndrome: The Nutritional Treatment of Henry Turkel, MD*.

We began with Aristotle and we shall finish with him:

> *Give me a child until he is 7 and I will show you the [wo]man.*
>
> Aristotle, Greek philosopher,
> 384 BC – 322 BC

References

1. Worrall G. Common Cold *Can Fam Physician* 2011; 57(11): 1289–1290. www.ncbi.nlm.nih. gov/pmc/articles/PMC3215607/
2. Hutchinson J. How many children have SEND? Education Policy Institute, 24 November 2017. https://epi.org.uk/publications-and-research/ many-children-send/ (accessed 28 November 2019)
3. Alliance for Natural Health. Half of all children with be autistic by 2025, warns senior research scientist at MIT. Alliance for Natural Health, 23 December 2014. www.anh-usa. org/half-of-all-children-will-be-autistic-by-2025-warns-senior-research-scientist-at-mit/ (accessed 28 November 2019)
4. Vaccinated vs. Unvaccinated. Children's Health Defense. https://childrenshealthdefense.org/?s=V accinated+vs+unvaccinated

Chapter 57
Haematology

Anaemia

The term 'anaemia' simply means not enough blood. With such, there is poor delivery of essential nutrients, including oxygen. So, anaemia presents with symptoms of poor energy delivery (see Chapter 5).

One can be anaemic either because of loss of blood through haemorrhage or because the bone marrow is going slow and not producing enough red blood cells. Both are potentially significant, and anaemia should always be taken seriously. It is easily diagnosed from a blood test and this can be easily done by your GP or on a DIY finger-drop sample of blood (see www.natural-healthworldwide.com).

Common causes of blood loss

Common causes of blood loss include:
- heavy periods
- bleeding in the gut: blood may not be easily seen in the stools and should be looked for in every case of anaemia. Ask

for faecal occult blood testing. This may be an early sign of cancer. Faecal calprotectin is a good test for inflammation in the bowel and may become a useful screening test for cancer.
- the red blood cells are breaking up too soon. This may be associated with haemolytic anaemia (e.g. sickle cell disease), thalassaemia, red cell membrane defects (due to poor antioxidant status), red cell enzyme defects (glucose 6 phosphate deficiency), autoimmunity, or hypersplenism (due to other disease such as cirrhosis of the liver).

Common causes of bone marrow going slow

The bone marrow may be going slow due to:
- **Poor energy delivery mechanisms:** At medical school I was intrigued by 'the anaemia of chronic disease'. This simply meant that many conditions were associated with anaemia, but no mechanism was mooted. Of course, it is obvious now – any chronic disease is associated either with poor energy delivery mechanisms and/or with a lack of raw materials (because they are needed elsewhere). The bone marrow is very busy – it normally replaces all blood platelets every eight days, white cells every 20 days and red cells every 115 days. It is full of fat to supply the fuel for this business and full of raw materials, including essential minerals – that is what

makes bone marrow the most delicious and nutritious food.

- **Lack of raw materials**: The commonest rate-limiting steps are lack of iron and/or vitamin B12.
- **Insufficient bone marrow** due to disease such as leukaemia, cancer, myelofibrosis etc.
- **Poisoning**: This may include prescription drugs, carbon monoxide, toxic metals such as lead, alcohol and pesticides.

The effects of smoking

Smoking causes an odd sort of anaemia. Carbon monoxide in cigarette smoke binds to haemoglobin and displaces oxygen. Consequently, we have red blood cells circulating which are not carrying any oxygen. The body tries to compensate by making more red blood cells, and as a result one can end up with too much blood (polycythaemia) whilst still showing the symptoms of anaemia. This type of anaemia may not be obvious on a blood test; it has to be suspected clinically.

Treatment for anaemia

As in other chapters, treatment is to:
- Identify the cause
- Start Groundhog Chronic interventions (Appendix C),
- Improve energy delivery mechanisms (Chapter 30).

Thrombosis

Thrombosis is when blood clots in the arteries and/or veins. It is an important subject because blood thinners are widely advocated to prevent such, but this is risky medicine because of the likelihood of bleeding. The key is to identify what results in sticky blood and address those factors. In order of importance we have:
- Sugar: This is sticky stuff and results in sticky blood. Do a PK diet (Chapter 21).
- Hugh's syndrome: This is an autoimmune condition and can be diagnosed with a blood test for antiphospholipid antibodies. It often presents with recurrent miscarriage.
- Vitamin K deficiency: Vitamin K has the highly desirable property of lining blood vessels so that if the blood vessel is intact it inhibits clotting, but when broken it promotes clotting. It is present in green leafy vegetable but is also synthesised by microbes in the gut.
- Damage to the lining of blood vessels which makes them sticky (see arteriosclerosis in cardiology Chapter 42)
- High homocysteine (again see Chapter 42: Cardiology)
- Smoking
- Lack of movement: This may be the result of surgery, enforced stillness (long journeys, workplace conditions) and bed rest.

Embolism

This is when those clots (thrombosis) break off to cause blockage downstream (see Chapters 49 Neurology and 42 Cardiology).

If the clots break off from the lining of the heart or the lining of arteries, then they can pass to any part of the body: head, gut, arms, legs. Clinically this presents with a stroke, acute gut ischaemia with severe pain or acute limb ischaemia with severe pain.

If the clot breaks off from the lining of a vein it passes through the heart and gets stuck in the lungs, causing a pulmonary embolus. Rarely it may pass through a hole in the heart resulting in stroke etc (as above).

Superficial venous thrombosis and thrombophlebitis

If such a blockage occurs in the arms, then there will be other serious pathology – see a doctor PDQ! However, it usually occurs in the legs because the pressure of blood in the veins is highest there. Blood clots in veins leave a tender, worm-shaped lump. Yes, this is uncomfortable, but the clot remains where it formed – this is not a medical emergency. However, it is a wake-up call – you have just had a lucky escape. Address your risk factors before they kill you.

Deep venous thrombosis (DVT)*

DVT is much more serious as there is potential for the clot to break off and travel to the lungs, causing a pulmonary embolus. It requires immediate diagnosis and anticoagulants to treat it. A typical clinical picture would be an immobile patient with the above risk factors, acute pain in a warm leg and 'pitting oedema' (swelling that occurs due to an accumulation of fluid), with swelling of the calf muscle.

I do not recommend dust from the stone of King Louis IX's tomb for DVTs but rather I see this as a wake-up call to do Groundhog Chronic. My guess is Raoul got more benefit from his long walk to the tomb!

Reference

1. Galanaud JP, Laroche JP, Righini M. The history and historical treatments of deep vein thrombosis. *J Thromb Haemost* 2013; 11(3): 402-411. doi: 10.1111/jth.12127. www.ncbi.nlm.nih.gov/pubmed/23297815

*Historical note: The first well-documented case of DVT is from 1271. Unilateral swelling and oedema were reported in the leg and ankle of Raoul, a 20-year-old Norman cobbler. Subsequently, a leg ulcer formed, and Raoul was advised to visit the tomb of King Louis IX of France to seek healing. Raoul did as he was told and rubbed dust from the stone covering the king's tomb into the wound. The wound healed, and Raoul lived for 11 more years.[1]

Chapter 58
Prescription drugs

– prescription drugs and prescribing doctors are dangerous
– my hates should be your hates

One of the first duties of the physician is to educate the masses not to take medicine.
Sir William Osler, 1st Baronet, FRS FRCP,
Canadian physician,
12 July 1849 – 29 December 1919

*Of the dreaded Sir Roderick Glossop, a doctor in New York, visiting a patient:
'a bald-domed, bushy-browed blighter, ostensibly a nerve specialist, but in reality, as everyone knows, nothing more nor less than a high-priced loony-doctor.'*
P G Wodehouse, English author,
15 October 1881 – 14 February 1975

Though the doctors treated him, let his blood, and gave him medications to drink, he nevertheless recovered.
Tolstoy in *War and Peace*, Russian author,
9 September 1828 – 20 November 1910

Drugs, and those who prescribe them, are dangerous because, with a few exceptions, they suppress symptoms. The patient is no longer alerted to serious malfunction and proceeds through life as if all is well. Red warning flags of disease are ignored because they can be. It is the old story: drugs afford short-term gain but long-term pain. When prescribed by a reassuring, highly paid professional, apparently backed by the latest hard-nosed science, it is difficult to resist. We then have the soft background noise of the media further herding us to short-term ease and apparent safety. We are being ushered to premature death by established institutions, great kindness and gentle professionalism.

In October 2010 I was suspended from the General Medical Council register because I stated on my website that doctors were dangerous. I was told that by doing so I was bringing the reputation of the medical profession into disrepute. Other reasons for such suspension were given but this was the only correct reason which, incidentally, I was rather proud of. I took this GMC decision to Judicial Review but, despite no new evidence being presented, the GMC reinstated my licence to practice before my case could be heard in the High Court.

These doctors and drugs are an illusion of treatment.

> *The most dangerous thing is illusion.*
> Ralph Waldo Emerson,* American
> essayist, lecturer, philosopher, and poet,
> 25 May 1803 – 27 April 1882

Red warning flags are meant to be uncomfortable because this motivates. Change is always difficult. A serious symptom such as pain does not half concentrate the mind and stimulate an action to avoid the cause. Perhaps the check list in Table 58.1 will make for such uncomfortable reading that you too will be inspired to make the difficult Groundhog interventions and wean yourself off these drugs. Remember you must put Groundhog in place first BEFORE you stop the drugs and monitor the effects.

Table 58.1: Commonly prescribed drugs, their risks and ways to mitigate the damage

Which drug	Why dangerous?	What does it increase the risk of	What you can do to mitigate in addition to Groundhog interventions
Statins	Blocks endogenous production of coenzyme Q10 thereby impairing energy delivery to all cells	Accelerates the ageing process	Co Q10 100 mg daily for life See Chapter 38 for how to slow the ageing process
Stomach acid blockers e.g. proton pump inhibitors (PPIs), H2 blockers, antacids	Stomach acid is essential to digest protein, absorb minerals and prevent upper gut fermentation and infections	Osteoporosis, infections, gut tumours Accelerate ageing	PK diet Vitamin C to bowel tolerance Digestive enzymes
Asthma inhalers Nasal sprays	Open up the airways so infection and pollutants get into the lungs Steroid inhalers suppress the immune system	Accelerate lung damage Chest infections	Saltpipe with iodine
Diabetic drugs	Risk of hypoglycaemia – to mitigate this risk, doctors like patients to run a higher than normal blood sugar	All disease, especially infections, arterial disease, dementia, cancer	PK diet – see our book *Prevent and Cure Diabetes*

*Footnote: Emerson suffered from dementia towards his final years but in typical fashion, when asked how he was, he would reply. 'Quite well; I have lost my mental faculties, but am perfectly well.'

Arthritis drugs e.g. NSAIDs... aspirin	Suppress the immune system so healing, and repair are blocked The gut lining is normally replaced every three days but NSAIDs slow this process. Consequently, holes appear resulting in leaky gut and bleeding. Disturb the microbiome	Degenerative disease so bleeding from the gut Increased risk of infection Arterial disease, kidney damage	See Chapter 47: Rheumatology
...and other immuno-suppressants e.g. steroids, and '-imabs'	As above but more rapidly and severely	Ditto	Ditto
Paracetamol	Kidney damage and death with remarkably small doses	Ditto	Glutathione prevents toxicity See below
Diuretics	Increase the loss of all minerals from the urine	All disease!	Sunshine salt to replace losses Vitamin C is a mild diuretic
ACE inhibitors e.g. captopril, ramipril Lisinopril	Slightly anti-inflammatory and so suppress the immune system	Increase risk of cancer, especially lung cancer	PK diet
Calcium antagonists	Big Pharma's substitute for magnesium Interfere with cell communication	Increase risk of cancer	PK diet
Major tranquillisers	Suppress energy delivery mechanisms Induce metabolic syndrome	Accelerated ageing	
SSRIs	Addictive	High risk of suicide, especially when first used	
Opiate-like painkillers, e.g. codeine, tramadol	Addictive Immunosuppressive	Increase risk of infection and cancer	

The Big Pharma story

Do not trust Big Pharma where profits are generally more important than patients.

The Pill and HRT story

My good friend and colleague Dr Ellen Grant recognised the serious side-effects of these hormones during the 1960s when she was working as a pathologist. We know they all increase the risk of cancer, arterial and heart disease, diabetes and probably dementia because they induce metabolic syndrome, are growth promoting, immunosuppressant and addictive. Big Pharma has invested trillions in covering these facts up. Why? Because there is a huge market. There is potential for every woman in the world to spend much of her life taking these hormones. Follow the money.

The paracetamol story

If paracetamol had been recently developed it would never have been licensed let alone made available as an over-the-counter drug. That is because the toxic dose is so low compared with its therapeutic dose. A small overdose kills. But this it largely preventable with glutathione and/ or methionine. Indeed, this is the antidote in the event of paracetamol overdose. Drug companies got their heads together and decided that all paracetamol tablets should contain methionine to render paracetamol completely safe. This never actually happened because this would increase the cost by a few pence per tablet. Follow the money.

The statin story

Statins reduce blood total cholesterol levels but as we know this has little to do with arterial disease (see Chapter 42: Cardiology). A compelling fact is that one would expect a dose-related response – i.e. that lowering the cholesterol should lower the risk of arterial damage – but this is not the case because cholesterol is a symptom of damage, not a cause of it. The effects of statins may be explained by their being vitamin D mimics and vitamin D is a great anti-inflammatory. I suspect statins could be safely replaced by vitamin D, and this is part of Groundhog. Worse, statins inhibit the endogenous production of co-Q10, and this accelerates the ageing process (see Chapter 38: How to slow the ageing process). Drug

companies got their heads together and decided that all statins should contain co-Q10 to mitigate such. This never actually happened because this would increase the cost by a few pence per tablet. Is this starting to sound familiar? Follow the money.

The Vioxx story

Vioxx was launched in 1999 as an NSAID that did not cause gut bleeding. Rheumatologists in Europe were offered a free first class return on the Orient Express to Venice where they were feted by Merck. Vioxx prescribing took off. I first heard of problems with it when reading the business section of the *Daily Telegraph*, which reported that Merck shares had fallen sharply as their wonder drug had been estimated to have killed 160,000 people through its promotion of heart attacks and strokes. In 2005 Vioxx was withdrawn from the market. Merck had known of these (underwhelmingly described) 'side effects' from a paper published in 2000,[1] but had kept schtum. Follow the money.

In December 2005, the *New England Journal of Medicine* issued an Expression of Concern regarding a paper by the VIGOR Study Group that had been the foundation of the drug's positive image.[1] This Expression of Concern[2] was with respect to three additional myocardial infarctions in the patients studied which were known to at least two of the paper's authors before the publication date and yet were not disclosed in the paper. In the Expression of Concern, the editors stated that: 'The fact that these three myocardial infarctions were not included made certain calculations and conclusions in the article incorrect.' This brought into question the validity of the VIGOR paper's conclusions about the safety of Vioxx upon which Bombardier et al had written favourably.[3]

The thalidomide story

The perfect safe drug for pregnancy anxiety and sickness was created in 1953 in West Germany by Chemie Grünenthal. The first case report of the serious birth defect phocomelia appeared in 1956. A further 10,000 cases appeared in Germany, all linked to thalidomide. Regardless, in 1958 the UK distributor Distillers brought thalidomide to the UK where a further estimated 2000 babies suffered. Worldwide, perhaps a total of 24,000 babies suffered. In 1961, the Australian Dr William McBride published his findings in the *Lancet*,[4] and the cat was out the bag and the drug banned. The drug companies already knew full well of the link but did not voluntarily withdraw the drug. Why not? Follow the money.

The Prozac story

Tryptophan, an amino acid, is an effective antidepressant and was widely used on NHS prescription during the 1980s. It is the precursor for serotonin and probably fermented in the gut to such. We know *E coli* does this. At last! A safe, effective, cheap, physiological treatment for low mood. You would think it impossible for Big Pharma to effectively abolish such a treatment? But tryptophan was a potential competitor to Big Pharma's new tranche of drugs – the SSRIs. A contaminated batch of tryptophan came onto the market from a single company in Japan, Showa Denko, and only this batch produced a side effect – namely, eosinophilic myalgic syndrome. Big Pharma pounced on this opportunity and the propaganda that followed resulted in the effective banning of all the known-to-be-safe tryptophan preparations from the pharmacopoeia. Why? Follow the money.

The homocysteine story

High homocysteine is a major risk factor for arterial disease, dementia and cancer. It is easily, safely and inexpensively treated with B vitamins (see Chapter 42: Cardiology). So why is this not standard medical practice? Why is homocysteine not the familiar word that cholesterol is in our language? Follow the money.

The Ro-Accutane story

First do no harm. The manufacturers of Ro-A pretend not to know its mechanism of action, but we can get a clue since Ro-A was developed for cancer chemotherapy because it permanently kills cells. It is also teratogenic. It is effective in acne by permanently destroying sebum cells, but it destroys other cells too. Ro-A was taken off the market in 2009 because of massive lawsuits involving depression, suicide, birth defects, severe persistent headache, psychosis and much more. It is still available as isotretinoin. Why still available? Follow the money.

The magnesium story

Intravenous magnesium was found to be such a brilliant drug to treat acute chest pain that it was in danger of becoming front-line therapy. It would be very safe for GPs and paramedics alike to use. It is a powerful vasodilator and clot buster so affords cheap and instant pain relief as well as preventing cardiac muscle death (myocardial infarction – MI). It is a great anti-arrhythmic and prevents serious complications, such as ventricular fibrillation (VF). This dysrhythmia is much beloved of hospital-based soap operas where VF and need for defibrillation are an essential for every plot. Magnesium would spoil their fun too.

Big Pharma suddenly became aware that cheap, safe, highly effective magnesium was about to expunge their profits, whoops, I mean their prescriptions. It sponsored a study to look at the benefits of magnesium in acute myocardial infarction. Hitherto, the dose of magnesium shown to be of optimum effect had been 80 mmol delivered over 24 hours. The study was set up using 120 mmol over 24 hours – known to be a toxic dose (he who pays the piper calls the tune). The magnesium toxicity effects mitigated its beneficial effects to produce a conclusion that magnesium was useless. This is research misconduct and was reported as such in the *Journal of Nutritional & Environmental Medicine* by Dr Downing.[5] But it was great news for Big Pharma: drugs for acute MI were back on the menu. Follow the money.

Dr Sam Browne taught me about intravenous magnesium and a very useful tool that has been.[6]

Postscript

I hardly dare submit the manuscript for this book to my lovely publisher Georgina because I keep thinking of new topics that I should have added, and Craig keeps coming back with more questions. I hope we have at least inspired you to ask the right questions and motivated you to make the difficult changes. We shall make updates whenever possible, but you must walk the path knowing that others too have struggled:

> *The only true wisdom is knowing you know nothing.*
> Socrates, Classical Greek Philosopher,
> died 399 BC

> *Curiosity is one of the most prominent in certain characteristics of a vigorous intellect.*
> Samuel Johnson, English writer,
> 18 September 1709 – 13 December 1784

> *Perfection is not attainable, but if we chase perfection, we can catch excellence.*
> Vince Lombardi, American football player, coach and executive,
> 11 June 1913 – 3 September 1970

Now we move onto some case histories that have occured during my medical practice. These cases demonstrate the principles that we have laid out in the book so far.

References

1. Bombardier C, Laine L, Reicin A, Shapiro D, et al. Comparison of upper gastrointestinal toxicity of rofecoxib and naproxen in patients with rheumatoid arthritis. VIGOR Study Group. *New England Journal of Medicine* 2000; 343: 1520-1528.
2. Curfman GD, Morrissey S, Drazen JM. Expression of Concern: Bombardier et al, 'Comparison of upper gastrointestinal toxicity of Rafecoxib and Naproxen in patients with rheumatoid arthritis. New Engl J Med 2000; 343: 1520-8. *New Engl J Med* 2005; 353: 2813-2814. DOI: 10.1056/NEJMe058314
3. Wadman M. Journal grows suspicious of Vioxx data. *Nature* 2005; 438: 899. doi:10.1038/438899b
4. McBride W. Thalidomide and congenital abnormalities. *Lancet* 1961; 278 (7216): 1358. doi.org/10.1016/S0140-6736(61)90927-8
5. Downing D. Is ISIS-4 research misconduct? *Journal of Nutritional & Environmental Medicine* 1999; 9(1): 5-13. www.tandfonline.com/doi/abs/10.1080/13590849961780
6. Browne SE. The case of intravenous magnesium treatment of arterial disease in general practice: review of 34 years of experience. *Journal of Nutritional Medicine* 1994; 4: 169-177.(Accessed on The Magnesium Web Site. www.mgwater.com/browne01.shtml, 28 November 2019).

PART VII
Case histories

Chapter 59
How to slow the ageing process and live to one's full potential

Performance-maximising case histories
Ketosis for marathon-winning performance
Super-ketosis for gold medals
Chronic fatigue syndrome (CFS) reversal

Introduction

Medicine is built up of single cases. Individual patients – single cases – are the essence of what medicine deals with. Every patient is important, and every case can be a lesson.
Gunver, 2012[1]

In caring for patients, clinicians constantly perform experiments. During a single week of active practice, a busy clinician conducts more experiments than most of his laboratory colleagues do in a year.
Alvan Feinstein, clinician, researcher and epidemiologist

So, here we present case studies from my medical career to date. These 'experiments' often have formed my first discovery of some new therapy, or intervention, and thereafter I have found application of these new interventions across different pathologies.

Dr Joseph Bell (Scottish doctor, 2 December 1837 – 4 October 1911) was a great believer in the power of individual observation and the case report. He is known as the 'real-life Sherlock Holmes'. Sir Arthur Conan Doyle met Dr Bell in 1877 while he was a medical student. Doyle observed in detail Bell's celebrated deductive abilities. For example, Bell could tell from the tattoos of sailors where they had sailed and so he was able to estimate the possibility of certain types of infections being present. He once concluded (correctly) that a man was an alcoholic by noting that he always carried a flask in the inside breast pocket of his coat.

And for those perhaps still clinging to the notion that 'objective' measures are superior to 'subjective'...

It is precisely the most subjective ideas which, being closest to nature and to the living being, deserve to be called the truest.
Carl Jung (26 July 1875 – 6 June 1961)

And finally, I appeal to the Ancients. The Ancient Egyptians practised the documentation of Case Reports meticulously as can be seen in the Edwin Smith Papyrus. They laid out each report in a pre-determined format for the ease of those that followed:

- Every case starts with the words 'information regarding...' suggesting the history of the disease.
- Then an examination follows and starts with 'if you examine a patient with...'
- Then the physician hypothesises the disease by writing one of the following expressions: 'I will treat [X]', and/or 'I will not treat [Y]'
- Finally, the treatment is described.

I trust that the reader will forgive me for presenting my Case Studies in a free-flowing style rather than this formal structure.

Ketosis for marathon-winning performance

Everyone's definition of fatigue is different, but perhaps the most interesting was from an elite athlete, Matt, who consulted me in the 1980s. His complaint was that he ran his marathons in 2 hours 28 minutes and that he felt he could do better. He ascribed his failure to live up to his full potential as a 'candida problem'. At the time, we clinical doctors were only just getting to grips with this issue. There are many candida species – a common, and perhaps the best known, one is 'candida albicans'. Interestingly this means 'white white' as candida derives from the Latin 'candidus' (meaning white) and albicans derives from 'albus' (also meaning white – think Albus Dumbledore, my daughter tells me – Craig). But this problem is remarkably common and follows from changes in diet.

With hindsight it is easy to see why we were starting to see epidemics of this problem. The Western world had chosen to follow the disastrous nutritional recommendations of the American physiologist Ancel Keys, who determined that the healthy diet was one high in sugar and starch. In fact, 'chosen' is being a little too lenient – people in general hadn't chosen at all; instead, they had sugar and starch thrust upon them in the supermarket. The result of this was that anyone with less than perfect digestion turned their clean upper gut into a fermenting one.

The upper gut (oesophagus, stomach and small intestine) should, of course, be near sterile to allow us to digest meat and fat. But for some, diets high in sugar and starch overwhelmed their ability to sterilise and digest. Their upper gut became colonised by yeasts and bacteria that enjoyed the perfect life – being kept snug and warm, and regularly fed with their favourite foods. Given the right substrate, these microbes can double their numbers every 20 minutes – so their sex life was great as well!

We are only now starting to understand the biochemical and immunological havoc created by the upper fermenting gut. Sugars are fermented to various alcohols, D lactate and other such, all of which poison the body. Indeed, D lactate acidosis is a well-recognised condition of cattle which arises when they eat too much carbohydrate. Clinically it may be indistinguishable from BSE ('mad cow disease'). Microbes in the gut are greedy for micronutrients; consequently, much of the goodness of food goes to nourish these unwelcome invaders, rather than us. They grab these delicacies because they are first in the queue, sitting in the upper gut. The immune system is activated in the gut to keep these microbes at bay and the resulting low-grade inflammation drives many pathologies, such as ulcer disease, inflammatory bowel disease and, almost certainly, cancer. Finally, these microbes get into the bloodstream with the potential to drive pathology at distal sites, resulting in arthritis, cystitis and much more.

In the 1980s, Biolab offered a wonderful test to demonstrate yeast fermentation in the upper gut. Blood tests were done for alcohol levels before and after a modest 5 grams / 1 teaspoonful-load of glucose. As the biochemists know, there are many alcohols to which sugar may be fermented, but fermentation to ethanol (the alcohol of beer and wine) is almost pathognomonic of (synonymous with) yeast fermentation. My patients were either horrified or delighted to be diagnosed with 'auto-brewery syndrome'. One even asked me if I would be an expert witness for him to escape a drink-driving charge. Auto-brewery syndrome occurs where intoxicating quantities of ethanol are produced through endogenous fermentation within the digestive system – put simply, 'fermenting gut'.

Matt's symptoms of fatigue (by his standards), foggy brain and abdominal bloating, could easily be explained by auto-brewery syndrome and we were able to confirm this with the Biolab test. So how to treat? An understanding of the mechanisms by which pathology arises, as described above, gives us clear management principles vis:

> starve the little wretches out with a sugar-free diet
>
> kill them with antifungal medicines, and
>
> replenish the micronutrient deficiencies with a good multivitamin and mineral.

Recently I have found that an excellent tool for killing yeast in the gut is vitamin C. It is a joy to use because it is completely safe, does not require a doctor's prescription and is easy to tailor dose-wise to the individual's need using Dr Robert Cathcart's bowel tolerance method (see page 31.3). However, during the 1980s I used a range of herbal preparations to good effect. Combinations worked best, such as garlic, caprylic acid (coconut oil) and grapefruit seed extract. Dr John Mansfield saw excellent results using pure nystatin powder.

One of the joys of working with athletes is that they are highly motivated. Make a minor suggestion and they turn it into a crusade. The word athlete derives from the Greek 'athlos' (ἄθλος), meaning 'contest', and an Ancient 'athlete' was always competitive in the extreme – in fact the Ancient Olympics (dating from 776 BC) were a form of war. The Greek city states had to declare a temporary truce so that the various athletes could travel to the games without fear of being killed on their journey by decidedly unfriendly neighbours.

Matt chose to do not just a sugar-free diet but a ketogenic diet. We now know that not only would this starve out the yeast but also any bacterial fermenters. Of course, he was delighted to see his gut symptoms and foggy brain disappear, but what was most interesting to him was how his athletic performance improved.

I have learned much about the ketogenic diet from such athletes. Being 'keto-adapted' improves performance for at least two reasons. Firstly, fuel is stored as fat instead of glycogen in muscle and liver. Glycogen carries an osmotic load of water, so immediately the power to weight ratio is better – the ketogenic marathon runner is 1-2 kg (2.25-4.5 lb) lighter than his carb-consuming contemporary. Secondly, the pantry is much bigger. The carb runners 'hit a wall' at 17 miles as they run out of fuel. The Americans call this 'bonking'!* (If, dear reader, you are American, bonking has a very different meaning in the UK!) These carb runners have to be fed sugar to keep going; typically, this would be sugar dissolved in water at the rate of 90 grams per hour. By contrast, the keto-adapted athletes

---

*Footnote: The earliest citation for the use of 'bonk' in the context as above (running out of energy) is a 1952 article in the *Daily Mail*. The use of 'bonk' as a verb for having sex is more recent, although this use is now going out of fashion. (According to the *Online Urban Slang Dictionary*, there are at least 195 words meaning to have sex.)

need no such sustenance for their marathons. Indeed, keto-adapted Michael Moreton holds the World distance record for running 172 miles in 24 hours.

And what about Matt? He ran the Potteries marathon and improved his personal best by 12 minutes. As he put it, 'I did not just break my personal best; I smashed it.' What a guy!

Super-ketosis for gold medals

During the first Gulf War of 1991, many troops were lost to friendly fire. A major cause of this had to do with food. Troops were told that during the initial thrust they must not expect any back-up supplies for five days. They had to carry all they needed for frontline action. Not surprisingly, they filled their rucksacks with survival essentials and many soldiers discarded rations for ammunition. Many went for some days without food. One of the effects of this was severe mental fatigue and it was notable that most deaths from friendly fire resulted from soldiers in a state of starvation. Dr Keira Clarke of Oxford University was commissioned by the US military to look at foods that could sustain a soldier most efficiently. The budget for this piece of research was $10 million.

When fats are metabolised as a fuel they are first converted into ketones. Dr Clarke experimented by manufacturing beta-hydroxybutyrate – a ketone that normally arises when the body is fuelled by fat. This was then fed to ultra-fit, world-class athletes, at the rate of 1.5 grams of beta-hydroxybutyrate per kilogram of body weight per day, spread out in three separate doses. This was supplied in the form of a drink which, apparently, tastes pretty disgusting. However, this had some interesting metabolic benefits. First, blood readings showed that glucose levels came down, as did triglycerides and cholesterol. Fatty liver was reversed. Essentially, metabolic syndrome was reversed.

On this ketone drink, athletes were not hungry, and all lost weight. But despite this, their performance increased on average by 7%. This, for an elite athlete, is an astonishing improvement and will make the difference between an 'also ran' and a 'gold medal' performance.

Prior to the Rio Olympics, Team GB set up a training camp in Belo Horizonte, Brazil. Much of the emphasis was on quality food. My guess is that the endurance athletes used the beta-hydroxybutyrate drink. This would not have been advertised for obvious reasons. This may explain why Team GB won more medals than ever before, coming second in the medals' table to the USA and knocking China into third place. Although the ketone drink cost £80 a day, it has been estimated that each medal won represents about £4 million of funding, so perhaps £80 a day represents good value.

Chronic fatigue syndrome (CFS)

Olivia, aged 18, first consulted me in 2016. She is one of those enviable people who is brilliant at everything – not just super-bright but also a gymnast and diver. She has won medals at many national and international competitions together with countless county titles. You can see her in action at www.youtube.com/watch?v=s7agPY9z6Eg.

Despite having access to the best doctors her health declined in a way best described by her:

The more severe fatigue started in 2012 with the inability to wake up in the mornings and my body was forcing me to fall asleep for 1-2 hours in the middle of every day and there was nothing I could do to stop it. I would also have an overall sense of fatigue and lack of energy every day. Each year it got much worse until the beginning of 2015 when it became so severe I became very limited and training became non-existent. I would sleep all day, go to diving, do a quick stretch and I would feel extremely tired and would go home; that was all I did all day. I was confined to my bed for most of the day, only getting up to eat and go to the toilet until eventually (December 2015) I was unable to move from my bed. I felt like someone was there knocking me with a sedation every time I woke up. I couldn't move, walk or get up, and couldn't take baths. My mum had to wake me up for food.

The history always gives the best clues. It was no coincidence that Olivia's fatigue followed Gardasil vaccination. It is my experience, and that of other 'ecomed' doctors, that the HPV vaccines are the most pernicious at triggering fatigue problems. She was eventually diagnosed with autoimmune hypothyroidism – the main risk factors for autoimmunity being vaccination, vitamin D deficiency and consumption of dairy products. Thyroxin only afforded modest benefits.

Clearly, we had to address energy delivery mechanisms and so we applied the tools of the trade as detailed in Chapter 30. She evidently had a pre-diabetic state with blood sugar once spiking to 12.8 mmol/l (3-6 mmol/l reference range) after a meal. Mitochondrial function tests showed that her mitochondria were functioning at just 42% of the lowest limit of reference range. This was largely due to deficiencies of magnesium, vitamin B3 and carnitine. They also showed

that ATP was not being used efficiently – I am now fairly sure this is an adrenal-thyroid issue.

Olivia did a brilliant job with the paleo-ketogenic diet. At the same time, we swapped her from thyroxin to natural desiccated thyroid and increased the dose according to the biochemistry and clinical parameters. She improved progressively and six months later she commented:

I have been following the regime you have given me, and I am doing really well and feeling much better. I also hope to resume diving this year. It seems like all my symptoms were interconnected. Thank you for helping me become a much healthier person. I have been keto for many months now and have lost over a stone in weight. I feel very good eating this way and will continue to follow a low-carb high-fat lifestyle for the rest of my life. I have much respect for you helping people get to the root of their illnesses; all other doctors wanted to do was palm me off on drugs and pills (which were probably making me worse), not even bothering to find the cause of my symptoms.

Olivia has now started diving again.

Reference

1. Gunver SK. Why medical case reports? *Glob Adv Health Med* 2012; 1(1): 8–9. doi: 10.7453/gahmj.2012.1.1.002

Chapter 60
How to fight infectious diseases

Infectious disease case histories
MRSA
Mumps
Orf

MRSA

The PK diet is the single most powerful determinant of health such that, without this important foundation stone in place, all else stands little chance of success. In the treatment of all Western disease, the PK diet is non-negotiable. With this in place, then natural remedies become so much more effective.

To illustrate this point, let's look at the case of Martha (aged 31). She presented to me six months before writing this with a large, infected, discharging, stinking abscess in her armpit (axilla). This began with a cyst in her axilla in 2006, which then evolved into a pilonidal ('nest of hair') cyst. These are usually located in the cleft of the buttock but may occur anywhere hairy. This inflamed cyst was excised in 2016 but this failed to clear the infection. She was treated with many courses of antibiotic, which reduced the inflammation somewhat but never cleared it. In 2017 she underwent even more extensive surgery under general anaesthetic to try to remove all the infected tissue, but again this was unsuccessful. By the time she came to see me she had received

multiple courses of antibiotics and had a large ulcerous hole in her axilla, surrounded by lumpy inflamed flesh. It was extremely painful and exuding pus. It was regularly probed, drained and dressed, but was not healing. The infection was a classical large carbuncle which would be caused by many microbes, but the main one would have been staphylococcus. Since antibiotics were ineffective, by definition she had an MRSA (multi-resistant *Staphylococcus aureus*) infection. Martha described her consultant as being 'concerned'. I was blooming terrified!

My special interest is in patients with chronic fatigue syndrome and ME. Increasingly it is becoming clear that for many there is a low grade chronic infection which is making them ill. This part explains the fatigue (much energy is going to the immune system to fight infection) and the inflammatory symptoms (which include pain, such as fibromyalgia). I have seen many patients who have been treated unsuccessfully with antimicrobials, even though they have had a proven infection; this started me thinking about how best to fight infection in the body. I have increasingly come to the view that life is an arms race – you and I are a free lunch for millions of microbes that would love to make themselves comfortably at home in our delicious bodies (and, indeed, Craig and I ended up writing another book about this very topic – *The Infection Game*).

Martha had become home to billions of bacteria that were enjoying an easy life in her warm body, being well fed, well watered and revelling in free sex – multiplying like the proverbial rabbits.* They were so comfortably ensconced that even the atomic bomb of antibiotics could not dislodge them.

I started to do some research and it quickly became apparent that all chronic disease, from cancer and coronaries to dementia and degenerative disorders, have an infectious associate. I suspect the link is not casual but causal. The penny dropped whilst chatting to one of my veterinary friends who reckoned the vast majority of domestic animal disease is driven by infection. So, what is it about modern Western life that is causing so much immune suppression that an apparently healthy young woman could become victim to an infection that was slowly eating her body away? And what can we do about it?

The immune system is an army and similar strategies apply. There are two proven mechanisms for fighting an invading army – starve them out with a scorched earth policy and shoot them down in as many ways as possible. So, I applied these principles to Martha.

Microbes can only survive on sugar and carbohydrates. Diabetics are particularly prone to infection because their high blood sugar levels feed invaders. The biological equivalent of scorched earth is a ketogenic diet. For Martha, this was the most difficult intervention because she was a 'fruit-oholic' – she had followed the NICE Guidelines' advice to eat her 'five a day', which comprised bananas, orange juice, pears, apples and grapes. Of course, fruit is a bag of sugar which is happily fermented by bacteria and yeasts. When my patients give me a doubting look on this score, I remind them that this is how cider and wine are made. Martha was convinced and changed to a PK diet to cut off supplies to MRSA and other microbes.

Having starved the microbes of their favourite food, the next strategy was to kill the little wretches with vitamin C to bowel tolerance. In this respect the dose was, and always is, critical – Martha needed 30 grams a day to get to bowel tolerance. Most people need between 4 and 15 grams for such and so this was a reflection of her high infectious load.

Then we used topical (on the skin) iodine oil ad lib so the flesh was permanently stained yellow.

Both iodine and vitamin C kill all microbes on contact – none are resistant, including MRSA. Importantly, neither are toxic and so healing and repair can progress.

What happened? Martha's gaping holes stopped discharging, the smell went and for the first time in 12 years she started to heal without antibiotics. Five months later the holes were gone, and the skin had healed over. And now, at the time of going to press (April 2020) Martha

---

Footnote: Rabbits were introduced into Australia in 1859, after a southern Australian farmer imported two dozen wild English rabbits and set them free on his land for hunting purposes. Within six years, the Australian rabbit population was around 22 million, and 2 million could be killed each year without any discernible effect. (Interested readers should see https://en.wikipedia.org/wiki/Rabbits_in_Australia.) This is a classic example of the power of unrestrained exponential growth. In the case of the Australian rabbits, we have the equation as below, and microbes are even quicker than rabbits:

$P(t) = P_0\,e^{r \cdot t}$ t is time, measured in months,

          P_0 is the initial population (24 rabbits), and

          r is the growth rate (19% per month).

$P(t) \approx 24\,e^{0.19t}$ models the exponential growth of the rabbits.

is still infection free and it looks like it will now continue to be the case. Phew – what a relief!

Mumps

For many, the effect of mumps vaccination (as part of MMR) is to postpone rather than prevent mumps. I have seen two young men, both MMR-vaccinated, in their early 20s, with severe mumps orchitis (testicular inflammation). The diagnosis was not difficult – I recall Nick walking in with the rolling gait of a professional jockey, bandy-legged in order to prevent any pressure on the throbbing grapefruits hanging between his legs. They had previously gone under the title of 'wedding tackle'. Thankfully he went on to recover and fathered two children, neither of whom underwent MMR vaccination! In the interim I learned some of the tools of the trade to treat acute viral infection in children. The key point to remember is that acute febrile illness in childhood is an essential part of immune programming. Not only does this train the immune system to respond appropriately, but it also prevents us ever getting the particular infection again and, it is now becoming clear, protects us against other diseases in life, such as brain tumours.

We now know that getting an acute febrile illness as a child reduces overall cancer risk and the more often this occurs the better. At the very least children should get rubella and chicken-pox (vaccination is no substitute) which are the most protective against cancer, but so too are infections with measles, mumps, pertussis and scarlet fever. The report on this from NVKP in the Netherlands references 54 medical papers,[1] while the article by Hoption Cann et al (2006) concludes that: 'Infections may play a paradoxical role in cancer development with chronic infections often being tumorigenic and acute infections being antagonistic to cancer.'[2] This latter study specifically references meningioma and glioma tumours of the brain.

The key is to use the tools of the trade (see Chapter 30) to reduce enemy numbers and strength, so the immune system has an easy and, consequently, effective fight.

The next time I saw a case of mumps, I was prepared. This arose in a neighbour who appeared at the back door looking like a greedy hamster. Over the previous 24 hours she had grown bilateral, half avocado-sized swellings of her parotid glands so the angle of her ear lobes was up and out. I oversaw her slugging back her first 10 grams of vitamin C in a pint of water (then 10 grams every hour to diarrhoea), slathered iodine oil over the avocado swellings and instructed her to keep applying it so her cheeks remained stained yellow. The result? Next day – yes, the very next day – all symptoms and signs had gone.

Orf

Orf is a pox virus acquired from handling sheep and goats. It is a common problem in farming communities. It usually appears on the hands, but Jan presented with a fast-enlarging lump on the bridge of her nose. She had been filling the sheep's hay cratch (feeder) when a gust of wind had blown its corrugated iron lid which fell and cut her nose, so allowing the virus in. Usually farmers apply purple foot-rot spray, but this was not convenient with a lesion so close to the eyes. Jan drizzled on Lugol's iodine 15% to keep the lesion stained yellow. So, yes, she had a funny-coloured nose for a few days, but healing was complete – she has a small scar but that was the result of the ragged cut, not the orf. Jan has remained orf free ever since.

References

1. Zandvliet HA, Wel Evd. Science: Increase in cancer cases as a consequence of eliminating febrile infectious diseases. Nederlandse Vereniging Kritisch Prikken (NVKP). (www.wanttoknow.info/health/cancer_link_vaccination_fever_research.pdf, Zandvliet et Wel, Nederlandse Vereniging Kritisch Prikken). This references 54 medical papers.

2. Hoption Cann SA, van Netten JP, van Netten C. Acute infections as a means of cancer prevention: opposing effects to chronic infections? *Cancer Detect Prev* 2006; 30(1): 83-93. (www.ncbi.nlm.nih.gov/pubmed/16490323)

Chapter 61
Ophthalmology/eye problems

Ophthalmology case history
Iritis with chronic lymphatic leukaemia (viral infection)

Chronic iritis

Carola (aged 80) had suffered from iritis (inflammation affecting the iris) ever since being pregnant with her son. Iris is the name of the Greek Goddess of the rainbow and the word came to be used to describe any brightly coloured ring, for example, the eyes of a peacock's tail. That her condition was named after a Greek goddess was of little comfort to Carola, who presented to me with pain and blurred vision. She had been treated for decades with steroid eye drops. Iritis has always been reckoned to be inflammation of unknown cause and steroids the standard treatment. What one has to be particularly careful about in this situation is a dendritic ulcer of the cornea because to apply steroids to such risks a perforation and blindness. So, iritis is always a job for a consultant ophthalmologist.

Besides her iritis, Carola had also consulted me for nutritional management of her chronic lymphatic leukaemia (CLL). Viruses have a clear role in many leukaemias and lymphomas, with the herpes viruses being particularly pernicious. Of course, we put in place Groundhog interventions (see Appendices 1–3), especially the ketogenic diet and vitamin C to bowel tolerance. She did extremely well. Despite having no conventional therapy whatsoever, her white cell count fell progressively. However, she continued to be troubled by recurrent attacks of iritis and I continued to be troubled by her need for steroid eye drops. Even with consultant input to prevent perforation, steroid eye drops are a risk factor for cataracts, glaucoma and central serous chorio-retinopathy.

She attended my surgery one day with a flare of her iritis. We decided to experiment. I prescribed the anti-viral drug acyclovir 800 mg to take five times daily, then off she trotted to see the consultant. By the time she arrived, the pain in her eye was a little less and her visual acuity was normal, so the consultant agreed to continue her prescription of antivirals and refrain from using steroids. Her eyes settled down completely. In consequence, the consultant was happy to prescribe low-dose acyclovir for the long term. Consequently, since 2015, Carola has taken 800 mg of acyclovir daily and has been free from iritis. Even more interesting, the rate at which her white cell count reduced has accelerated – we know she has CLL but it would no longer be suspected from a blood test since her lymphocyte count is now in the normal range.

During pregnancy one is slightly immunosuppressed. This is an essential to prevent Mother rejecting Baby as a foreign body – of course, Baby genetically speaking is half Dad. (Craig's mother used to refer to this half as the 'Alien Half'!) This immune suppression results from the high levels of female steroid sex hormones. But immune suppression is a dangerous business and in Carola's case this allowed a herpes virus to make itself at home in her eye; there it remained (and will do so for life), occasionally flaring to cause iritis. I suspect this wretched virus also got into her bone marrow and triggered her leukaemia.

Chapter 62
Endocrinology/ hormone problems

A case of hypothyroidism and dementia

Aged 45, Jo first came to see me in 2012. She had three issues. The biggest problem was that her mother and grandmother had both developed dementia in their 50s and she wanted to know how to avoid this. Secondly, she was fatigued. Thirdly, she was overweight. Indeed, this latter problem was such an issue that in 2007 she had undergone gastric bypass surgery.

It was clear from blood tests that she was hypothyroid. Her free thyroxin (T4) level was just 7.5 pmol/l. My lab's reference range is 12-22 pmol/l. Astonishingly, some NHS lab reference ranges are 7-14 pmol/l; this may explain why her NHS GP refused to prescribe thyroid hormones. I started her on thyroxin and we built the dose up slowly. Clinically, this was ineffective. On thyroxin, her free T4 came up to 17, but her TSH was high at 4.27 mlU/l (lab reference range: 0.27-4.2 mlU/l). Jo was told by her GP that 'this was normal and the problem was in her head'. Jo, being convinced she had a thyroid problem, consulted with Dr Skinner. Dr Skinner was an NHS consultant virologist at Birmingham and inevitably saw patients with post-viral chronic fatigue

syndromes. He cured hundreds of patients with thyroid hormones through the simple principle of treating the patient instead of the blood test. Because his methods did not accord with the views of conventional endocrinologists, he was hounded by the General Medical Council (GMC – yes, sigh, I know the feeling).

Dr Skinner prescribed natural desiccated thyroid (Armour), up to 3.5 grains (210 mg), which was also ineffective, so he swapped Jo to pure T3 and gradually increased the dose to 180 mcg – this is high-dose therapy; a normal dose would be 20-40 mcg. But Jo started to see real results clinically which paralleled the escalating dose of T3. She never developed any symptoms of overdosing with thyroid hormones (being a midwife she was well able to monitor things closely). Her weight started to come off and her energy levels and foggy brain started to improve. We can only explain this in terms of thyroid hormone receptor blocking – but what could have been causing this? I suspect it has something to do with metabolic syndrome, which is the starting point of diabetes. We are seeing epidemics of type 2 diabetes in which one would expect to see low levels of insulin, but not so – insulin is either normal or high. This is called 'insulin-resistant diabetes'.

I suspect that whatever was blocking the insulin receptor was also blocking the thyroid receptor.

Dr Skinner died, bless him; undoubtedly the stress of the GMC contributed. Consequently, Jo came to see me. We then had the dementia problem to consider. There are two threads here – vitamin B12 deficiency and metabolic syndrome are both major risks for dementia. Many of my ME patients respond well to B12 injections. Jo was already deficient because gastric bypass surgery results in malabsorption of vitamin B12 and she was on injections every three months. She had iatrogenic (medically caused) pernicious anaemia. However, I know three-monthly injections are totally inadequate. So many patients report an initial boost with each B12 injection, which then runs out rapidly. Jo was no exception. So, she started to inject herself – once a week was inadequate as she was fatiguing after a few days. Daily injections resulted in further improvements in both physical and mental fatigue.

A second major cause of dementia is metabolic syndrome. I told Jo about the Bredesen study 'Reversal of Cognitive Decline'.[1] Dale Bredesen is a Californian Consultant Neurologist who took 10 patients with Alzheimer's disease for his study. He prescribed a ketogenic diet – one in which the patients fuelled their body with fat and fibre instead of a typical Western metabolic syndrome diet of sugar and starch. Nine of the 10 patients reversed their disease, with six returning to employment. The one patient who did not improve was unable to keep to the diet. Now, had this been a drug trial, it would have been covered by every national paper in the World. Indeed, the ketogenic diet is of proven benefit in many neurological conditions, with the best documented being epilepsy. The *New Scientist* recently reported the case of a young man with a malignant brain tumour who cured himself with a ketogenic diet.[2]

Having divulged these bits of information, we arrived at a tipping point. Jo quickly picked up on the rationale for a ketogenic diet and before I could say Jack Robinson* the information flow was in the other direction. She was educating me. Fuelling the body with fat and fibre is evolutionarily correct. Jo turned her body from that of the hibernating bear (cold, sleepy and lethargic) to the lean hunter-gatherer (warm, active and creative). Indeed, the paleo-ketogenic (PK) diet is the starting point to treat almost absolutely everything.

These three threads – correction of thyroid function, a ketogenic diet and high-dose vitamin B12 by injection – have transformed Jo. At her worst, she weighed 120 kg (19 stone). She is now 61 kg (9 ½ stone). Her energy levels are restored, she is working long hours and is out on her Harley Davidson motorbike with her gorgeous new partner. She is regularly tested for cognitive function and there are no signs of deterioration – in my language, she is a sharp as a tack!

Jo has taken the PK diet to its logical conclusion and now the only food she eats is 800 g to 1 kg of the best organic ribeye steak daily – no veg, no fibre. She is never hungry. Reviewing this and her supplements I wondered about iodine. People who are not taking iodine are invariably deficient. 'Let's do the test,' said Jo. I was fully expecting to see a deficiency… and was flabbergasted to see a completely normal result. So that is another thing she has taught me…

One final challenge to my thinking… Jo points out that her gut function is entirely normal on her fibre-free diet. The Native Americans of the Great Plains, the Inuit Eskimos and the Maasai and Samburu tribes of Africa consume

---

*Footnote: Many derivations of the phrase 'faster than you can say Jack Robinson' exist but perhaps the most memorable is that of the officer commanding the Tower of London in the late 17th century, one Sir John (Jack) Robinson. The swiftness with which he carried out beheadings led to 'Jack Robinson' being associated with speed of execution (literally).

fibre-less diets, yet they too are free from digestive ills and modern diseases. Cripes Myhill – back to the drawing board; I had better start researching fibre… And as a final update, at the time of going to press (April 2020) Jo continues to eat only 800 grams of the best rib eye steak she can find daily.

References

1. Bredesen DE. Reversal of cognitive decline. *Aging* 2014; 6(9): 707-717. http://www.drmyhill.co.uk/drmyhill/images/0/07/Reversal-of-Cognitive-decline-Bredesen.pdf .
2. Hodson H. Ketogenic diet's reputed anticancer credentials put to test: Did a low-carb, high-fat diet aid Andrew Scarborough's recovery from a brain tumour? *New Scientist* 2016, 24 February. www.newscientist.com/article/2078558-ketogenic-diets-reputed-anticancer-credentials-put-to-test/ (accessed 11 July 2019)

Chapter 63
Cardiology/ heart problems

Cardiology case histories
Arterial disease (HDL:LDL ratio as a marker; high homocysteine)
Atrial fibrillation (lead poisoning)
Heart failure (statins)

When am I going to die? Diagnosing arterial disease

Arterial disease damages and kills so many Westerners, but it takes years for this disease to manifest clinically. Persuading patients to change their ways is the most difficult aspect of life for the ecomed doctor. 'I have eaten like this for years and I feel okay now,' is the usual refrain. Accountants tell us that with respect to financial matters, past performance is not an accurate indicator of future results. Somehow, my patients do not translate this maxim easily to health matters. So how can I show my patients that their arteries are diseased? Many are disinclined to respond to the rantings of an old crone like me. But give them a test that tells them for sure something is amiss, and I have a powerful tool of persuasion.

Cholesterol is a good test, when correctly interpreted. Doctors routinely get it wrong in two ways. Firstly, they believe that high cholesterol causes arterial damage – WRONG. Secondly, they ignore the friendly high-density lipoprotein (HDL) cholesterol. Let me explain. Cholesterol is not a cause of arterial disease but a symptom of such. The two major causes of damage to arteries are sugar and high blood pressure. High blood pressure results in turbulence of the flow of blood within the arteries and this damages their delicate lining. It is no coincidence that arterial damage starts where turbulence is greatest, at

*Footnote: Perhaps the earliest written reference to a 'knight in shining armour' dates from 1790, in the British journal *The Monthly Review*, in a poem called 'Amusement: A Poetical Essay', by Henry Pye (English poet and MP for Berkshire, 10 February 1744 – 11 August 1813):

No more the knight, in shining armour dress'd
Opposes to the pointed lance his breast

Henry Pye was the first poet laureate to receive a fixed salary instead of the historic *tierce* (around 35 Imperial gallons) of Canary wine, and he needed it. His father died in 1766, leaving him nothing but a debt of £50,000, and the burning of the family home further increased his financial difficulties.

points where arteries divide. Even in the blood-stream, sugar is sticky stuff and it sticks to the arterial wall, compounding the damage.

Cholesterol, our knight in shining armour,* comes to the rescue to heal and repair this arterial damage. It is HDL which is used up during this process. What this means is that the proportion of HDL to total cholesterol is a very useful, non-invasive measure of arterial damage. Anyone can get their HDL measured either by their NHS GP or on a private DIY finger-drop sample of blood. The 'acceptable' figure is that HDL should make up at least 20% of total cholesterol, but the higher the result the better. Low levels of HDL mean that it (HDL) is being used up in healing and repairing arteries, which in turn means that there must be a lot of such healing and repairing of arteries to be done – that is, lots of damage! My patients eating good paleo-ketogenic (PK) diets can get an HDL of up to 40% of their total cholesterol. I have two patients in my practice, both in their late 90s, whose HDLs are 64% and 38% respectively. Both are healthy, with excellent brains.

Measuring HDL is therefore an excellent tool to screen for arterial disease, to monitor response to treatment and, consequently, to look for causes of arterial disease. Sugar and blood pressure are not the only causes of such. A 69-year-old man, Mark, consulted recently with fatigue and a family history of dementia, stroke and heart disease. He was eating a pretty good PK diet and his blood pressure was normal. I ran his bloods to discover that the proportion of HDL to total cholesterol was just 16%. This meant his HDL was being used up to heal and repair his arteries, so we had to ask the question: What was damaging them?

A greatly overlooked cause of arterial damage is homocysteine. This is an amino acid, normally present in the body, which forms part of the methylation cycle. Methylation is an essential biochemical tool which multitasks in the business of reading DNA, detoxification, healing, repair and much more. If homocysteine is high, we can infer poor methylation and all the aforementioned processes go slow. No wonder a high homocysteine reading is a marker for many disease processes.

Mark had a very high homocysteine of 26.10 umol/l. (I like to see this below 10.) A tendency to high homocysteine runs in families and so this explained why his mother and grandmother both died with dementia. All Mark's first-degree relatives needed screening so along trotted his two daughters – one had a perfect level of 5.1, but the other was slightly raised at 12.2 and needed treatment.

At this point my now learned readers will be asking why homocysteine screening is not routinely done in NHS practice. The answer is simple – it can be treated easily with vitamins. This is a major problem for Big Pharma for three reasons. Firstly, Big Pharma does not like the use of cheap vitamins because no profit can be made. Secondly, it does not want cures because cured people do not need drugs. Thirdly, damage to arteries is the best possible investment for shareholders since this guarantees the future prescription of statins and blood pressure, heart and dementia drugs.

Mark's daughter, Katie, took this message on board enthusiastically. In addition to her standard multivitamin, minerals and essential fatty acids she took methylated B12 3 mg sublingually, methyl-tetrahydrofolate 800 mcg and pyridoxal-5 phosphate 50 mg daily. What was so interesting was that not only did her homocysteine level come down, but her energy levels came up. She had not realised until that moment that she had been so fatigued – she had simply assumed that was normal for her natural self.

Mark was sceptical about the supplements and did not take them because his NHS GP had never heard of homocysteine and never seen it measured or treated. Big Pharma propaganda had done a cracking good job here. Let's hope

Mark's lesson in nutritional medicine does not arrive in the form of a fatal heart attack. In the meantime he still refuses to take on board the message, while Katie continues to do very well.

Atrial fibrillation (AF) cured by detoxing

We are seeing epidemics of cardiac dysrhythmias (or 'arrhythmia') – that is, any condition in which the heartbeat is irregular, too fast or too slow. Atrial fibrillation (irregular and often abnormally fast heartbeat) used to be an uncommon problem, occasionally seen in elderly people and often associated with heart failure. I am now seeing young, fit people switching into AF… but why?

Ned was one such. In 2014 he was a fit, slim 51-year-old who prided himself on his ability to walk long distances and keep up with the best. He suddenly found he could not do this. He struggled with hills, becoming acutely short of breath. If he really pushed himself, he developed chest pain. The diagnosis was easy and achieved simply by feeling his pulse. One's pulse should be about 70-80 beats per minutes and regular. It quickens very slightly on inhalation and slows with exhalation. The commonest cardiac dysrhythmia is 'ventricular ectopic beats'. In this case, the pulse at the wrist is regular, but then suddenly a beat is missed, before continuing regularly. If one's hand is over the heart, one perceives a double beat. Sufferers tell me this feels as if their heart has done a somersault! This pulse is a regularly irregular pulse.

Ned's pulse was different again. It was irregularly irregular. Not only was the rhythm all over the place, but so was his blood pressure. With experience, this is an obvious feel.

When the heart beats normally there are two phases. First the atrial chambers of the heart accept blood returning from the body via the veins, fill and then contract to send a dollop of blood down into the ventricles. Dollop is a technical term – I learnt it at the university of life! The ventricles are the real powerhouses of the heart. Once filled, they contract powerfully to send a pulse of blood through the arteries. A series of valves ensures blood flows in the right direction. As one can imagine, timing is everything. This is achieved by the pacemaker – so first the atria have to contract whilst the ventricles relax… then vice versa.

In AF the atria lose their rhythmical contraction. They wobble like a jelly. There is no regular dollop of blood streaming into the ventricles, and no regular filling. The ventricles contract at random, sometimes to eject too much blood, sometimes too little. The heart no longer works efficiently and cardiac output falls, on average by 20%. That means physical performance will also reduce by at least 20%. No wonder Ned could not keep up with his walking friends. Until recently, the relationship between cardiac output and oxygen consumption had generally been thought of as being linear, but studies have shown that this may not be the case, so Ned probably did 'lose' more than 20% of his performance.[1]

We always have to ask the question 'why?', so, why does the pacemaker fail, leading the atria to fibrillate? One common, and greatly overlooked, cause is poisoning by toxic metals. Ned was far too young and far too fit to explain his AF in terms of poor blood supply to his pacemaker (the usual reason in old age) – there had to be another reason.

We live in such a polluted world that we all unwittingly carry a toxic load which may include toxic metals. This is compounded where there are deficiencies of friendly minerals, such as zinc and selenium. This is because if, for example, the body is in need of zinc, but its diet is deficient in such, then it will grab something that 'looks' like zinc, such as lead. Thus lead gets incorporated into body tissues – typically the heart, brain, bones and kidneys – where it gets stuck, sometimes for decades. What this means is that a simple blood or urine test will not show up any toxicity. I have yet to find a patient willing to undergo a brain or heart biopsy! Chelating agents have come to our rescue. The word 'chelate' comes from the Greek word for claw. They literally grab the toxic metals and pull them out in our urine – so we have a test for heavy metal load. This test has a well-established scientific foundation.

So, Ned emptied his bladder, took 15 mg per kg of body weight of DMSA (in his case, 900 mg) and collected his urine over the next six hours. A sample of that was sent off to the lab. We are 'allowed' to have 2.2 micromol of lead per mol of creatinine. Ned's result was 37.17. There are many ways one can reduce one's toxic metal load, such as vitamin C to bowel tolerance, taking iodine and/or taking zinc 30 mg at night followed by glutathione 250 mg. However, DMSA is of proven benefit and I wanted to get Ned's lead down as low as possible as quickly as possible because he was on the waiting list for cardioversion. To my mind it is daft to cardiovert (i.e. apply an electric shock to the heart to restore sinus rhythm) without treating the underlying cause because the patient will simply revert to AF for the same reason it began in the first place.

Ned took a weekly dose of 900 mg of DMSA for 16 weeks and we rechecked the urine test – the lead had come down to 3.63. Subsequent cardioversion was successful. Here we are seven years later, and Ned is fit and well, taking no prescription medication and back to walking faster than I can. Dammit!

Finally, where did the lead come from? Probably from lead water pipes in the Victorian house in which he lived as a child.

Heart failure reversed

The two big killers of Westerners are heart disease and cancer. Coming a close third are the consequences of Western medicine. Dr Barbara Starfield of the Johns Hopkins School of Hygiene and Public Health published a paper in the *Journal of the American Medical Association (JAMA)* on this topic.[2] The death rate figures per annum for the USA were:

> 106,000 deaths from prescription medication
>
> 80,000 deaths from hospital-acquired infections (like MRSA)
>
> 20,000 deaths from other errors in hospitals
>
> 12,000 deaths from unnecessary surgery
>
> 7000 deaths from medication errors in hospitals

The most shocking fact is that the deaths from drugs arose from those prescribed in 'normal' doses. Many people are not told that a death is drug related and the following case history illustrates the multiple problems suffered by a patient as a result of well-intentioned, NICE 'guideline-informed', but ultimately dangerous prescribing.

Arthur consulted me in 2012, aged 77, because he had developed heart failure accompanied by severe fatigue and breathlessness on exertion. The problem with drugs for heart failure is that they do not address the root cause of the failure. He did not have valve or ischaemic heart disease and initially his symptoms were controlled by diuretics. However, as he worsened, other drugs were added in and by the time he consulted me he was on a shopping list of long-term medications which included furosemide, spironolactone, amlodipine, bisoprolol, isosorbide mononitrate, lisinopril, atorvastatin, bisoprolol, clopidegrol and omeprazole. Arthur comes from a generation that does not question doctors and so he naturally assumed that the prescription medication he was taking was doing him good.

The sort of heart failure that Arthur was suffering from results when the heart muscle cannot beat powerfully enough, which leads to low cardiac output. This happens to be my special area of interest because my chronic fatigue syndrome (CFS) patients are also in a state of mild heart failure. Like Arthur they too suffer all the symptoms of low cardiac output – fatigue, exercise intolerance, poor cognitive function, poor circulation and so on. The mechanism of this has to do with mitochondria (see Chapter 5) – muscles can only beat powerfully if they are well supplied with energy; cut off the energy supply and they immediately weaken.

Arthur was taking statins. These drugs are prescribed mindlessly by so many doctors for so many conditions whenever the word cholesterol is mentioned. But they have a very serious side effect. They block the body's own production of co-enzyme Q10, which is an absolute essential for good mitochondrial function. I think of co-Q10 as the oil of our mitochondrial engine. Without co-Q10 we cannot get energy to our bodies. The first department to fail is our muscles, including heart muscle. Indeed, I rarely see a CFS sufferer who can tolerate statins – statins cause severe muscle pain, fatigue and weakness. If energy delivery is further impaired the muscle will die – this is called rhabdomyolitis and may lead to death.

I advised Arthur to stop the statins and instead to take the package of supplements that we know are effective in improving the poor mitochondrial function of CFS. He started on co-enzyme Q10 200 mg, magnesium 300 mg, acetyl-L-carnitine 1 gram, niacinamide 1500 mg slow release, and D-ribose 5 grams, three times daily.

Heart failure normally carries a very poor prognosis – 50% of sufferer are dead within two years. By contrast, Arthur immediately started to improve. Within days of stopping statins he felt better. I reckon it takes about four months of supplements to really impact on mitochondrial function; during this time Arthur improved progressively. When this happens, pathology too goes into reverse and this had two fascinating consequences.

His kidney function became so much better that the diuretics he was taking became much more effective. His cardiologist insisted he continue to take diuretics (because cardiologists do not expect heart failure patients to recover). Diuretics work by inhibiting renal absorption of sodium – as sodium is peed out it pulls water with it – hence the diuretic effect. However, one must replace the sodium (and sometimes the potassium) salts lost in this way. Arthur had not been told to do this – indeed, worse than that, he had been advised to avoid salt! When he was admitted to hospital for a minor surgical procedure, he developed epileptic-like convulsions. Blood sodium levels were found to be 123 mmol/l (normal range 133-146 mmol/l) and this was the cause of his fits. He was cured by taking Sunshine salt 5 grams daily. He no longer takes diuretics because he does not need them.

Having improved heart function so much, Arthur's blood pressure came back up to normal. Again the cardiologist insisted that he continue with his medication for high blood pressure, which he had been taking for years… read on.

A further problem arose through taking a stomach-acid blocking drug, omeprazole, together with the over-zealous prescription of drugs for blood pressure. We need an acidic stomach to absorb minerals – without minerals we cannot make healthy bone. So, acid blocking drugs cause osteoporosis. Arthur's blood pressure was over-treated and he ended up with blood pressure that was too low, which caused him to have dizzy spells. During one such episode he fell and suffered a fractured pelvis because he had osteoporosis, as caused by the acid-blocking drugs. It took major surgery and 10 months of rehabilitation to start to recover. However, Arthur was left with severe hip pain… but his surgeon did not want to operate because of past heart problems. I wrote a detailed letter to the surgeon explaining the problems of medication, the success of nutritional supplements and suggestions for anaesthesia. The hip replacement then went very well under no sedation but rather simple local anaesthetic. Arthur experienced no pain and after a morning of surgery he enjoyed a good lunch!

Arthur is now 86, can potter about his house and go out for trips. He is pain free. His brain is active and sharp – he keeps me on the ball with his incisive questions. He eats a paleo-ketogenic (PK) diet and takes several nutritional supplements. He is now on no prescription medication other than thyroxine. He has cheated death at least three times. Good man! I expect him to do well.

References

1. Beck KC, Randolph LN, Bailey KR, Wood CM, et al. Relationship between cardiac output and oxygen consumption during upright cycle exercise in healthy humans. *J Appl Physiol* 2006; 101(5): 1474-1480. DOI: 10.1152/japplphysiol.00224.2006

2. Starfield B. Is US health really the best in the world? *Journal of the American Medical Association (JAMA)* 2000; 284(4): 483-485. www.jhsph.edu/research/centers-and-institutes/johns-hopkins-primary-care-policy-center/Publications_PDFs/A154.pdf (accessed 11 July 2019).

Chapter 64
Gastroenterology/ gut problems

Crohn's disease cured

Crohn's disease, named after Dr Burrill Bernard Crohn,* is a really nasty bowel inflammation with the potential to kill. As with many Western diseases, the conventional approach fails to ask the question 'why?'. Conventional treatment consists of symptom-supressing medication, immune suppressants and, if it all goes pear-shaped, intravenous steroids and perhaps surgery. This is not a good prospect when you are a girl aged 13.

Carol's mum brought her to see me in 2001. At that time, I was very familiar with the work of Dr John Hunter at Addenbrooke's hospital, who had shown that diet was central to the treatment of Crohn's disease. His Stone Age (paleo) diet for acute Crohn's was as effective as hospital in-patient treatment with intravenous steroids. Of course, diet is also much safer than hospitals and steroids. What was more important is that those patients who stuck to the diet greatly

reduced their risk of relapse. So, the first step for Carol was such a diet, which cut out the major allergens – namely gluten grains, dairy and yeast. This afforded improvements so great that she was able to stop her Crohn's prescription medication. She also felt so much better.

However, her mother, understandably, wanted a cure. It just so happened that I had attended a lecture by Professor John Hermon-Taylor of St George's Hospital, London. He was primarily a surgeon specialising in Crohn's disease, but he was also a talented microbiologist and had discovered a new microbe associated with Crohn's – namely, *Mycobacterium avium paratuberculosis* (MAP). As the name suggests, this is a TB-like microbe and, indeed, the pathological lesion of Crohn's shares many characteristics with TB. This is the very same microbe that causes Johne's disease in cattle. I knew about this microbe because it is a particular problem for Welsh Black cattle, who seem especially susceptible to Johne's disease. That too presents with a chronic

***Footnote:** Crohn's disease is named after Burrill Bernard Crohn (13 June 1884 – 29 July 1983), an American gastroenterologist who decided to become a doctor so that he could help his father with his terrible indigestion. Crohn was also a painter of note (watercolours) and a scholar of the US Civil War. He practised medicine until he was 90 years old.

inflammation of the gut, diarrhoea and failure to thrive. Indeed, Professor Hermon-Taylor had some fascinating epidemiology to reveal. He had found a higher than background incidence of Crohn's in the Taff Valley of South Wales. Behind lie the Brecon Beacons – rough hills where the tough Welsh Blacks thrive. The MAP microbes were found in water samples from the River Taff… which then supplied local residents.

MAP passes from the cow into her milk. My GP father always used to state that milk was one of the most dangerous liquids one could drink. Correct, Dr Dansie – coronaries, cancer and now Crohn's! Being a tough microbe, MAP is not killed by pasteurisation. Indeed, Hermon-Taylor reckoned that 10% of UK bottled milk tested positive for MAP. Of course, not everyone drinking milk would develop Crohn's disease, but if the gut defences were down for reasons of either allergy or abnormal gut microbiome (fermenting gut), then there would be potential for MAP to make itself at home in the gut wall.

Great theory, but I was primarily interested in the practical application. Hermon-Taylor published a paper in 1997 where he described his experience of treating Crohn's with antibiotics. In total, 46 Crohn's patients were treated with a 'TB look-alike' regime of antibiotics. Great improvements were documented objectively with colonoscopy and blood tests for inflammatory markers. Of 19 steroid-dependent patients, only two required steroids once the treatment was established. The conclusion overall was 'substantial clinical improvement'.[1]

Train tickets to London were purchased by Carol's mum and off they went to see Prof Hermon-Taylor.[†] A package of antibiotics was started. I insisted that Carol stick to her paleo-ketogenic (Stone Age 'plus') diet. This was essential. Not to do so would set up the very conditions that allowed her to get infected in the first place. Obviously, she had to avoid all dairy products because there was a risk she might consume those containing MAP. She had to remain on a very low-carbohydrate diet, or an abnormal gut microbiome would result.

Bless her – she did it. Not easy as a teenager when temptation abounds. But fear is a driving factor and it worked. All her gut symptoms settled down and her energy levels were restored. But was this a cure? It depends how one defines cure. If 'cure' means was it safe for her to return to the wicked ways of modern Western diets was she free of Crohn's? Then no, she will never be cured. But that applies to all diseases. Can she look forward to a long and healthy life if she sticks to the prescribed regimes? Yes, of course.

Here we are 16 years on. Recently Carol presented again with poor energy. She had slipped on the diet and was clearly fermenting in her upper gut again, so I had to crack the whip to get her back on track. Interestingly, she had developed hypothyroidism and correcting this made the world of difference.

Reference

1. Gui GP, Thomas PR, Tizard ML, Lake J, Sanderson JD, Hermon-Taylor J. Two-year-outcomes analysis of Crohn's disease treated with rifabutin and macrolide antibiotics. *J Antimicrob Chemother* 1997; 39(3): 393-400. www.ncbi.nlm.nih.gov/pubmed/9096189

[†]**Footnote:** I always ask my patients if they are happy to share their story. Carol got back to me with 'Reading this brought back memories of Mum and I on that train to London. I will never forget meeting Professor Hermon-Taylor. What a character! Never mind his life-changing treatment! Without which, and also your help, I quite likely wouldn't be skiing in Canada and living the life I do!'

Chapter 65
Dentistry and its hidden problems

Dentistry case histories (contributed by Dr Shideh Pouria and Dr Jose Mendonça)
Cardiac dysrhythmia and asthma
Neurological problems and chronic fatigue
Inflammatory arthritis

Dental amalgam is such toxic stuff that I routinely advise that we should all get rid of it. If you have the money, and/or are sick, then this needs to be done properly by a well versed 'mercury-free' dentist. If you do not have the money and are not too ill, then get the fillings removed with standard dentistry. You may have a temporary spike in mercury toxicity (which can be mitigated by the detox techniques detailed in Chapter 34) but for the rest of your life you will be much better off.

I learned the above early on in my career and so, with money being a precious resource, I did not insist on toxicity or sensitivity tests for mercury because I knew what the result would be. Much better to invest in treatments. I was always worried that my recommendations for an expensive intervention had the potential to result in the complaint, 'Well, that was a waste of money', but this has never happened. In Chapter 45 you can read about Craig's experience with the removal of dental amalgam.

The other way dental health impacts our general well-being is through infections relating to the teeth. This is a well-known fact pertaining to

periodontal disease where various conditions, such as heart and brain disease, are linked to it. Yet the concept of dental root infections as a source of inflammation and chronic disease remains controversial and few such patients are assessed in this respect. At a recent peer supervision group meeting my colleague Dr Pouria presented a number of cases she had treated together with our surgical colleague Dr Jose Mendonça. Here are the case histories, in their words, of three patients with complex medical problems treated successfully.

Case 1: Cardiac dysrhythmia

A 56-year-old man with a history of asthma, nasal polyps and palpitations was referred originally to the clinic for recent episodes of recurrent upper respiratory tract infections, sinusitis, and two episodes of pneumonia resulting in three incidences of punctured lung. He had a number of risk factors for respiratory disease, including occupational exposure to solvents, mould, dust, red wine and smoke allergy, as well as iron overload from a genetic disorder of iron metabolism. He required regular inhalers from his chest physician and blood-letting to reduce his iron load. His cardiologist had ruled out any underlying cardiac reasons for his occasional dysrhythmias. His dental history revealed the presence of 11 amalgam fillings. He was also exposed to pesticides sprayed on golf courses and surrounding farms. He was a non-smoker who enjoyed moderate amounts of caffeinated and alcoholic drinks. There was a strong family history of early and fatal stroke.

Preliminary investigations confirmed the presence of dust and mould allergy. His blood tests revealed a very high load of occupational volatile organic compounds and pesticides and the presence of toxic metals from the dental materials used. He had very poor antioxidant protection and was very depleted in key minerals, such as zinc and magnesium, as well as vitamin D3.

Over the ensuing months and years, he applied the lifestyle, dietary and treatment regimens of ecological medicine and his condition consistently improved, with better asthma control, energy, resilience and no further infections. Three years later, he developed persistent palpitations following a course of antibiotics; these improved on a course of antifungal medications, but when he relapsed, he was referred to the cardiologist when he was found to be in fast atrial fibrillation (AF). He was treated unsuccessfully with DC cardioversion (electric shock), blood thinners and beta-blocker drugs to slow down his heart rate, which caused severe fatigue and shortness of breath, and a short-lived episode of unexplained loss of memory.

We discussed the underlying risk factors for cardiac dysrhythmias, and these included: exposure to mercury,[1] low magnesium levels, poor antioxidant function, alcohol, dysbiosis and latent infections, such as viruses and dental infections. A panoramic dental X-ray of his jaws showed infected cavities related to an extracted right upper 3rd molar and 15 large mercury fillings. He was treated supportively and referred for oral surgery and removal of all his mercury fillings and replacement with more biocompatible materials (in this case zirconia). He was deemed to be at high risk for surgery given his dysrhythmia and being on blood-thinning drugs. However, the surgery went very well with debridement of infected bone in his jaw and removal of the mercury fillings. His symptoms all disappeared the day after surgery. At a recent follow up, two years later, the patient no longer suffered with any infections nor had he had any episodes of dysrhythmias and was off all medications, including his inhalers for asthma.

Discussion

This case is an example of the non-pharmaceutical treatments which may help patients with dysrhythmias and demonstrates the phenomenon, which is often described in ecological medical practice, that there are many potentially modifiable factors that impact cardiac function and rhythm. The main factors found to be important in the management of such patients with dysrhythmia are:

1. The presence of a dysbiotic (imbalanced) microbiome may cause a systemic metabolic disturbance predisposing the patient to, or triggering, dysrhythmias. Multicellular organisms live in close association with microbes, and humans are no exception, where populations of colonic micro-organisms co-exist in true symbiosis with the host. When this ecosystem is disturbed, 'dysbiosis' develops, where one or more potentially harmful micro-organisms dominate the ecosystem. This creates a gut ecology predisposing to both local and systemic disease. The presence of an imbalanced

microbiome, especially in the presence of a higher proportion of fungal species due to antibiotic resistance of these species, leads to the exposure of higher amounts of specific fungal waste metabolites (often alcohols) which are readily quantifiable in urinary organic assays.

2. Palpitations are a well-recognised symptom of food intolerances. One of the key effects of dysbiosis is impaired protein digestion leading to the absorption of partially digested short-chain polypeptides which may mimic various hormones. Some of these short-chain polypeptides may have catecholamine-like function, leading to dysrhythmias. Sometimes exclusion diets are necessary to seek out the foods which trigger palpitations. Re-introduction of offending foods will highlight which foods need to be excluded to avoid palpitations. Many patients treated for dysbiosis by clinical ecologists find that symptoms of palpitation disappear on achieving a more normal microbiome through appropriate dietary measures and a course of anti-fungal drugs and probiotics.

3. Exposure to toxic metals, chemicals and xenobiotics have the potential for causing inflammation, immune activation and free-radical damage in every tissue in the body, including cardiac tissue; mercury in particular, through the inactivation of catecholaminei-0-methyl transferase, increases serum and urinary epinephrine, norepinephrine, and dopamine levels. This effect may result in high blood pressure and predispose to dysrhythmias.

4. Magnesium deficiency: Intravenous magnesium has been used to prevent and treat many different types of cardiac dysrhythmia because of its many electrophysiological actions on the conduction system of the heart. Magnesium supplementation therefore constitutes an important tool in managing cardiac dysrhythmias, something that is neglected by cardiologists.[2]

5. Increased risk of cardiac disease through low vitamin D levels.

6. Role of alcohol in dysrhythmias: Animal studies have shown varying and apparently opposite effects of alcohol on cardiac rhythm and conduction. Chronic heavy alcohol use has been incriminated in the genesis of cardiac dysrhythmias in humans.[3] Electrophysiological studies have shown that acute alcohol administration facilitates the induction of tachydysrhythmias, such as idiopathic AF and ventricular tachydysrhythmias. The basic dysrhythmogenic effects of alcohol may relate to subclinical heart muscle injury from chronic alcohol exposure, producing patchy delays in the electrical signal conduction. The hyperadrenergic state of drinking and withdrawal may also contribute, as may electrolyte abnormalities arising from excess loss of magnesium and other minerals. Most of what we know about alcohol and dysrhythmias relates to heavy drinking. The effects of alcohol from dysbiotic microbiome on cardiac tissue have not been investigated and may represent an interesting avenue for future research.

7. Role of infections in dysrhythmias: Whilst the precise aetiology of AF is uncertain, it is clear that the condition is associated with the presence of inflammation. C-reactive protein (CRP), a sensitive biomarker of systemic inflammation, has been reported to be significantly higher in patients with AF compared with controls.

A variety of possible inflammatory triggers have been considered, including a role for latent dysrhythmogenic infections. One publication from 2004, studied 100 randomly selected patients with idiopathic paroxysmal AF through a structured questionnaire.[4] The results showed that in 22% there was an association with infection; 34% of patients cited alcohol as a trigger, of which red wine and spirits produced significantly more episodes of dysrhythmia than did white wine (p = 0.01 and 0.005 respectively). Specialist neuronal cells may also be induced by chronic stealth/intracellular infections to boost the sympathetic nervous system activity, triggering or enhancing electrical instability in patients with other predisposing factors, such as mineral imbalances. One such example is bartonellosis. Bartonella is a well-recognised cause of sub-acute cardiac myocarditis where Bartonella DNA has been detected in the cardiac tissue.[5] Silent myocarditis may lead to electrical instability triggering dysrhythmias. Another study showed that herpes viruses had a significant relationship to patients with AF compared with normal. This has been noted in other infections, such as toxoplasmosis too.[6] Therefore, patients with AF with no underlying cardiac or thyroid disease, should be screened for an inflammatory or infectious cause before being considered for more invasive or pharmaceutical treatments, such as anti-dysrhythmics, long-term anticoagulation and cardioversion with potential for serious side effects.

In summary, this case demonstrates that addressing dysbiosis through dietary measures of reducing carbohydrates, avoiding alcoholic drinks and increasing nutrient density, plus use of antifungal medications and probiotics may help in the treatment of palpitations and the symptoms of cardiac rhythm disorders. Likewise, supplementation with appropriate vitamins and minerals can help control intractable and treatment-resistant dysrhythmias. Given the toxic effects of heavy metals and chemicals on cardiac tissues and function, it is important to seek out the load of toxins on patients with dysrhythmias and reduce any such load through avoiding exposure and safe supporting of the body's own detoxification pathways, in particular in patients with dental exposure to mercury. The identification of stealth organisms and latent dental infections associated with root canals, cavities and other infections may make a crucial difference when treating these patients. Cone Beam CT scanning technologies have transformed the diagnosis of hitherto hidden dental infections, allowing doctors to collaborate with dentists much more effectively in confidently treating patients with underlying dental issues and AF.

Case 2: Neurological symptoms resolving with dental intervention

A 34-year-old woman was referred to the clinic with a one-year history of severe fatigue, cognitive and memory deficits and left sided weakness in her arms and legs which became worse at night. She also complained of fasciculations and twitching in both legs, which was worse on the left. She experienced tingling and heaviness with poor balance, headaches and pressure in her skull. She had also noted some muscle wasting in the muscle groups which felt weak. She complained of occasional palpitations and reported severe sugar cravings, disorientation and agitation in between meals.

The onset of her neurological symptoms was

chronologically preceded by dental treatment to a failed root canal in the right upper 6th molar. In March 2015 she developed pain in the tooth which had not been treated successfully and her endodontist repeated the procedure in April of the same year. Following on from the treatment she became dizzy, feverish, nauseous and extremely fatigued. It was after this that she experienced difficulty in walking, reduced cognitive function and brain fog but neurologists found no abnormalities on an MRI of the brain. She had symptoms of gut dysbiosis, in particular bloating and alternating constipation and loose stools for which she had been treated with metronidazole, to which she had severe neurological reactions, as well as a number of herbal antimicrobial treatments which she did not tolerate either, especially as they triggered severe mental problems, including psychosis and suicidal tendency.

She had been suspected to have neuro-borreliosis despite negative serology for Lyme disease on the basis of one mosquito bite to which she had reacted with infection tracking up her leg. On another more recent occasion, two weeks after being bitten, she had experienced progressive hand and leg weakness accompanied with confusion in time and space, tinnitus, twitching and pain under her feet. Her legs were burning and she had buzzing in her head and numbness in her hands. She experienced pain behind her eyes, pressure in her head and severe fatigue. She reported poor coordination leading to falls.

Her past medical history also included exposure to mould having lived in a damp house during which time her whole family had felt unwell. She had also been scratched by a sick cat that had subsequently died but had not been investigated for either toxoplasmosis or Bartonella both of which may be associated with neurological disease.

On examination she had no visible fasciculation (twitching in her muscles) and no focal neurological signs other than universally brisk reflexes and muscle wasting in her left arm and leg despite which she had normal and equal power in all muscle groups. There was evidence of thoraco-lumbar scoliosis to the right. She had cold extremities, multiple dental crowns and an extracted molar.

Her risk factors for neuro-inflammation included:
- five heavily infected root-filled teeth
- a dental abscess
- likely fungal dysbiosis
- a mercury filling in the extracted tooth
- a family history of neurological disease
- possible Lyme/co-infection or a viral myopathy
- mould exposure.

Given the clear chronological link between her dental treatment and the onset of symptoms she was referred for a panoramic X-ray of her teeth as a prelude to assessment by an oral surgeon. This showed the presence of five devitalised and infected teeth for which she had had root canal treatment. There was evidence of severe bone loss and the tips of the root canal had breached the sinus floor, with infection extending into the sinus cavity.

She underwent extensive oral surgery, having seven extractions, debridement and insertion of zirconia implants. Shortly after the surgery, the muscle weakness disappeared as did the pressure in her head. Her overall health and well-being improved significantly with abundant energy. She claimed she could do 'anything' she wanted. Her balance came back and she no longer tended to fall over. She suffered a minor relapse in her symptoms when she had a viral infection. Given that she had had many courses of antibiotics, her GI symptoms were continuing to trouble her and a close family member had been diagnosed with threadworm and flukes, so she was treated with a course of tinidazole followed by fluconazole for fungal dysbiosis. These treatments alongside a better diet made a significant impact on her symptoms. At a recent follow up appointment she reported to have been completely well with respect to her neurological symptoms, on a good diet and with appropriate supplementation.

Discussion

This case demonstrates the various factors that may contribute to neuro-inflammation and ultimately neurodegeneration.[7, 8] In the case of this patient, there was not only a family history of early death from brain disease, but she had had multiple exposures including moulds (neurotoxic), pesticides, possible infectious agents such as viruses[9] and stealth organisms[10] like Bartonella and toxoplasma from cat scratch. Vector-borne infections may also be transmitted via mosquito bites. She also had extensive chronic dental infections which required dental surgery. As in Case 1, the advent of cone beam CT scanning has allowed greater precision in identifying hitherto difficult-to-diagnose dental infections. The treatments offered to this patient not only prevented the development of possible life-threatening neurological disease but also, via the comprehensive systems approach, led to significant improvement in her general health and quality of life.

Case 3: Rheumatoid arthritis

A 40-year-old woman presented with a diagnosis of rheumatoid arthritis (RA) affecting all her joints, but in particular her knees and ankles, inability to lose weight, severe constipation, generalised bloating, dependent oedema, especially of the face, and headaches. Her initial diagnosis of RA was in January 2013, with high markers for such. She was started on Plaquenil at that time and had taken it for three months. Following a second opinion she was advised to stop the Plaquenil and commence on disease-modifying drugs.

Other relevant history included: diagnosis of autoimmune thyroid disease, raised BMI, multiple courses of antibiotics for multiple infections, predisposing her to dysbiosis and immune dysregulation. On average she would have one or two courses per annum. She had symptoms of dysbiosis with severe bloating, constipation, and sugar cravings. She often suffered from low mood. She had noted that her joint symptoms deteriorated with increased carbohydrate intake and with dietary chicken and egg intake.

Her dental history revealed multiple fillings with mercury amalgam.

She had had three children delivered by Caesarean section. During each pregnancy she had had severe hyperemesis gravidarum which resulted in damage to her teeth and many of her amalgam fillings falling out. Two years prior to her presentation, one of her large old mercury amalgam fillings had fallen out which had been promptly replaced with further mercury amalgam. She had required orthodontic treatment with prolonged use of braces. She had also had root fillings which were performed in late 2001.

On examination she looked fatigued, with low mood. She was overweight and had considerable facial swelling with some ankle and hand swelling also. She had amalgam fillings and metal-bonded crowns, as well as candidiasis in her oral cavity. There was no palpable goitre. Apart from a large abdominal scar, the rest of her examination was unremarkable.

Given her history, we decided to rule out infections and dysbiosis as well as assess her nutrient status and toxic load. She was started on the fungal dysbiosis diet and on a course of an antifungal treatment with nystatin. Her investigations showed she had severe vitamin D deficiency with low levels of minerals, in particular zinc and magnesium. Her blood tests also revealed raised total load of nickel, chromium (VI), mercury, vanadium and palladium, all of which would have been part of her dental fillings or braces. She also had evidence of poor antioxidant function.

A comprehensive stool analysis did confirm the growth of *Candida lusitaniae* that was fully sensitive to nystatin and all azole antifungals

Over the course of the following months she adhered to a nutrient-dense diet and took nystatin. Her digestive symptoms improved, she lost 3 kg in weight, and her oedema reduced. She started a course of targeted supplementation. Her energy picked up, she was able to restart exercise, and she described her cognitive function as having a clear mind and excellent memory. She continued to have flares in her arthritis, either in response to carbohydrates in her diet or as a result of a die-off reaction to the antifungal medications.

At a follow-up consultation, she mentioned that she had a broken crown on a root-filled tooth. A screening panoramic X-ray of both jaws revealed severe infection in her jaw. When reviewed by a consultant oral surgeon, he felt that this could explain the on-going facial swelling and chronic inflammation. For this reason, she underwent oral surgery as well as having all the metal removed from her teeth. This involved the removal of the infected molar and an impacted wisdom tooth and all amalgams. Later on, a further molar with a metal crown and amalgam underneath had to be extracted as the tooth and surrounding tissue were necrotic. She required debridement, periodontal ligament removal, ozone therapy to the bone underlying the extracted infected, necrotic teeth and postoperative antibiotics. Given the size of the defect she also required local grafting of plasma progenitor cells to repair her jaw. Subsequently, she has fully recovered from the surgery and her symptoms of RA have completely resolved.

Discussion

This case of chronic, inflammatory arthritis is one of a number of cases which have responded to dental surgery, antibiotics, and nutritional interventions. Rheumatoid arthritis (RA) is a chronic inflammatory disorder that leads to joint damage, deformity, and pain. It affects approximately 1% of adults in developed countries. It is associated with significant morbidity and mortality.

An infectious aetiology for rheumatic conditions has been quoted in the medical literature for decades. Despite 3000 years of history demonstrating the influence of oral health on general health, it is only in recent years that the association between dental diseases such as chronic periodontitis and systemic conditions such as atherosclerosis, bacterial endocarditis, diabetes mellitus, respiratory disease, preterm delivery, rheumatoid arthritis,[11] and, more recently, osteoporosis, pancreatic cancer, metabolic syndrome, renal diseases and neurodegenerative diseases such as Alzheimer's disease, has been acknowledged. Furthermore, the so-called focal dental infection theory fell into oblivion as endodontics established itself in the main-stream of dental interventions. Focal dental infections have been attributed to dental pulp pathologies and periapical infections in teeth with both treated and untreated root canals. In recent years, their role has continued to be dismissed even though increasing interest is being shown in the relationship between periodontal infection and systemic diseases.

A review of the literature found no studies on the role of focal dental infections in RA even though, in medical practice, a definite role is acknowledged for infections in some types of arthropathies, such as Lyme disease. Even though the dental and medical literature admits that periodontal pathogens and their products, as well as inflammatory mediators produced in periodontal tissues, might seep into the bloodstream, causing systemic effects and/or contributing to systemic diseases, the same consideration is denied to the potential risk of focal infections. Various mechanisms, such as common susceptibility, systemic inflammation, direct bacterial infection and cross-reactivity, and molecular mimicry have been used to explain this phenomenon.

From a medical perspective, this case suggests that in intractable progressive joint disease, dental infections when identified and treated, may lead to the resolution of the systemic arthritis. Further follow up of these patients is required to assess long-term benefits of this approach. Furthermore, a close liaison with dental and surgical colleagues in managing rheumatoid patients to identify such aetiologically relevant infections and their prompt treatment can save much pain, morbidity, cost and mortality among this cohort of patients.[12, 13, 14]

Conclusion

In summary these cases demonstrate that in addition to: 1. addressing dysbiosis through dietary measures (reducing carbohydrates, avoiding alcoholic drinks, increasing nutrient density) and treatment with antifungal agents and probiotics, 2. supplementation with appropriate vitamins and minerals, 3. seeking out and reducing toxin load; the identification of stealth organisms and latent dental infections associated with root canals, cavitations and other infections may make a crucial difference to patient health. Since the advent of CBCT technologies, the diagnosis of hitherto hidden dental infections has been transformed and allows doctors to collaborate with dentists much more effectively in confidently treating patients with underlying dental issues and systemic symptoms which may seem unrelated at the first glance. This will not only reduce the burden of morbidity and mortality in patients, reduce the need for pharmacological interventions and their side effects, but it will also save on costly interventions.

References

Case 1

1. Houston MC. Role of mercury toxicity in hypertension, cardiovascular disease, and stroke. *J Clin Hypertens* 2011; 13(8): 621-627.

2. Ho KM. Intravenous magnesium for cardiac arrhythmias: Jack of all trades. *Magnes Res* 2008; 21(1): 65-68.

3. Balbão CE, et al. Effects of alcohol on atrial fibrillation: myths and truths. *Ther Adv Cardiovasc Dis* 2009; 3(1): 53-63.

4. Hansson A, et al. Arrhythmia-provoking factors and symptoms at the onset of paroxysmal atrial fibrillation: A study based on interviews with 100 patients seeking hospital assistance. *BMC Cardiovascular Disorders* 2004; 4: 13. www.biomedcentral.com/1471-2261/4/13

5. Wesslen L, Ehrenborg C, Holmberg M, et al. Subacute Bartonella Infection in Swedish Orienteers Succumbing to Sudden Unexpected Cardiac Death or Having Malignant Arrhythmias. *Scandinavian Journal of Infectious Diseases* 2001; 33(6): 429-438. https://doi.org/10.1080/00365540152029891

6. Leak D, Meghji M. Toxoplasmic infection in cardiac disease. *Am J of Cardiol* 1979; 43(4): 841-849. https://doi.org/10.1016/0002-9149(79)90087-0

Case 2

7. Filipini T, et al. Clinical and Lifestyle Factors and Risk of Amyotrophic Lateral Sclerosis: A Population-Based Case-Control Study. *Int J Environ Res Public Health* 2020; 17: 857. DOI: 10.3390/ijerph17030857

8. Olsen I, Singhrao SK. Can oral infection be a risk factor for Alzheimer's disease? *J Oral Microbiol* 2015; 7: 29143. DOI: 10.3402/jom.v7.29143

9. Liang Li, et al. Viral infection and neurological disorders – potential role of extracellular nucleotides in neuro-inflammation. *ExRNA* 2019; 1: 26. DOI: https://doi.org/10.1186/s41544-019-0031-z

10. Coughlin JM, Yang T, Rebman AW, et al.

Imaging glial activation in patients with post-treatment Lyme disease symptoms: a pilot study using [11C]DPA-713 PET. *J Neuro-inflammation* 2018; 15(1): 346. DOI: 10.1186/s12974-018-1381-4

Case 3

11. Detert J, et al. The association between rheuma-toid arthritis and periodontal disease. *Arthritis Research & Therapy* 2010; 12: 218.
12. Scammell A. *The New Arthritis Breakthrough* Evans Publishers ISBN: 0-87131-843-1
13. Tilley BC, et al. Minocycline in rheumatoid arthritis. A 48-week, double-blind, placebo-con-trolled trial MIRA Trial Group. *Ann Intern Med* 1995; 122(2): 81-89.
14. Adwan M HQ. Tetracycline Antibiotics for Treating Rheumatoid Arthritis: A Systematic Review and Meta-Analysis [abstract]. *Arthritis Rheum* 2009; 60(Suppl 10): 406.
15. Wu MK1, Dummer PM, Wesselink PR. Consequences of and strategies to deal with residual post-treatment root canal infection. *Int Endod J* 2006; 39(5): 343-356.

Contributing authors

Dr Shideh Pouria, MB BS BSC MRCP(UK) PhD CMT

Dr Pouria qualified in 1991 from King's College School of Medicine, London, and has worked in numerous clinical and academic posts within the National Health Service, UK. Most recently she held a consultant post in Renal Medicine at Guy's Hospital. She has extensive experience in general and specialist medicine as well as in medical research in the field of mucosal immunology and glycobiology of IgA. It was through her PhD project in mucosal immunology that she became interested in the role of environmental factors in health and disease. She embarked on her training with the British Society for Ecological Medicine in 2006 and was the Medical Director at the Burghwood Clinic for Allergy, Environmental and Nutritional Medicine until 2013. She has continued to work in private practice since, treating patients with complex, chronic, inflammatory problems. She has held a visiting research Fellowship at King's College, is the vice-president of the British Society for Ecological Medicine, and served on the scientific advisory board for the Allergy Research Foundation until 2018. She is the author of a number of peer-reviewed papers and has written chapters in books on nutritional and ecological medicine.

Dr Jose Mendonça Caridad, MD DMD PhD

Jose Mendonça Caridad is the director of the Head and Neck Surgery Unit, Adult Stem Cell Therapy Unit, at POLUSA Hospital in Galicia, Spain, where he is involved in both clinical practice and research. He is president of the NGO Surgeons of the World, focusing on the development and practice of Head and Neck Surgery in Africa.

He received his medical degree from Santiago University in Spain where he later completed a Master's degree in microbiology, continuing with stomatology residency at the same university (DMD). After some time as a rural physician he followed a fellowship in Maxillofacial Surgery at UCLA with a special interest in orthognathic and reconstructive surgery and research into facial biomechanics. As a result of this he was awarded 'Cum Laude' in his doctoral thesis (PhD). He has been a university lecturer in oral surgery for both pre- and post-graduate programmes and has lec-tured and published extensively on the topic of metal-free regenerative surgery. He pioneered adult stem cell therapies in head and neck sur-gery and published the first paper on stem cells for advanced diseases such as radio-necrosis and tissue regeneration.

He is a member of such notable medical asso-ciations as the American Association of Oral and Maxillofacial Surgeons, the International Society of Metal Free Implantology and British Society for Ecological Medicine, amongst others. He is also a consultant in aeronautical medicine.

Chapter 66
Respiratory medicine

Respiratory case histories
Bronchiectasis (milk allergy and fungal infection)
Chronic obstructive pulmonary disease (chronic infection)
Chronic sinusitis (fungal infection)

Bronchiectasis

Thelma first consulted me in 1997. She had suffered asthma since the age of 3 that was so severe she missed most of her school years until 13 when she was prescribed steroids. At the time these were very helpful and allowed her to get back to school and college. She continued to survive until 1987 when, aged 33, she deteriorated. Thelma is a tough character; she continued to push on at work, but then collapsed, coughing up blood. She was admitted to hospital with a presumptive diagnosis of tuberculosis. Investigations showed she had a collapsed lung and lung abscess. Thankfully she recovered, but the lung infection became chronic and she was diagnosed with bronchiectasis.

Bronchiectasis was known of in Ancient Greece and Hippocrates is known to have recommended wine to such patients because it was thought that alcohol reduced sputum – indeed, pure ethanol is a moderately effective, but only transient, bronchodilator and symptom suppressant.[1]

Thelma was prescribed a different form of symptom suppressant – blue and brown inhalers for life, but even so, every winter she suffered worsening infections needing antibiotics and steroids. By the time she consulted me she was also deaf in one ear and anosmic – she had no sense of smell. Since smell is closely related to taste, food was no longer a pleasure.

I have to say that in 1997 I did not know then what I know now. Consequently, the full package of effective treatment for Thelma took nearly 20 years to evolve and I now better understand her history in the light of her response to treatment. Symptoms that date from childhood almost always have an allergic component. Dairy allergy is such a common problem and associated with mucus and catarrh. I recommended cutting out all dairy in 1997 but Thelma was a dairy addict and it took 20 years before she really cut out all dairy.

Within three days of giving up dairy her nose unblocked, her sense of smell returned and she was turning the TV and radio down.

A further breakthrough came in 2006 when antibiotics started to make her worse. I prescribed a systemic antifungal with which not only was her chest greatly improved but her energy levels were better – Thelma told me she could go skipping without getting short of breath! This flagged up the possibility of a fungal infection in her chest. Indeed, it transpired that the house in which she had lived between

1984 and 1997 was full of mould – she had even had mushrooms growing inside! I persuaded her NHS consultant to do a RAST blood test for aspergillus, but this was negative. However, the clinical history is always more important than tests and it was essential for her to take antifungal drugs every time she needed antibiotics. Eventually in 2014 she had a skin test for aspergillus which was strongly positive, and she was diagnosed with such.

My mind has been greatly concentrated recently as many of the patients I see with ME have an infectious trigger to their ME and continue to suffer from flu-like infectious symptoms. Often, they come with diagnoses such as Lyme, chlamydia or chronic Epstein-Barr. How could I treat these people safely, affordably and effectively? Many have been diagnosed with multiple infections and been treated with various antibiotics, antifungals or antivirals, with perhaps temporary, but not lasting, benefit. There were many parallels with Thelma's case.

Life is an arms race, as I repeat many times in this book. You and I are a free lunch for bacteria, yeast, viruses and other microbes, aching to make themselves at home in our very comfortable bodies. We are already losing that arms race. Judy Mikovitz, who showed that XMRV virus is one likely cause of ME, states that 15% of our DNA is comprised of retrovirus. The general principles of treating any infection are therefore:

to starve the little wretches out and

kill them in as many different ways as safely possible.

What distinguishes human cells from microbes is that microbes can only fuel themselves with sugars and starches. Human cells can run on fat and fermented fibre (short-chain fatty acids). So, the starting point for treating any person with any infection is a paleo (no dairy or gluten) ketogenic (very low carbohydrate) diet in order to starve the little wretches out. The next phase is to use vitamin C. Vitamin C contact-kills all microbes – indeed, it is used as a food preservative for that very reason. But vitamin C is harmless to humans.

After years of prevarication, Thelma changed to a paleo-ketogenic (PK) diet. Nowadays I am much tougher about diet – I refuse to compromise on this. As I say to all my patients: 'My job is to get you well, not to entertain you'. Indeed, Craig and I have written *The PK Cookbook* so that people can do this diet on their own. This diet is for everyone – for the well to stay well, as much as for the sick to get better. Being a carb-addict, Thelma suffered the expected withdrawal symptoms. In parallel with this she took vitamin C to bowel tolerance – eventually getting up to 15 grams a day. This was combined with an iodine salt pipe – another clinical tool that is of proven benefit and a major part of my armamentarium. Infection can be killed with a pincer movement – iodine from the outside and vitamin C from the inside.

The result? Thelma has since been infection free. No chest infections, no winter flu, no need for vaccination. Antibiotics and antifungal drugs were only needed following a dietary holiday hiccup. Her energy levels are much improved at the time of writing. Only occasionally does she need to use the blue and brown inhalers. Now that is what I call a result!

'Bronchiectasis' is defined in the medical books as an *irreversible*, chronic enlargement of certain bronchial tubes, implying the condition can only worsen with time. Once again, the prescribing of symptom suppressants had led to chronicity and a progressive deterioration. Thelma is living proof that 'irreversible' conditions can be reversed and that life can be good again when time and effort are focused on addressing the root causes of illness.

Chronic obstructive pulmonary disease

Since first writing Thelma's case history for this book I now have three further patients with COPD who have been able to remain infection free and reduced their use of inhalers since applying these Groundhog Chronic interventions (see Appendices 1–3).

Chronic sinusitis

Luke, 41, is a friend and neighbour. He must be the fittest and strongest person I know – the other day I watched him pick up a water-sodden railway sleeper and carry it under one arm. He has never missed a day's work in his life, but he did occasionally mention his sinusitis, which presented variably with blockage, inflammation and, most notably, severe frontal sinus pain. Indeed, it was this that prevented him pursuing one of his hobbies – namely, scuba-diving – as the water pressures involved were excruciating. A course of antibiotics would sometimes afford improvement, but what worked best for him were NSAI (non-steroidal anti-inflammatory) drugs, such as ibuprofen. I really did not like him taking those because in my view that amounted to symptom suppression.

It is of no reassurance to patients to tell them that I learn most from those whose symptoms I struggle with, but with the right questions in the forefront of your mind it means that when you stumble over an answer you do at least see it! Thank you, Margaret, for pointing me at mycotoxins, and thank you Dr Costantini for excellent clinical detective work – you have now plugged a large gap in my knowledge.

Look at life from the point of view of a fungus. Having found a comfortable spot to live, it does not want other microbes homing in on the act. Key to survival is to produce toxins that kill competitors. Fungi produce mycotoxins to kill bacterial competition, and these toxins include penicillin, cephalosporin and streptomycin – these we know as antibiotics (the names are a giveaway). But there are many other mycotoxins, and Dr Costantini (formerly the Director of the World Health Organization (WHO), Mycotoxin Collaborating Center at the University of Freiburg, Germany) has shown that many diseases have a fungal, mycotoxin-driven aetiology:

> *Mycotoxins are known to drive hepato-cellular carcinoma, oesophageal cancer, lung cancer, colon cancer, kidney cancer, breast cancer, colon cancer, endometrial cancer, leukaemia, lymphoma, astrocytoma and Kaposi's sarcoma. The autoimmune diseases appearing to have a fungal/mycotoxin origin are: scleroderma, diabetes mellitus, HLA-related disease, rheumatoid arthritis, Sjogren's syndrome, psoriasis and systemic lupus erythematosus. All of the drugs effective in the treatment of these diseases possess antifungal or anti-mycotoxin activity. This includes all NSAIDs.*[2,3]

Bingo! We have an explanation for Luke's chronic sinusitis and its response to NSAIDs. But these drugs have a systemic effect – I wanted a local effect. In the full knowledge that he was generously acting as another of my human guinea pigs, Luke started sniffing with the iodine salt pipe (see Chapter 32). The results were miraculous. Sinus pain, inflammation and blockage gone within a few days of sniffing. Normally a cold would result in days of misery, but the salt pipe nipped these in the bud too. I did very well out of the situation too – I received a free delivery of 10 tonnes of firewood… and for a pyromaniac like me that is some gift!

References

1. Sisson JH. Alcohol and airways function in health and disease. *Alcohol* 2007; 41(5): 293–307.
2. Costantini AV. The Fungal/Mycotoxin Connections: Autoimmune Diseases, Malignancies, Athero-sclerosis, Hyperllpldemias, and Gou. October 11, 1993. 28th Annual Meeting New Horizons in Chemical Sensitivities – State of the Art Diagnosis and Treatment. http://arthritistrust.org/wp-content/uploads/2012/10/Fungal-Mycotoxin-Connection.pdf (accessed 6 June 2019).
3. Costantini AV. The Fungalbionic Book Series. www.fungalbionicbookseries.com (accessed 6 June 2019).

Chapter 67
Nephrology/kidney and urinary tract problems

Nephrology case histories
Chronic renal failure (multiple toxicity)
Kidney stones and renal colic (organophosphate poisoning)
Interstitial cystitis and incontinence (allergy to gut bacteria)

Chronic renal failure

Joe was referred to me in 2005 for treatment of his Gulf War syndrome. The two Gulf Wars fought were the most toxic wars in history. All the pro-inflammatory infectious and toxic problems of modern Western lives were compressed into a few months. Young men, who were not allowed to become soldiers unless they were 100% fit and well, were rendered sick for life. Joe told me that he and others were subjected to a combination of extensive vaccination (up to 14 different vaccines on one day), toxic chemicals (including pesticides like organophosphates and pyrethroids, plus dioxins, flame retardants, tributyl tin and so on), chemicals from burning oil well fires, contaminated drinking water, radiation exposure from depleted uranium used in warheads and, probably, microbes that were part of stealth biological warfare, notably *Mycoplasma incognitus*. (Professor Garth Nicolson demonstrated that *Mycoplasma fermentans*, of which *Mycoplasma incognitus* is a strain, was used as biological warfare in the Gulf.)[1, 2, 3]

All the above factors would be expected to accelerate the rate of degeneration and switch on autoimmunity, allergy and cancer. Not surprisingly, Joe had a complex clinical picture (combination of symptoms and signs) which included, in order of severity:

Scleroderma – both his forearms felt solid, like lumps of wood
Scleroderma in the lungs, which clinically presented with obstructive pulmonary disease
Chronic fatigue syndrome, with such poor energy delivery mechanisms that he was in heart failure
Multiple chemical sensitivity and food allergies
Rosacea
Irritable bowel syndrome

Where there is such a complex clinical picture, it is almost impossible to tease out the different threads of mechanisms. Indeed, when one mechanism goes down so do others. Resources were limited, but Joe wanted to prove a poisoning had been involved: a fat biopsy in 2005 showed the presence of organophosphates, tributyl tin, PCBs, lindane and DDD (an organochloride insecticide). The DNA adducts test (page 19.2) showed high levels of benzene and tin with very low levels of zinc. In this case we simply had to put in place all the Groundhog interventions that were possible. Joe did it all because he had no choice.

In 2006, before the benefits of the above could be fully realised, and possibly because of a detox reaction, Joe got worse. His scleroderma started to manifest as malignant hypertension, with encephalopathy and renal failure. He spent 14 days in intensive care, and was unconscious for five days. He was treated with high dose steroids, antibiotics, anti-hypertensives, warfarin and anti-epileptic drugs. It was extraordinary that he survived – he should have died then.

On discharge he was taking a shopping list of medication. He was on the waiting list for renal dialysis with a creatinine level of over 300 micromol/l (normal range 52-96 micromol/l) translating to a glomerular filtration rate of 19 ml/min (normal range >90). This was late stage renal failure.

Once home, Joe was able to reinstate his regime of diet, nutritional supplements, thyroid/adrenal prescriptions and detoxification. His energy levels were much better when taking doxycycline, prescribed for a sinus infection. This squares with him having picked up a chronic mycoplasma infection in the Gulf War. We continued doxycycline 100 mg daily long term.

Joe made great progress. His scleroderma improved to the extent where the skin of his forearms became soft again. His rheumatologist was disbelieving – she told Joe that she must have got the diagnosis wrong in the first place because scleroderma has an inevitable downhill

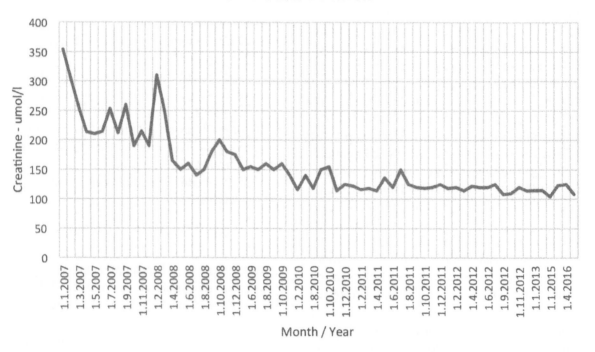

Figure 67.1: Joe's improving creatinine levels showing improvement in his kidney function

progression. His blood pressure normalised and we were able to stop much of his medication. But what was most unexpected was the improvement in his renal function as charted by his creatinine levels in Figure 67.1:

There have been additional tools put in place as I have learned more – namely:

Tools for the fermenting gut – Joe suffered very much from abdominal bloating despite doing an excellent Stoneage diet. We decided to cut out all carbohydrates ruthlessly – he had to swap from powering his body with carbs to powering it with fat. This had some interesting effects. Joe lost 10 lb of weight in less than a week – much of this was allergic oedema. His bloating ceased as did his noisy rumbling gut. His rosacea improved markedly. This can be explained by allergy to microbes from the fermenting gut.

Intravenous magnesium bolus injections greatly improved his energy and well-being.

So Joe got to the stage when the only prescription medications he was taking were inhalers for his COPD and doxycycline. Although we had clearly improved the manifestations of scleroderma in his skin and his arteries, his lung function worsened so he needed continuous oxygen. I suspect his inhalers were to blame since Joe was doing so well in all other respects. We had started the salt pipe with iodine but too late – he could not stop the inhalers. He was on the waiting list for a lung transplant but died in 2017 before a donor could be found.

Renal stones

John came to see me primarily with chronic fatigue syndrome secondary to organophosphate poisoning. Indeed, he was one of the worst contaminated patients that I had even seen. He had worked in the Scottish salmon farming industry and it is a fundamental problem of any intensive farming system that infections and parasites move in. Salmon grown intensively in Scottish lochs are susceptible to sea lice, *Lepeophtheirus salmonis*. John was a diver and would swim down to the fish cages with a back-pack of organophosphate chemicals. One day when swinging the container onto his back it burst, showering him with its contents. At the time the seriousness of the incident was not recognised, so he did not undergo proper decontamination. Organophosphates readily pass through the skin. This is how Ronald Maddison was killed at Porton Down in 1953 – within 45 minutes of 200 mg of sarin being applied to his forearm, he was dead.

Leading Aircraftsman Ronald Maddison, who was 20 years old at the time, had been offered 15 shillings and three days' leave for volunteering to take part in the study. He agreed and planned to use the money to buy an engagement ring for his fiancee, Mary Pyle. A full post mortem was carried out and an inquest was held in secret before the Wiltshire Coroner, Harold Dale, who returned a verdict of misadventure. Ronald's father was allowed to attend the inquest but he was also warned that if he disclosed any details of the inquest to anyone, including his own family, he would be prosecuted under the Official Secrets Act. Ronald's body was delivered (by the Ministry of Defence) to his family in a steel coffin with the lid bolted down. Body parts, including brain and spinal cord tissue, skin, muscle, stomach, lung and gut were retained without his family's knowledge or permission, and these body parts were used over several years in toxicology experiments. Ronald's father, John, received £40 to pay for the funeral costs. Subsequently, the Maddison family led a campaign and, through their efforts,

Ronald's death became the subject of a police investigation, named Operation Antler, which ran from 1999 to 2004. The then Lord Chief Justice, Lord Woolf, overturned the original inquest verdict in November 2002 after a hearing in the High Court. This led to a new inquest which opened on 5 May 2004. This turned out to be the longest inquest ever held in England and Wales, at that time, with around 100 witnesses giving evidence over 50 days. Finally, on 15 November 2004, the inquest jury returned that Ronald had been unlawfully killed and his family received £100,000 compensation, a far cry from the £40 they had previously received for his funeral expenses.

As we started treatment, John developed renal colic. I don't think this was a result of the treatment since it takes some years for renal stones to form. Renal colic is one of the most agonising pains one can suffer. It illustrates how painful muscle spasm can be. The colic was due to a kidney stone being stuck in his ureter (the tube from kidney to bladder) and the pain resulted from the ureteric muscle spasm trying to move it on. He managed to pass that stone but X-rays showed the presence of many other kidney stones. John started to suffer recurrent attacks of severe pain every time another stone moved on.

There are three narrowings in the ureter, between the kidney and the bladder, where stones tend to stick. The surgeons tried a 'Dormia basket' to fish out a stone stuck where the ureter comes into the bladder. Lithotripsy was also tried in an attempt to shatter the large calculus stuck in the renal pelvis (the centre of the kidney). But none of these interventions prevented John's repeated attacks of pain.

At that time I was only just beginning to appreciate the properties of vitamin C. The prevailing wisdom at the time was that vitamin C, as ascorbic acid, might cause renal stones. This did not seem biologically plausible to me. John and I both did some research and, with his full knowledge and understanding of the possible issues, John started on vitamin C to bowel tolerance (see Chapter 31). The result? John has had no further attacks of renal colic. Interestingly, a recent X-ray showed he still had a large stone in his kidney, but it is smaller. Vitamin C is slowly dissolving it away.

Interstitial cystitis

The following is another increasingly common clinical picture. Carol, 64, paints the scene. She presented, in a recent November, with a first episode of cystitis – the urgent need to pee, pain on micturition, small volume and frequency. She assured me, smiling, that this was not honeymoon cystitis. She was describing the symptoms of an inflamed bladder. The GP had diagnosed a urinary tract infection (UTI), sent off a mid-stream urine (MSU) sample and prescribed trimethoprim. So far so good. At a follow-up visit, the MSU sample was back showing no infection and the course of antibiotics completed. However, the symptom of cystitis was only slightly better and now Carol had become incontinent of urine. It was not the sort of incontinence that arises when the perineal floor is weak/wanting so urine leaks with running or jumping. It was the sort of incontinence when the urge to pee is so great that the urine leaks out before one can get seated on the throne. It was no respecter of situation – it occurred anytime, anyplace. The GP could prescribe a bladder calmer in the form of VESIcare, which helped a little, but the mainstay of management was a liberal supply of inco-pads. Carol faced a life-sentence of nappies.

Carol is bright and picked up on my suggested mechanism at once. She was eating a typical high-carbohydrate Western diet. As we age, we get less good at digesting foods (many comment they cannot manage large meals) and there is a tendency for them to be fermented. Numbers of microbes in the gut build up and so more than expected spill over into the bloodstream. These pass through the kidneys into the urine to be peed out. This means normal, healthy urine does contain some microbes – indeed, the definition of a UTI is more than 10,000 microbes per ml of urine. (On this basis, should Carol's urine test hold 9999 microbes per ml she would be told there was no infection.) However, should she sensitise to microbes, inflammation would be switched on. Effectively she had a bladder that had become 'allergic to microbes'. Remember, the symptoms of inflammation driven by allergy are the same as those driven by infection (page 16.1).

We had another clinical clue. Why should she have suddenly presented with allergy to gut microbes? She had recently had an annual flu vaccination – we know these are good at switching on allergy – perhaps this was the trigger? Vaccination, by definition, provokes an immune response, and whenever this is done, one risks an allergic or autoimmune reaction because both allergy and autoimmunity are immune responses. By way of example, a study by Swedish doctors showed that children who went to anthroposophical schools (Steiner or Waldorf schools) were less prone to eczema (an allergic response). Vaccination rates are lower in children whose families follow an anthroposophical way of life.[4] We also have an American study by Enriquez et al which found lower rates of self-reported atopic illnesses among children whose families refused vaccines.[5] A review of 'Vaccine allergies' by Chung (in 2014) discusses possible mechanisms of allergic responses and specifically references the influenza vaccination.[6] Chung takes a more 'conventional' approach, citing allergic responses to ingredients within the vaccination, such as egg protein, but he does go on to admit

the possibility of other mechanisms.

It is easy to switch the immune system on, much more difficult to switch it off. So, what to do? We had either to get rid of the allergic incitant (the gut bacteria in Carol's bloodstream) or to reduce it to such low numbers that her immune system felt safe ignoring it.

Thankfully, we found that another antibiotic, cephalexin, abolished her incontinence completely. However, this would never make for a long-term solution because of the risk of a cephalexin-resistant strain emerging. We had to treat her fermenting gut and this we did by starving the little wretches out with a PK diet and killing them with vitamin C to bowel tolerance. My rule of thumb is that one needs a peaceful war-zone for at least six months to re-educate the immune army. So, I kept Carol on full dose cephalexin 500 mg three times daily for two weeks, then tailed the drug off very slowly so that by six months she was on 250 mg three times a week. During this time her bladder function was perfect with no incontinence. We stopped the cephalexin with no problem.

I impressed on Carol the importance of keeping to the PK diet and vitamin C to bowel tolerance for life – the threat of a return to nappies has been more than enough to keep her on course.

References

1. Nicolson GL. Gulf War Research. The Institute for Molecular Medicine. www.immed.org/illness/gulfwar_illness_research.html (accessed 6 July 2019)
2. Nicolson GL, et al. Chronic Mycoplasmal Infections in Gulf War Veterans' Children and Autism Patients. *Medical Veritas* 2005; 2: 383-387.
3. Nicolson GL, et al. High Prevalence of Mycoplasmal Infections in Symptomatic (Chronic Fatigue Syndrome) Family Members of Mycoplasma-Positive Gulf War Illness Patients. *J*

Chronic Fatigue Syndr 2003; 11(2): 21-36.
4. Flostrup H, Swartz J, Bergstrom A, Alm JS, et al. Allergic disease and sensitization in Steiner school children. *J Allergy Clin Immunol* 2006; 117: 59-66. www.jacionline.org/article/S0091-6749(05)02128-7/pdf
5. Enriquez R, Addington W, Davis F, Freels A, et al. The relationship between vaccine refusal and self-report of atopic disease in children. *J Allergy Clin Immunol* 2005; 115: 737-744. www.jacionline.org/article/S0091-6749(05)00026-6/pdf
6. Chung EH. Vaccine allergies. *Clinical and Experimental Vaccine Research* 2014; 3(1): 50-57. www.ncbi.nlm.nih.gov/pmc/articles/PMC3890451/

Chapter 68
Rheumatology/bone and joint problems

A case of bunions

'I look great in wellies but terrible in sandals': an odd start to a consultation. A bunion was the problem. My immediate reaction was to refer to an orthopaedic surgeon. But hang on – I am supposed to be an ecological doctor asking the question 'Why?' I had never been impressed with the usual answer which blamed bunions on poor footwear. This was not biologically plausible – there had to be another cause.

Only too often a consultation starts with no real idea of where it is leading. However, Sue gave a typical history of dairy allergy. Her mother had told her she was a terrible baby with screaming colic for the first three months, despite being breast-fed. She later suffered eczema, recurrent coughs and colds and glue ear. Her teenage years were blighted by migraine followed by irritable bowel syndrome. This is the typical progression of the dairy allergic child in which the cause remains the same but the target organ changes.

I declared my thoughts and started to recommend a dairy-free diet. With devastating logic, she replied, 'Yes, but if this was a dairy allergy would not both big toes be equally affected?' A cursory examination showed a perfectly normal left foot but an 'orrible bunion on the right. I could not explain this but because I did not know what else to suggest she did in fact do a dairy-free diet. Fascinatingly, her bunion settled down over the ensuing weeks. Her toe remained distorted, but the inflammation and pain disappeared.

So, what was the mechanism of this? During the 1980s I worked with the wonderful Dr Honor Anthony who used to say: 'All arthritis is allergy'. I did not believe her at the time, but I now know she was absolutely right. Sue clearly had an allergic bunion. But why was it that one toe joint sensitised to dairy products but no other joint in the body was affected? It is odd what it is that gives one sleepless nights, but this was one such – a eureka moment at 2:00 am proved instructive. I was lucky because I was awake at the time. Many eureka moments come during sleep – Friedrich von Stradonitz said that the ring structure of benzene came to him in a dream and Craig reads difficult maths problems before going to sleep, only to wake with answer 'written out' in his head. Some eureka moments follow a bang on the head, which is ironic given that the word bunion is derived from the French *buigne* ('bump on the head')!

My current hypothesis is as follows: The bunion joint, the proximal metatarsal, is particularly susceptible to injury in at least two ways. This is the joint that is most susceptible when kicking, stumbling or slipping. It is also the joint most susceptible to crushing – if you, like me, keep horses you will know this. My friend Angie had a horse Lad who seemed to delight in treading on her toe. When tissue is damaged there is bruising and when this happens blood comes in direct contact with tissues, which is, of course, not meant to happen. Blood should be separated from tissues by a blood vessel wall. With bruising, there is potential for that injured tissue to sensitise to whatever is in the bloodstream at the time. This may be a food antigen – most commonly milk protein, but it may be gluten or yeast. However, it may be a microbe. At medical school, we were taught that the gut forms a near impervious barrier to foods and microbes, only permitting the miniscule products of digestion into the bloodstream. We now know this is not true. The gut is porous to bacteria. Indeed, even brushing your teeth allows bacteria in your mouth to flood into your bloodstream. This is called bacterial translocation and is the reason why patients with heart disease need to take antibiotics with any dental procedure – to prevent infective endocarditis.

I am now confident that this is the underlying mechanism of many chronic pain conditions. The patient ascribes the pain to an injury, such as a whiplash or fall. This may be the trigger for the pain, but pain should melt away as the damage heals. I think that any on-going pain and inflammation are maintained by allergy – allergy to foods or allergy to gut microbes. This problem is now greater than ever before because so many people carry an abnormal gut microbiome. Why so? In order of importance I reckon:

> high-carbohydrate diets which feed un-
> friendly microbes
> low-fibre diets which starve the friendlies
> the ever-increasing use of antibiotics which
> impact on friendlies and unfriendlies and
> the lack of live fermented foods in Western diets.

This list illustrates the point that the most profound effects on the gut microbiome are driven by diet. However, the gut does need to be seeded with the right microbes and this should happen at the point of birth when the near sterile infant gut is inoculated with the mother's gut microbes and fed by her breast milk. Caesarian sections and bottle-feeding are further contributing to the decline of gut microbiome quality. As my daughter put it, 'This is bad shit'.

Having hypothesised the mechanism, I then had to put it to the test. This meant a two-pronged approach – a diet that both cut out the major allergens (one possible area of concern), and was also very low in carbohydrates, high in fibre and rich in fermented foods (another area of concern). As is often the case, ONE intervention multi-tasked and addressed more than one area of concern; in this case that intervention was the PK diet. This diet, the paleo-ketogenic (PK) diet, has been remarkably successful in treating many chronic pain syndromes – not just chronic arthritis ('It's my age, doc'), but chronic muscle pain (fibromyalgia) and nerve pain (neuralgia). These conditions are typically treated with paracetamol, NSAIDs, antidepressants, gabapentin, morphine-like drugs, steroid injections and sometimes major surgery. How satisfying to cure these patients with a PK diet! And all this came from a case of bunions.

Polymyalgia rheumatica*

We seem to be seeing epidemics of polymyalgia rheumatica (PMR), a nasty inflammatory condition for which the medical profession can only offer steroids and NSAIDs. Steroids work extraordinarily well, with complete relief of symptoms within 24 hours. Indeed, a short trial of steroids – that is, prednisolone 30 mg daily for three days – can be the most efficient way to diagnose this condition. The problem is that the conventional medical detective work stops at this point, with the result that the patient is left on steroids, often high dose, sometimes for months or years, with all the side effects that result.

Table 68.1: Diagnosis of polymyalgia rheumatic

Clinical picture of polymyalgia rheumatica	Diagnosis	Notes
Muscle pain and stiffness of the shoulders and hips in the mornings. It is very debilitating. These symptoms settle as the day progresses only to recur the next day	Blood tests for inflammatory markers such as: CRP (C-reactive protein) ESR (erythrocyte sedimentation rate) Plasma viscosity	But the test can be normal – normal tests do not exclude the diagnosis

All the fun and interest of medicine results from working out the underlying causes. All diagnosis is hypothesis – it is the response to treatment that is critical for a positive confirmation of our first guesses. We know from the dramatic response of PMR to steroids that this is a disorder of the immune system, but what is the immune system doing wrong?

This is the hypothesis: I suspect PMR and its increasing incidence arise from modern Western high-carbohydrate diets. Too much carbohydrate in the diet can overwhelm our ability to digest it – instead, these carbohydrates are fermented in our gut by microbes. These microbes are miniscule compared with human cells and easily pass through our gut wall into our bloodstream – indeed, this is a well-recognised phenomenon and is called bacterial translocation (Chapter 11). We can be allergic to anything, not just foods, pollens, drugs and other chemicals, but also microbes. So, for example, rheumatic fever is allergy to streptococci and many cases of eczema result from allergy to staphylococcus.[3, 4] Increasingly I am seeing that many cases of arthritis are due to 'allergy' to gut microbes. Indeed, Dr Alan Ebringer, consultant rheumatologist at the Middlesex Hospital, demonstrated how ankylosing spondylitis is caused by 'allergy' to klebsiella bacteria from the gut.[2] Perhaps PMR is allergy to gut microbes? Let us put that hypothesis to the test.

*Footnote: Polymyalgia rheumatica was isolated as a disease in 1966 by a case report on 11 patients at Mount Sinai Hospital.[1] It takes its name from the Greek 'polymyalgia' which means 'pain in many muscles'.

Case history: Jo's polymyalgia rheumatica

Jo is a friend and fellow Team Chaser (horse racing in teams over cross-country fences). She had been fit and well until 2005 when, aged 57, she developed PMR. She had a raised ESR of 34 mm/h which rose further to 97 mm/h. She was prescribed high dose steroids, which immediately improved her joints but made her feel muzzy-headed and spaced out. She had to stop the steroids but her joint symptoms immediately returned, so she was unable to ride and was reduced to hobbling around on foot.

I suspected allergy to gut microbes and so she did a Comprehensive Digestive Stool Analysis to look at her gut microbes. This showed the presence of six additional species of bacteria that I would not expect to find, all at high levels. Therefore, she started on a very low-carbohydrate, ketogenic diet. After her third week on this diet,

Jo sent me an email: 'The result is nothing short of miraculous. The muscle pain is very much better!' Three months later Jo's PMR aches returned and her ESR spiked up to 48 mm/h. She confessed that she had lapsed on the low-starch diet because new potatoes, carrot and beetroot had been introduced into her diet. They had arrived in the market and she couldn't resist. She toughened up, got back onto her low-carbohydrate diet and her muscle aches disappeared. By the autumn of 2012 she was able to ride and start competing again at Team Chasing.

Jo was also diagnosed with borderline osteoporosis. This responds very well to nutritional supplements. She was already taking a good multivitamin and minerals and so we added in high-dose vitamin D (50,000 iu weekly) and strontium (250 mg daily). As a result of these interventions, her bone density scans results were as shown in Table 68.2.

Table 68.2: Bone density results before and after high-dose vitamin D and strontium

21/01/2011	28/03/2013
Lumbar spine 0.895 gm/sq cm	Lumbar spine 0.950 gm/sq cm (increase of 6%)
Femoral neck 0.751 gm/sq cm	Femoral neck 0.779 gm/sq cm (increase of 4%)

Doctors expect bone density to decline with age. The regimes recommended have increased Jo's bone density simply by taking nutritional supplements. I have now collected 23 patients who have had bone density scans done before and after these regimes of supplements and I know them to be effective. This is such a joy because so many people are intolerant of the bisphosphonate drugs conventionally prescribed.

This case illustrates the power of nutritional medicine. Patients may moan about the difficult diets, but my response is, as ever: 'My job is to get

you well, not to entertain you!' Sometimes I have to be cruel to be kind.

Osteoporosis: beware of doctors and drugs

The starting point to treat osteoporosis is often NHS prescribed calcium and vitamin D which, for the reasons as outlined in Chapter 47, are ineffective. Time is wasted and osteoporosis progresses. Ricki's back became even more C-shaped and following an episode of acute back pain, vertebral collapse from worsening osteoporosis was diagnosed. HRT, bisphosphonates or monoclonal antibody drugs may be prescribed and, in Ricki's case, she received the monoclonal antibody. Although in the short term there may be an increase in bone density, these drugs cannot be stopped because to do such results in greatly accelerated osteoporosis and so you end up where you may have been had you never taken the drugs.

Back to Square One,[†] as they say. All went swimmingly for some months, but then Ricki developed a urinary tract infection which progressed to septicaemia and she jolly well nearly died. Why? Monoclonal antibodies are immunosuppressive. Ricki is now left with the hideous choice of staying on the drug and risking life-threatening septicaemia, or stopping the drug and risking agonising vertebral collapse.

This clinical picture of drug treatments with short-term gain but long-term pain is all too common. Dependency or addiction result, and a miserable, undignified slide into the grave ensues. This is not how I am going to die. Reread Chapters 38 and 47 for effective, risk-free prevention and cure.

Allergic muscles and 'stiff man' syndrome

Allergy never ceases to surprise and amaze me for the multiplicity of symptoms that it can cause. It is now clear to me that any part of the body can react allergically. Irritable bowel syndrome

is allergy in the gut (to foods or gut microbes), migraine is allergy in the brain, asthma is allergy in the lungs, so why not allergic muscles? The more I look for this condition the more I find it, and it is obvious when you look for it.

The natural progression of allergy is for the allergen to remain the same but the target organ to change. The classical history through the life of the dairy allergic would be, as noted in relation to Sue's bunions (page 68.1), to start with colic as a baby, then move on to other manifestations, such as toddler diarrhoea, catarrh, ear infections and sore throats, irritable bowel syndrome, migraine, arthritis and so on. Being dairy-allergic myself, I recognised the progression early on. However, it took me some months to realise that the severe, lancinating back pain I started to experience was a further allergic manifestation. Through collaboration with some of my willing guinea-pig patients, we came up with the following mechanism. This hypothesis has so far survived the clinical tests of time.

What seems to happen is that muscles become sensitised as a result of mechanical damage. Muscle and connective tissue are separated from the bloodstream by a blood vessel wall. Tearing or bruising means muscle comes in direct contact with blood, which may be carrying food or microbial antigens. The hypothesis is that allergy is switched on at that time, but the pain which follows the muscle damage, and which persists for the long term, is misattributed to damage, whereas actually it is allergic sensitisation. So, a torn muscle in the back from, say, lifting a heavy load could sensitise to, say, dairy products, and it

[†]**Footnote:** Back to Square One – There are two main ideas as to where this phrase derives from and probably both are correct and mutually reinforced by each other. Firstly, it could derive from football radio commentaries in the 1930s. The football pitch was divided into numbered grids and each grid described the position of play. 'Square one' was in front of the home team's goal. As the number increased, so the areas moved up the pitch. When there was a goal kick by the home team, play could be described as being 'back to square one'. This system is also used by football supporters to describe play to fellow blind supporters at some football clubs these days. The second possibility is that this phrase describes the long slide down the biggest 'snake' in *Snakes and Ladders*, back to square one.

is the consumption of dairy subsequently which keeps the problem on the boil.

The diagnosis is made more difficult because we often see delayed reactions, which start 24 to 48 hours after allergen exposure and last for several days. Muscles can only react in one way, which is to contract, and this can vary from a low-grade cramp to muscle tics or jumping, to acute lancinating pain. I suspect the type of reaction depends on how much of the food is being consumed – regular consumption results in chronic low-grade spasm and cramp, but the odd inadvertent exposure in somebody who is normally avoiding that food can cause acute lancinating pain so severe that the sufferer literally collapses. Typically, this just lasts a few seconds. When I dropped on my kitchen floor having triggered such a spasm, this was greeted by howls of laughter from my daughters who thought I was putting on a terrific act for their personal entertainment!

As soon as the spasm goes, the pain vanishes and all is well. Mother finds herself branded a hypochondriac. 'What was all that fuss about then, eh?' It happens to Craig, the lovely editor and co-author of all my writings, who was 'diagnosed' by his NHS GP with sciatica, but who never suffers this pain when he keeps off the crisps (99.9% of the time). However, when he relapses and munches his way through a bag of chips, sure enough the sharp pain returns.

Acute pain is triggered by stretching the affected muscle. Initially any stretch will cause it; then, as things settle down, only a sudden stretch will do so. The sufferer protects him/herself from the pain by moving slowly. Other muscles in the vicinity of the allergic muscles may also go into spasm to protect against sudden inadvertent stretching, and this causes a more generalised muscle spasm and stiffness. Because muscles can only react in one way, through contraction, this produces further symptoms, such as cramp, restless legs, jerking muscles, twitching muscles and fasciculation (flicker of movement under the skin). Some of these muscle contractions

will be accompanied by pain. There is a further complication because, if muscles contract inappropriately, they can damage themselves literally by pulling themselves apart (and, indeed, this is the mechanism that athletes employ to get fitter – if you damage the muscles slightly, this stimulates the production of more muscle). Further pain develops because the blood circulation through muscles is disturbed and there is a build-up of toxic metabolites, in particular lactic acid. Lactic acid causes pain. We then see a particularly vicious cycle, with allergic muscles causing spasm, spasm causing build-up of toxic metabolites, toxic metabolites causing more pain and the muscles reacting to pain with further spasm. Indeed, I have two patients with 'stiff man syndrome' who have been cured – in the one case simply by avoiding dairy products and, in the other, through doing a paleo-ketogenic diet. My guess is stiff man syndrome is an extreme version of allergic muscles.

Typically, the problem is much worse in the morning and improves as the day progresses. Often there are good days and bad days. Gentle regular exercise, such as walking, is very helpful and, indeed, some patients find that they have to exercise very intensely and very regularly to keep the problem at bay (if the allergen has not been recognised). Heat, hot baths and gentle massage all help to relax the muscle in the short term, as does keeping the body in one particular position, but the first movement after these interventions has to be done carefully or the pain will come straight back again. Relaxants, such as alcohol, afford relief, but this is not sustainable medicine. It's the old story – diet is central to recovery. Just do it!

Pain after orthopaedic surgery

Carwen (see Chapter 74) has a chronic lymphatic leukaemia, the progress of which we can monitor by measuring the number of lymphocytes in her blood. Levels had been falling nicely since 2009, but having reached lows of 5-6 x 109/l (healthy range, 1.5-4.0 x 109/l), numbers started to creep up again to 7.5. Why?

In March 2018, Carwen underwent surgery to place a metal implant in her foot to straighten her toe. The surgery was beautifully done – there was an excellent cosmetic result and she recovered well – but at four months she still had marked tenderness at the operations site and confessed to persistent discomfort extending up her leg. We could not explain this in terms of local infection or poor surgical technique. Her symptoms were typical of inflammation (and reduced by anti-inflammatories), so what was going on?

I wondered about metal allergy and so we did lymphocyte sensitivity testing – a measure of the activity of lymphocytes in the presence of certain metals. Carwen had large positive reactions to chromium, titanium and nickel – the very metals used in her foot. This was a biologically plausible mechanism for her ongoing inflammation and pain. The treatment, of course, is to address the cause. We now have another battle on our hands – persuading the surgeons to un-pick their handiwork and remove the offending metals. The surgeon has yet to agree to do this, but since Carwen's pain is increasing I cannot see any other option. It will be interesting to see if post-op the pain goes and the lymphocyte sensitivity and counts fall.

References

1. Davison S, Spiera H, Plotz M. Polymyalgia rheumatic. *Arthritis & Rheumatism* 1966; 9(1): 18-19. doi.org/10.1002/art.1780090103
2. Ebringer A. The relationship between Klebsiella infection and ankylosing spondylitis. *Baillieres Clinics in Rheumatology* 1989; 3(2): 321-338. www.ncbi.nlm.nih.gov/pubmed/2670258 (accessed 7 July 2019).
3. Cunningham MW. Streptococcus and rheumatic fever. *Current Opinion in Rheumatology* 2012; 24(4): 408-416. doi:10.1097/BOR.0b013e32835461d3
4. Gong JQ, Lin L, Lin T, Hao F, et al. Skin colonization by Staphylococcus aureus in patients with eczema and atopic dermatitis and relevant combined topical therapy: a double-blind multi-centre randomized controlled trial. *British Journal of Dermatology* 2006; 155(4): 680-687. www.ncbi.nlm.nih.gov/pubmed/1696545

Chapter 69
Dermatology/skin problems

Dermatology case histories
Acne (dairy, high-carb diets, vitamin B12)
Eczema and asthma (food sensitivities)

Acne – when drugs are more dangerous than disease

When you are young, appearance is everything. I learned this from my daughters. One wet winter, the river rose so the track up to my house was blocked. Yippee! The girls could not get to school, but neither could my patients get to me. All were postponed bar Rosemary, who was desperate for her B12 injection. I suggested she come and I would find some way of crossing the river. I decided the best method would be a pair of shorts and trainers, so that I could wade across. There would be minimal drag, and so I would not be sent downstream in the waist-deep flood. On seeing Rosemary arrive I trotted upstairs for my running gear and appeared in the kitchen. 'No, no,' chorused my girls, 'you can't possibly go!' Flattered by their obvious concern for my welfare I started to explain my thinking. But that was irrelevant to their line of thought. 'Mum,' Claire explained, 'you haven't shaved your legs.'

Acne is a miserable, disfiguring, ego-sapping, painful affliction largely of Western teenagers. Sufferers and their parents will go to great lengths to get this treated. It is generally felt that there are at least two factors that contribute to acne and this has resulted in two nasty, toxic treatments. During puberty there in an increase in the production of sebum onto the skin. The idea is that this gets infected, which results in the inflamed spots and pustules which are so disfiguring. Big Pharma has come up with two treatments. Firstly, one can kill the infection with antibiotics. Whilst this is effective in the short term, as soon as the antibiotic is stopped the problem returns. Young people may end up taking antibiotics for many years. This has potentially disastrous effects on their gut microbiome.

Another drug used is isotretinoin (the trade names is Ro-Accutane, often known as Ro-A) to block sebum production. The necessary vocabulary to describe this drug and its use in otherwise healthy young people cannot be used in polite society. (Maybe Craig's friend Wodge from Chapter 1 would be the best person to describe it!) In private I can revert to effing and blinding. I have seen so many lives destroyed by Ro-A, which was developed for cancer chemotherapy. It also causes birth defects. I see many patients whose chronic fatigue syndrome was triggered by Ro-A. Hoffmann-La Roche has paid out millions in compensation to patients with Ro-A-induced inflammatory bowel disease. I see a young man who has suffered unremitting headache for 18 years since taking a course of the drug. I have seen two other young men who both committed suicide shortly after taking Ro-A. Neither had ever suffered any previous psychiatric history. Effectively, they died from zits.

Why use such poisons when we all have to hand a cheap and effective treatment which has no side-effects? Read on. The problem, as always, is persuading young people to make the changes. But vanity is a great driver of change.

> *vanitas vanitatum omnia vanitas* – '*vanity of vanities; everything [is] vanity*'.
> **Vulgate Bible**, Ecclesiastes 1:2; 12:8

We have to start by asking the question 'Why?' Acne afflicts up to 95% of adolescents in Western societies. By contrast in a study of 1200 Kitavan people examined (including 300 aged 15-25 years), no case of acne (grade 1 with multiple comedones or grades 2-4) was observed. Kitava is one of the four major islands in the Trobriand Islands of eastern Papua New Guinea. The Kitavan diet is uninfluenced by the modern Western diet. Of 115 Aché people examined (including 15 aged 15-25 years) over 843 days, no case of active acne (grades 1-4) was observed. These simple observational studies tell us that Western lifestyles are to blame. The Aché are an indigenous people of Paraguay; they are hunter-gatherers.

I know, from my clinical experience, there are at least three important players. The starting point is to cut out all dairy products. I am not sure of the mechanism by which this works, but work for some it undoubtably does. If that fails, then the next step is to follow a ketogenic diet. I suspect the mechanism here has to do with blood sugar levels. If these run high, then sugar spills into all our secretions. Bacteria love sugar. As readers by now have doubtless discerned, the paleo-ketogenic (PK) diet is the starting point for preventing and treating all diseases of Westerners.

There is another fascinating trigger for acne; it is a known side effect of vitamin B12 injections. Light was thrown on a possible mechanism by an organophosphate-poisoned farmer whose acne was greatly improved by daily injections of vitamin B12. But Bert, aged 57, developed the most awful acne. He prized his energy levels higher than his looks and insisted on persisting with the jabs. Four months later his skin healed completely... so what was going on?

We know chloracne is a result of organochlorine poisoning – that is to say, toxins may cause acne. Vitamin B12 is very helpful for detoxing through its effect on the methylation cycle. I suspect the B12 mobilised toxins, which were excreted though the skin, driving the acne en route. Once detoxed, Bert's energy and skin recovered fully.

Throughout the centuries many 'cures' for acne have been put forward, showing just how serious this condition is. For example, the Ancient Egyptians, who thought acne was caused by telling lies, treated it with sulphur. Whilst the causal relationship is wrong, there is some evidence for the treatment,[1] but remember we are always looking for the causes of disease, rather than to suppress the symptoms, and so the PK diet trumps sulphur.

Eczema and asthma

Andrew first visited me aged 4 with severe eczema, asthma, hyperactivity, enuresis (bedwetting) and failure to thrive, in October 1987. He had been seen by the local paediatrician and standard symptom-suppressing treatments had been tried with no success. These included a range of steroid creams for the eczema and bronchodilators and steroid inhalers for the asthma. In the previous year Andrew had been prescribed 10 courses of antibiotics.

Andrew's mother had become interested in food allergy and had relieved many of his symptoms by avoiding symptom-provoking foods. By the time Andrew came to see me first, she had uncovered sensitivities to dairy, beef, soya, chocolate, sugar, honey (severe diarrhoea), strawberries, wheat, eggs, cod, margarine, grapes and oranges. He also reacted to zinc and calcium supplements. A combination of his severe respiratory symptoms and skin problems meant he rarely attended school.

At that time, I had no method of desensitisation available to me. Furthermore, in the 1980s I had not yet woken up to the fermenting gut issues. So, I started him on foods that he rarely ate, vis: lamb, sweet potato, rice, carrot, peas, sunflower and safflower, banana, apple, mango and pineapple. He ate these foods only for two weeks during which time all his symptoms cleared, and he became a well child. Clearly, we were lucky that Andrew's case was pure food allergy. Had he had a fermenting gut issue then he would not have improved so much.

Other foods were then reintroduced, one at a time, and, over the next five months, his weight increased by 3.18 kg (7 lb) to 18.14 kg (2 stone 12lb). However, this diet was unsustainable, partly because it was socially difficult, and partly because he started to sensitise to new foods. As a result, his eczema and asthma flared, although his bed-wetting and hyperactivity never returned. So, in March 1988 I started Andrew on enzyme-potentiated desensitisation (EPD). He was given the low dose EPD – that is, X theta.

EPD was given on the following dates:

March 1988 – first dose of X theta

June 1988 – second dose – this was followed by a flare of his eczema, thought to be due to inadvertent exposure to chrysanthemums

Sept 1988 – skin better; no tummy aches; able to reintroduce chips and sweet corn

Dec 1988 – clinically better, but still not tolerating any supplements

April 1989 – skin itchy but no eczema; asthma also improved; no antibiotics for six months

Sept 1989 – missed appointment

March 1990 – long gap – eczema flared in past month; off dairy, otherwise pretty normal diet

March 1991 – well; no asthma or eczema; off dairy; care with white fish and beef; only ever gets eczema on hands and feet.

Then Andrew attended once a year until 1998 since when I have lost touch. At that time, he was eating a normal diet but still could not tolerate any supplements. He had the occasional flare of eczema, largely controlled by Fucidin ointment. Andrew's Mum sent me a Christmas card in which she told me that in 2002 Andrew achieved Gold standard for swimming and a Gold Duke of Edinburgh Award. He was at university studying pharmacy (an irony seeing as the drugs did not work for him).

Reference

1. Wilkinson RD, Adam JE, Murray JJ, Craig GE. Benzoyl Peroxide and Sulfur: Foundation for Acne Management. *Can Med Assoc J* 1966; 95(1): 28–29. www.ncbi.nlm.nih.gov/pmc/articles/PMC1935555/

Chapter 70
Neurology/ nervous system problems

Neurology case histories
Dementia (high-carb Western diets and nutrient deficiencies)
Multiple sclerosis (mycotoxins)

Dementia

At the Middlesex Hospital Medical school in the 1970s I can remember the excitement of the consultant neurologist when a group of us medical students sat in on his outpatient clinic. 'You lucky people,' he said. 'You are about to see a remarkable, once-in-a-lifetime case.' In trotted Alf and has wife Vera, aged 78. The consultant started talking to Vera. All seemed well. He repeated his questions and she answered as if she had never been asked them before. Clearly, she had no short-term memory. When he challenged her with this she said, after a pause, 'Oh well, I had a very late night. I was away at a party and I expect I am still a bit hungover.' Her husband, Alf, sitting next to her rolled his eyes and looked into the middle distance – he did not bother to correct or question her statement. Clearly, she was confabulating again. Vera had fabricated a story to explain a lapse in memory and logic (confabulate derives from the Latin, *fabula* – story). Apart from this curious exchange, Vera seemed physically fit and well. The neurologist had no treatments or suggestions for management other than supportive therapy as Vera would

(inevitably, without nutritional therapy) decline.

After the couple left, the consultant asked us what we thought the diagnosis was. We had no idea, this being completely outside our experience of both life and medicine to date. He leant back with a look of superiority. 'I think this is a case of dementia, probably due to Alzheimer's disease. Remember that name. If you can hold that in your head for Finals, then you will impress your examiners.' We returned home repeating the word 'Alzheimer's', so it would stick in our memories.

Alois Alzheimer (1864–1915), was a German psychiatrist and neuropathologist. Whilst working at the Frankfurt Asylum in 1901 he met, and became obsessed with, a patient called Auguste Deter. This 51-year-old patient had strange behavioural symptoms, including a loss of short-term memory. When questioned she would often repeat the words: *'Ich hab mich verloren'* ('I have lost myself.'). Upon Auguste's death, Alois investigated her brain and found amyloid plaques and neurofibrillary tangles. Auguste is credited as the first person to be diagnosed with Alzheimer's disease.

From this single diagnosis in 1901, Alzheimer's is now the commonest cause of death in Westerners and has become a household word. Why should that be? There has to be an environmental explanation – indeed, the World Health Organization tells us that disease is 5% genetic, 95% environmental. Of course, doctors like myself know full well the reasons because we have been asking the question 'why?' for decades. Moreover, if one knows the 'Why' of a disease then it gives us the 'How' to prevent and treat it.

One such 'Why-asking' doctor is consultant neurologist Dr Dale Bredesen of the Mary Easton Centre for Alzheimer's Disease Research, Department of Neurology, University of California. Los Angeles, USA. Dr Bredesen recognised the many and various causes of Alzheimer's. He set up a study of 10 patients (age range 55 to 75) in which each was given personalised therapy. Alzheimer's disease is now sometimes called 'type 3 diabetes'. Indeed, having type 2 diabetes is a major risk factor for Alzheimer's – so, the most difficult, but perhaps the most important, aspect of Bredesen's treatment plan was a ketogenic diet, as it is for type 2 diabetes. All food had to be consumed within a 12-hour window of time that included no food three hours prior to bedtime. This, together with melatonin, improved sleep quality and along with various supplements this was an essential part of his treatment. This squares with the work of Matthew Walker who has demonstrated that it is during sleep that the brain 'self-cleans' via the glymphatics, potentially clearing amyloid from the brain. Walker has shown that poor quantity and quality of sleep are also major risk factors for dementia.[1]

Because Western diets are so deficient in micronutrients, Dr Bredesen's patients were given a basic package of vitamins, minerals and essential fatty acids, a package to improve antioxidant status and a package to improve mitochondrial function. All patients undertook 30-60 minutes of exercise a day and on four to six days a week, they received stress reducing therapies such as yoga, meditation or music and were encouraged to exercise their brains. Those with high homocysteine levels received vitamins to reduce levels below 7. Those who were hypothyroid or had poor adrenal function were also treated. Those with heavy metal toxicity received chelation therapy.

Bredesen's results were astonishing. Six of the patients whose cognitive decline had had a major impact on job performance were able to return to work or continue working without difficulty. Three more saw substantial improvement in memory and cognitive function. Only one patient declined, perhaps because she was the most severely afflicted at the start of the trial, with a rapidly progressing dementia and extensive amyloid on scans. If a drug trial had achieved such a result it would have made headline news. Bredesen had reversed the cognitive decline.

I rarely see dementia patients, but the patients I do see with CFS/ME suffer marked cognitive dysfunction. They too suffer poor short-term memory, inability to multitask and a tendency to procrastinate with intellectually demanding tasks. The regimes to treat them are essentially the same. One of my patients measured his recovery by the time it took him to complete the *Daily Telegraph* cryptic crossword puzzle – he got back to his usual 30 minutes (albeit in three separate sessions). My colleague and writing partner Craig celebrated his return of cognitive function one summer by writing out solutions to all the questions of the Oxford University Entrance Paper for Mathematics between the years 1962 and 2011, and continues to keep his collection up to date each year, hoping one day to compile them all in a book. In his darkest days he forgot how to count to 10. Dear reader, do not wait to be diagnosed with Alzheimer's. At the first sign of any cognitive decline, put the regimes in place before it is too late.

Multiple sclerosis (MS)

Angela has suffered from MS since the age of 32. She is now 72. I first saw her when I was an NHS GP in the early 1990s. The starting point to treat all disease is to hypothesise a biologically plausible mechanism for the underlying pathology because that gives us clear indications for treatment. The problem with MS is that at that time I did not have such a hypothesis. Even without such one can deliver treatment in the form of Groundhog interventions (Appendices 1–3). But these demand major lifestyle changes, and many people are resistant to such. When, in addition, they fly in the face of conventional medical advice and, perhaps worse, family perceptions of what a healthy lifestyle should entail, compliance with Groundhog is not easy. What helps greatly is the intellectual imperative to make these changes and this I could not furnish Angela with. Despite this, she worked hard at the Stoneage – now the PK (paleo-ketogenic) – diet, took the recommended nutritional supplements, tried high dose B12 injections and put in place a regime to tackle chronic viral infection. But none of these interventions turned things around. She has continued to deteriorate, albeit slowly, over the 25 years we have known each other.

We now have a good hypothesis for MS which could turn things around for Angela. MS may be a mycotoxin-driven disease.[2] In Angela's case this makes great sense. She worked as a farmer and in the area of cattle and sheep, and so she would have been in daily contact with hay and straw. Wet Wales means that these crops may be rained upon before storage and this allows fungi to flourish. All farmers know what mouldy hay looks like – as you gather it and stuff it into haynets or cratches, a dense cloud of mould spores flies out which often provokes sneezing and coughing. Indeed, many farmers develop 'farmer's lung' – an inflammatory condition characterised by allergy to mould and infection with moulds. So, exposure to moulds raises the possibility of inoculation of the sinuses, airways and, possibly, gut with fungi – a chance for them to find another comfortable home in our delicious, warm, moist and, for many, sugar-soaked tissues. There they happily ferment to produce mycotoxins which poison us. It may be no coincidence that fungi in the sinuses surround the olfactory nerve and maybe their hyphae penetrate directly. Since the olfactory nerve is a direct extension of the brain, mycotoxins will be pouring into the base of the brain.

There are two further clues. Angela also has pseudo-gout and mild renal failure. Both can be explained by mycotoxins. Dr Joseph Brewer developed a test for mycotoxins that is easily done on a urine sample. Of course, a normal result should be zero; however, sick people, especially those with chronic fatigue, often show positives and so Brewer established a range for common positives. It is not often a test result comes back that makes me leap out of my chair and pace up and down the room, but Angela's did. The results were so astonishing I have repeated them in full in table 70.1.

Table 70.1: Mycotoxin test results – Angela with MS, pseudo-gout and mild renal failure

Mycotoxin	Comment	Common range of positives (results should be zero)	Source
Ochratoxin 228.52	Wow! This is a record high by a mile – 10-fold higher than the common range of positives	3.5 to 20	From aspergillus and penicillium families Nephrotoxic, immunotoxic and carcinogenic Mainly from water-damaged buildings May drive Alzheimer's and Parkinson's
Sterigmato-cystin 118.92	Another record high	0.2 to 1.75	From aspergillus, penicillium and bipolaris families Closely related to aflatoxin Carcinogenic in gut and liver
Mycophenolic acid 1740.19	Cripes – you are well and truly poisoned! No-one could tolerate this sort of toxic stress	5-50	From penicillium Immunosuppressant Associated with miscarriage and congenital malformations
Zearalenone 892.62	Another record high	0.5-10	From fusarium Hepatotoxic, haemotoxic, immunotoxic and genotoxic Mainly from water-damaged buildings Oestrogen mimic

The treatment of course is to kill the little wretches by:

- starving them with a PK diet (Chapter 21)
- killing them using an iodine salt pipe, systemic antifungal, gut antifungal (vitamin C to bowel tolerance and nystatin powder)
- mopping up mycotoxins in the gut using clays (Chapter 34).

Angela has only just started on this regime. I can imagine her being pretty fed up with me for taking 25 years to arrive at a logical package of treatment* and I shall understand entirely if

*Footnote from Craig: I have yet to meet a patient of Sarah's who is fed up with her. In fact, the opposite is true. She never gives up on them. I was honoured to attend a portion of Sarah's considerable 60th birthday celebrations – she is truly at middle age now, aiming for 120! At that gathering, my wife, Penny, gave a speech on behalf of patients and also of sufferers, some of whom have never met Sarah, but who nonetheless have benefited from her work and website. Penny presented a very large poster with pictures of patients and sufferers and their words of thanks to Sarah. My Facebook Group co-admin, Kathryn Twinn, and I had arranged for an online 'Thank You' card to be done. This 'card', which grew so large that it morphed into an AO-plus sized poster, soon reached the limit of 250 patients and comments. Then we had to close it to further comments. When I took it to be printed, the chap in the print shop said, 'She's a popular lady then?' I just smiled.

compliance is low... but how exciting if she recovers! Watch this space.

For more about this, interested readers should see 'Multiple Sclerosis: A Chronic Mycotoxicosis?' at www.mult-sclerosis.org/news/Jul2003/MSA ChronicMycotoxicosis.html and related books.[3]

References

1. Walker M. *Why We Sleep*. Penguin Books, 2017.
2. Purzycki CB, Shain DH. Fungal toxins and multiple sclerosis: a compelling connection. *Brain Res Bull* 2010; 82(1-2): 4-6. doi: 10.1016/j.brainresbull.2010.02.012 www.ncbi.nlm.nih.gov/pubmed/20214953
3. Kaufmann D. *The Fungus Link* (2001), *The Fungus Link* vol 2 (2003), *The Fungus Link* vol 3 (2008). Media Trition.

Chapter 71
Psychiatry/mental health problems

Post-traumatic stress disorder (PTSD)

All disease states of Westerners can be largely explained and treated through attention to two pathological drivers – namely, energy delivery mechanisms and inflammation. These are both involved in that most complex of conditions, myalgic encephalitis or ME. This is characterised by poor energy delivery mechanisms *and* inflammation. However, some PWME (people with ME) also have, as I describe it, an emotional hole in their energy bucket and often this is a result of PTSD. How do we tackle this?

Dorothy is an ME patient. She is a qualified nurse who first consulted me in 2004, then aged 43. She had become so ill that she was bedbound, too ill to sit up and requiring full time care. With great determination and application, she put in place all the difficult things I ask my patients to do with respect to my standard work-up. She improved somewhat but this was not really cutting it. It was only then that her appalling history of childhood abuse and bullying came to the fore. It appals me what some parents are capable of – only yesterday I spoke to a 70-year-old who described living in fear of her violent mother.

When Dad was away, she spent the night sitting with her back against the bedroom door holding a knife to protect herself. She did not realise it but, of course, she too was suffering from PTSD. Both she and Dorothy had been hard-wired for hypervigilance for life. This wrecks sleep and is a risk factor for much pathology. They had both experienced a trauma, in the true sense of its Greek derivative – a 'wound', and their wounds had remained unhealed for years.

But I can hear readers say, we all have skeletons in the cupboard. Why do we not all suffer from PTSD? I think the answer lies with sleep.

We all have a sleep cycle that repeats through the night and lasts about 90 minutes. It is characterised by rapid eye movement sleep (REM) and non-rapid eye movement sleep (non-REM). REM sleep is about the future when we dream, and problem solve, whereas non-REM sleep is about the past, when the brain deals with the experiences of the day, remembers those experiences that are important and chucks out the rest. What we need is to sleep in a safe, kind, warm, comforting environment in which the brain can chuck out those damaging memories, shut them away safely and not be troubled by them. However, if we sleep in an unsafe, uncomfortable and stressed state, then those memories are re-lived in an adrenalin-fuelled state, reinforced with nightmares and flashbacks in an unforget-table and disturbing way.

How do we know we are doing this? Dorothy, clever girl, equipped herself with a heartrate monitor, to discover that throughout sleep her heartrate was highly variable, ranging from a normal of 70 bpm (beats per minute) up to 140 bpm. Clearly this was adrenalin-fuelled. She had a vicious self-perpetuating cycle of terrifying dreams, with outpouring of stress hormones to reinforce those vile memories. This was some-thing over which she had no conscious control.

Sleep is a vital part of good health. The World Health Organization has classified shift work as a probable carcinogen. Sleep deprivation is a greater risk for accidents than being drunk. It even impacts on natural killer cells and immune function. So, for Dorothy, the question was, how could we change her sleep in such a way as to allow her brain to discard these destructive memories?

Simply taking hypnotics was ineffective. Although she could be rendered unconscious by such, she did not get proper sleep. We know this because her pulse continued to spike whilst knocked out. What we needed was an adrenalin blocker. So, we decided to try a tiny dose of the adrenalin-blocker propranolol. Dorothy started to improve. She found she could sit up for longer.

After 20 years of speeding heart, especially in the morning, 10 mg of propranolol meant she could get to 11:00 am and do all her jobs that needed her to be more upright. So, we tried a further hike and more improvements followed. From being bedbound for 20 years she managed a weekly excursion without relapsing. She went on a cruise. She did some more research and read that adrenalin stimulated alpha-receptors as well as beta-receptors, and so we decided to add in an alpha-blocker – namely, clonidine 25 mcg, building up to 200 mcg. Further improvement followed. Now in the day her maximum heart-rate is 90 bpm and she is the best she has been in 25 years. The improved sleep achieved by the alpha– and beta-blockers was the mechanism by which Dorothy's 'wound' was being healed, at long last.

We seem to be seeing epidemics of PTSD. I think this has much to do with Western diets where we fuel our bodies with sugar and carbs. The hormonal response to this is an insulin spike followed by an adrenalin spike. Adrenalin com-pletely disrupts sleep and so prevents the brain from rationalising and tucking away nasty expe-riences. We know that the average Westerner is chronically sleep deprived 'time-wise', but in ad-dition Western diets result in poor sleep quality. We should be as disciplined about our sleep as our diet; indeed, the two are inextricably linked. If Dorothy can… so can you. Just do it!

Chapter 72

Immunology/allergy problems

Silicone implants

It is not often that I see a patient who suffers all of the complications of silicone implants, but Kitty was one such case. She consulted me in 1997. She'd had a mastectomy in 1983 for cancer with local lymph node excision and radiotherapy. She had recovered very well and got back to a full life; being very fit she swam daily. Unfortunately, she was advised to have an implant. 'You will be as good as new,' she was told. This was when her life started to fall apart.

Silicone is a material foreign to the body which perceives it as such. The immune system tries to expel the implant for the foreign body that it is. It employs the scar tissue method by laying down a tough layer of such tissue around the implant, which then contracts in order to squeeze the object out. This is highly effective for getting rid of splinters. Indeed, when I was working amongst the mining community of Newstead in Nottinghamshire, we had one man who had been crushed in a mining accident. He would appear in the surgery every few months as another lump of coal worked its way out through his back accompanied by much pus and serous fluid. But oh, the triumph of digging it out in its final

journey and the relief that afforded!

In Kitty's case, her body worked similarly hard to extrude her foreign lump of silicone. However, the immune system, as expected, formed a uniform wall around her soft implant and then started to contract. Her implant became rock hard and painful. What to do? A standard technique then was external capsulotomy. This is a posh name for a brutal technique – the sadist, whoops I mean surgeon, crushes the breast and implant until it ruptures. Major ouch! I often wonder if this procedure would have become acceptable had the surgeon been female in the case of a patient with a testicular silicone implant. External capsulotomy may leave the patient with a cosmetically acceptable soft breast, but the implant has been ruptured, the silicone has been dispersed and all the other problems associated with silicone are magnified.

Silicone leaks out from implants from the day they are inserted. As medical students we were – and are – taught that this is an inert plastic that is non-toxic. Whilst that may be true in the chemical sense, we now know it is not the case in the immunological sense. It is an immune adjuvant – so it switches on the immune system. Indeed, silicones were once used in vaccinations to ensure a good immune response to whatever was in the vaccine. We also see inflammation in biopsies of tissues around implants where the immune system tries to 'wall off' leaking molecules of silicone. Pathologically these are known as silicone granulomas – they have a tuberculosis-like appearance. But silicone leaks all over the body, where it can drive inflammatory reactions. This is a biologically plausible explanation for the diseases following silicone implants in the many women I have seen. These include autoimmune disease, such as multiple sclerosis, inflammatory arthritis and autoimmune disease. This condition now has a proper name – ASIA or 'autoimmune/ inflammatory syndrome induced by adjuvants'. As ever, science is slowly – too slowly for patients – catching up with clinical experience. Two papers, recently published (Soriano et al, 2014; Colaris et al, 2017) explore these issues.[1, 2]

Clinically, these patients present with fibromyalgia and chronic fatigue syndrome. What is so characteristic is these poisoned women use the adjective 'burning' to describe the nature of their pain. I find it fascinating how the subconscious brain communicates with the conscious brain, so it delivers the precise word that explains the symptom. 'Burning' is the meaning of 'inflammation'. Kitty clearly had inflammation confirmed by blood tests, which showed a persistently raised C-reactive protein, above 20 mg/l (reference range <5 mg/l).

Kitty's silicone migration accelerated after the capsulotomy. She suffered the widespread pain of fibromyalgia. The silicone migrated into her armpit and the inflammation irritated the brachial plexus leaving her with a weak and painful arm. Surgery was impossible because of the risk of further neurological damage. It looked, and felt, as if someone had stuffed a bunch of grapes into her armpit – it was full of silicone nodules with inflammatory scarring round each one as the immune system continued its attempt to extrude these foreign bodies. This was confirmed by MRI scanning. Kitty developed a widespread

inflammatory arthritis, worse in her feet, so she could barely walk. She also suffered severe fatigue because of what I describe as the immunological hole in her energy bucket. The immune system, like the brain, is greatly demanding of energy. Because of the inflammation throughout her body, Kitty's immune system was demanding more than its 'fair share' of the available energy and so, with the energy equation in deficit, no wonder Kitty became severely fatigued.

What to do? The problem with silicone is that it cannot be broken down by any biological enzyme system. It is a plastic – it is stuck in her body forever and there is no known detox technique to get rid of it. So, treatments are aimed at reducing the 'useless' inflammation. For Kitty this included a paleo-ketogenic diet (sugar and carbs are pro-inflammatory) and antioxidant minerals and vitamins to damp down the inflammatory fire – especially high-dose vitamin B12 (5000 mcg daily) and vitamin C to bowel tolerance (see page 27.2).

Kitty is a fighter. Her positive mental outlook has been an essential part of recovery. She can now attend eight yoga classes a week and swims regularly. She tells me that her butterfly stroke and tumble turns are not as good as they could be, but she is encouraged to hear they are much better than mine!

References

1. Soriano A, Butnaru D, Shoenfeld Y. Long-term inflammatory conditions following silicone exposure: the expanding spectrum of the autoimmune/inflammatory syndrome induced by adjuvants (ASIA). *Clin Exp Rheumatol* 2014; 32(2): 151-154.
2. Colaris MJL, de Boer M, van der Hulst RR, Tervaert JWC. Two hundred cases of ASIA syndrome following silicone implants: a comparative study of 30 years and a review of current literature. *Immunol Res* 2017; 65(1): 120–128.

Chapter 73
Spotting the new killers

New killers – case histories
Paralysis (diet coke addiction – aspartame)
Motor neurone disease (aspartame, cycad, organophosphates)

Paralysis

Avril, aged 26, swung her way into my surgery. By this I mean she used a pair of crutches to move. She was so weak from the waist downwards she was unable to walk, but she could just about bear her own weight.

'My neurologist has diagnosed me with ME because all the tests are normal, and he cannot explain my symptoms,' she told me. It was clear from a cursory examination that the weakness was not global, but confined to her back and legs. Despite this, she was not fatigued; indeed, she could 'walk' as fast as any normal person. Clearly, she did not have ME. As I have said many times before, 90% of diagnosis comes from taking a good history and diet is central. No doctor had enquired about her diet up until now, but it took less than a minute to elicit the fact she was drinking up to 3 litres a day of diet coke. She had seen no need to volunteer this information previously, which, I suspect, was a measure of her addiction. I suspect coke was so named because it contained cocaine. As recently as 2016, a French Coca Cola factory was found with 370 kg of cocaine in store.[1] Perhaps it is no wonder Coca Cola and Pepsi Cola are the most consumed soft drinks in the world.

However, what we do know for sure is that all brands of diet coke are sweetened with aspartame.

This is broken down in the liver to phenylalanine and formaldehyde. I first came across formaldehyde when I worked in Uganda. Meths (methanol for the chemists) was sometimes used by the Kampalans as an alcohol substitute. This too is broken down in the liver to formaldehyde and I saw some poor fellows who used meths to become blind drunk one day, woke the next day blind and remained blinded for life. I knew formaldehyde was neurotoxic.

Avril stopped her diet coke. Three weeks later she walked into my surgery cured. She had started jogging. Not often one achieves such a satisfying result in such a short time. A few weeks after this I bumped into my local MP Roger Williams who was running a campaign to raise awareness of the toxicity of aspartame and I told him Avril's story. Two weeks later he had Trevor McDonald on the case, we had all been interviewed, the TV documentary was prepared and listed for the Friday. We all queued up for our moment of fame only to find that the programme had been postponed to Monday evening. By the time Monday came around, it had been scrubbed. Why? 'Coco Cola was going to sue us.' My opinion of the integrity of ITV fell.

Michael J Fox, star of the *Back to the Future* films, and *Spin City*, was a paid spokesman for Diet Pepsi, and you can see him swigging it in the aforementioned films – a textbook example of 'product placement'. It has been widely reported that he became addicted to Diet Pepsi, drinking many cans each and every day. Fox was diagnosed with Parkinson's disease aged 30 and went public seven years later.

Motor neurone disease

A few months later, Jacky (aged 39) wobbled into my surgery. She had been diagnosed with motor neurone disease. I was immediately shocked – MND is a disease of older people. Stephen Hawking aside, this was the youngest case I had ever heard of. Of course, I wanted to know why and immediately asked about sheep dipping, agricultural sprays, cattle pour-ons, fly control in the milking parlour and the usual suspects. All negative. We sat for a moment in silence whilst I thought. Then Jacky tentatively offered an explanation: 18 months previously she had resolved to lose weight and chose a slimming programme whereby she simply added water to packets of powder (which was described as 'food'). These slurries were variously described as main course and pudding. Bless her, she had lost 25.4 kg (4 stone) in weight, but we calculated that she had consumed over a kilogram of aspartame during the process. In the absence of any other explanation it was biologically plausible that aspartame had switched on her MND.

The best documented environmental cause of MND comes from the Island of Guam in the South Pacific, where the staple food used to be cycad. This seed contains a toxin which has the ability to switch on MND. Before this was known, MND caused the death of 10% of inhabitants.

A feature of the Gulf War veterans is that they too experienced an increased risk of MND.

In my view the likeliest cause were the organophosphate chemicals (OPs) they were exposed to. OPs were extensively used in chemical attacks and for control of sand flies (the soldiers' tents were sprayed) and parasites (the uniforms were drenched). One veteran told me that the OP chemical alarm systems were constantly going off and the only way they got any sleep was to switch them off.

MND is a nasty, progressive prion disorder. I think of prion disorders as 'protein cancers'. Like cell cancers, these proteins start life as normal, desirable and essential to nerve function. However, they become twisted by toxic insults (such as cycad, OPs, and perhaps viruses and mycotoxins) into proteins that cannot be broken down by the body and, with a 'rotten apple' effect, distort other normal proteins. The prognosis for MND is very poor. Poor Jacky did not survive two years. Everywhere now we are surrounded by poisons and chemicals that are 'new' to our bodies and immune systems. We are not adapted to deal with them, and we cannot eradicate them completely from our lives – they are too pervasive. But what we can do is to minimise our exposures. Life is an arms race and the 'chemical war' that is being waged against us is one part of that race – by staying alert to potential danger areas, we can stay ahead of the game.

Reference

1. Telegraph Foreign Staff. 370 kg of cocaine found in Coca-Cola factory in France. *Daily Telegraph* 1 September 2016. (www.telegraph.co.uk/news/2016/09/01/370kg-of-cocaine-found-in-coca-cola-factory-in-france/ – accessed 15 January 2020).

Chapter 74
Oncology/cancer

Oncology case histories
Chronic lymphatic leukaemia (CLL) (viral infection during pregnancy)
Oesophageal cancer (fermenting upper gut)

Chronic lymphatic leukaemia (CLL)

Carwen first presented at my surgery in January 2004, then aged 69, with a droopy left eyelid. I was so pleased with myself (I told you I was a cocky little sod) in diagnosing a nerve palsy called Horner's syndrome. This was confirmed by a consultant neurologist and routine bloods demonstrated she also had chronic lymphatic leukaemia, with a high lymphocyte count of 11.04 x 109/l (reference range 1.5-4.0 x 10^9/l). This diagnosis was then confirmed by a consultant haematologist. The white cell count was not sufficiently high to merit chemotherapy. She was prescribed steroids for her Horner's syndrome, which thankfully resolved, and her lymphocyte count dropped to 6.49 x 10^9/l. She was also noted to have a right-sided cataract. Blood also showed borderline hypothyroidism with a free T4 of 8.6 pmol/l (reference range 12-22 pmol/l). So, I started her on thyroxin.

With any tumour I like to have a tumour marker so that one can assess progress. In CLL the lymphocyte count is such a marker. This meant we were able to closely monitor Carwen's response to nutritional and detoxification therapies.

Carwen started the basic package of treatment PK (paleo-ketogenic) diet, nutritional supplements, exercise), combined with monthly vitamin B12 injections. Cancer cells can only live on sugar while healthy cells can live on fats and short-chain fatty acids from fibre, so a low-GI (glycaemic index) diet was critical. Dairy products contain natural growth promoters and so these too were cut out. It was not, and is still not, easy! Carwen was a keen member of the local Women's Institute and every function was accompanied by breads, cakes, biscuits, pastas, pies and quiches, all of which were now forbidden foods.

Despite sticking to the diet, and gradually losing weight, Carwen's lymphocyte count continued to creep up.

In September 2005 we tested for DNA adducts. This is a test for substances 'stuck onto DNA'. Of course, nothing should be 'stuck on' to DNA – it should be pristine! We found the presence of lindane 'stuck on' to Carwen's DNA at 17 ng/ml. This was a breakthrough. Lindane is a known carcinogen and a problem for at least two reasons. Firstly, it may block genes or up-regulate them: carcinogenesis could result from blocking genes that control growth, from blocking genes that control the synthesis of proteins responsible for DNA repair, or from other mechanisms. Secondly, lindane has oestrogenic-like properties – and oestrogen is a growth promoter.

Where there is chemical insult, we have to

ask both where the chemical came from and also how it can be removed from the body. In Carwen's case, lindane probably came from treating inherited furniture for woodworm in 1977. Since then lindane has been banned as a timber treatment because it is so toxic.

I have done some sort of test of toxicity on over 30 patients before and after some sort of heating regime (sauna, Epsom salt baths etc) and I know that levels of pesticide and VOC come down reliably well with this regime. Because Carwen was not a fatigue syndrome patient and we had a local facility, she started traditional sauna-ing techniques on a twice-weekly basis.

In March 2006 we repeated the DNA adducts test and there was still 11 ng/ml of lindane present. Carwen increased her sauna-ing to three times a week and in September 2006 DNA adducts showed just a trace of lindane present. This was commented on by the lab as 'excellent progress'. The enzyme responsible for healing DNA is zinc dependent. In Carwen's original biopsy, zinc levels were just 27 ng/ml, but this had now come up nicely to 44 ng/ml (reference range 21 – 44 ng/ml).

During the course of the above regimes, Carwen progressively lost weight from 98 kg (15 stone 7lb) to 78 kg (12 stone 5lb).

During this time, we plotted lymphocyte counts and graphed them and that graph is shown in Figure 74.1. The normal range for

Figure 74.1: Carwen's lymphocyte count (CLL)

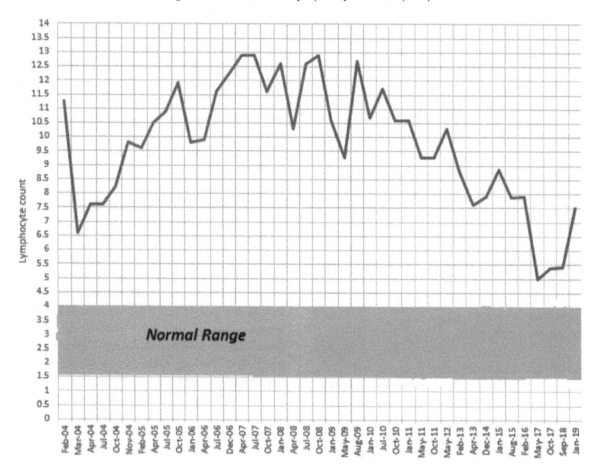

lymphocytes (1.5-4.0 x 109/l) can be seen as a grey band on this graph.

The lymphocyte count increased progressively from 2004, reaching a peak in 2007. During this time, Carwen had lindane on her DNA which could have acted as a growth promoter. Furthermore, she really struggled to do the diet and it was not fully established until 2007. Her lymphocyte count stayed fairly constant until 2009, since when it has fallen progressively. This fall was initially achieved with no conventional therapy, just a paleo-ketogenic diet, avoiding dairy products and carbohydrates, vitamin B12 injections, increasing exercise and, of course, the detox sauna-ing. Essentially, we put Groundhog Chronic (see page A3.1) in place.

Although the diet was hard work, Carwen felt so much better in herself she did stick to it eventually. Her energy levels improved, her falling asleep at functions disappeared (narcolepsy is commonly caused by intolerance of gluten grains), her chronic catarrh disappeared (probably dairy allergy) and her intolerance of sunlight improved so she no longer needed to wear dark glasses. A recent trip to the optician showed that her cataract had not become any worse. Interestingly, her optician reported that her visual acuity had improved by 3 dioptres and commented that it was most unusual for that to happen. I am now fairly sure that the reason for this is the vitamin C to bowel tolerance – I suspect because it improved the elasticity of the lenses (my sight has similarly improved).

However, during the above time Carwen continued to suffer the odd flare of her long-standing problem of iritis (inflammation of the iris of the eye), with a flare in May 2012. This had originally started following the birth of her only child and she had suffered recurrent attacks since. Her lymphocyte count spiked a little, which I thought was probably a viral response, so partly because of this and partly out of scientific curiosity, I decided to start her on the antiviral drug aciclovir

(800 mg five times daily) and referred her back to her consultant ophthalmologist. What was so interesting was that not only did her iritis clear up very quickly, but she felt so much better again, over and above previous improvements. When we repeated the lymphocyte count it had dropped to as low as it had ever been – to 8.7 x 10⁹/l. More recently it fell again to 7.4 x 109/l and you can see from Figure 74.1 that levels have dropped even lower than that subsequently. On the advice of her consultant ophthalmologist, we decided to continue with long-term, low-dose acyclovir (400 mg daily).

At her last visit to the haematologist, the doctor said to Carwen, 'I am puzzled as to why you are so well'!

As I explain separately in Chapter 68, I suspect that Carwen picked up a virus during her pregnancy and that it had caused her problems for years, initially with iritis, possibly as a cause of her Horner's syndrome and, more recently, as one factor driving her CLL. This illustrates the point that pregnancy may result in mild immunosuppression, with a chance for viruses to become established. It may well be that CLL has a viral element and that taking antiviral drugs over and above the other interventions has been additionally helpful. We do know a great many tumours are driven by infection.

It is also worth noting that Carwen has reported that she continues to feel extremely well in herself, indeed much fitter than most of her peers who are disbelieving when she informs them that she is suffering from leukaemia. Carwen is a singer – with acyclovir she found her singing voice much improved as previously she had lost clarity and pitch.

However, I know the battle is not over – it is a war, well fought, that Carwen is winning. She is now 83. She feels as fit as she has ever been and intellectually as sharp. Most importantly she is highly motivated and, with a bit of kicking from me (metaphorical, rather than actual, I hasten to add), sticking to the regimes. I see no reason why she should not continue to do well.

Update June 2019 – The observant will see that Carwen's lymphocyte count has started to rise again. She had a metal implant placed in her foot (see Chapter 68) in March 2018 and the rise followed this. I suspect this is causal. We are currently trying to persuade the orthopaedic surgeons to remove the metal from her foot... Watch this space!

Oesophageal cancer

The incidence of oesophageal cancer is rising faster than any other tumour. It is a nasty one to get as it often presents late, with dysphagia (trouble swallowing), by which time it is too big to operate and difficult to treat with radiotherapy without collateral damage. We have a clue as to why oesophageal cancer has become so common – it is preceded by Barratt's oesophagus, a pathological diagnosis made on the basis of a biopsy sample taken at endoscopy. Patients are told this is a pre-malignant lesion and advised to have regular checks by endoscopy to screen for cancer.

No wonder then that patients ask me what can be done to reverse Barratt's. The main symptom of this is painful acid reflux, which occurs when stomach acid regurgitates up on to an inflamed oesophageal lining. Standard medical treatment is acid blocking drugs such as proton pump inhibitors (PPIs), such as omeprazole. You and I now know that this simply accelerates the under-lying pathology. So, what to do?

Most cancers have an infectious driver (see our book, *The Infection Game*). We know that *H. pylori* is a risk factor for stomach cancer. So, let us hypothesise that the upper fermenting gut is a risk factor for Barratt's and oesophageal cancer. I have now seen three patients, all with the pathological diagnosis of Barratt's. All three did the PK diet and took vitamin C to bowel tolerance. All three were able to stop their acid-blocking drugs

without difficulty. All three were shown to have cured their Barratt's at follow-up endoscopy. Two had the audacity to ask their consultant why their Barratt's had resolved, only to be told, 'We must have got the diagnosis wrong in the first place because Barratt's never remits.'

Since 1990, I have seen three patients with oesophageal cancer. The first was an NHS patient who simply did a Stone Age diet – at that stage I did not appreciate the pernicious nature of carbohydrates in cancer. He saw me in the February, by May his dysphagia had gone and at his December appointment with the oncologist was greeted with the words, 'Why are you here? You should be dead.' This patient survived his tumour but went on to develop a form of dementia some years later.

The second was another man who again reversed his severe dysphagia through diet. He moved away and I lost touch with him. The third, and most recent, Barbara, consulted me in August 2017; she too had an oesophageal cancer that was inoperable, and so treated with a stent (to bypass the obstruction) and chemotherapy. This had not worked, she was deemed too ill for further treatment and given an appalling prognosis. This time I knew to put in place the Full Monty of Groundhog Chronic (page A3.1) and a few months later received the following email: 'Hi. Working very hard on diet, finding it quite difficult for all the same reasons, especially taking the vitamin C – YUK. Had good news on my scan as my tumour is stable and I am feeling really well. Thank you again for the opportunity you gave me. Fred has lost a stone as he is following the diet also so it's all good. Hope to see you soon. Love Bxx.'

The next communication I received the following August from Fred. Barbara's consultant had deemed that she had recovered so well that she would now be fit enough for more chemotherapy. But chemotherapy was very toxic to her heart and she died during treatment from a heart attack.

Chapter 75
Women's health

The premalignant cervix

There is a general acceptance of a one-way progression of premalignancy to malignancy to tumour growth and metastasis that can only be halted by surgery, chemotherapy and/or radiotherapy. Occasionally a window of opportunity arises when a willing 'victim' (Sarah means volunteer*) can put in place a novel intervention which does not interfere with the conventional treatment progression. Nancy was one such pioneering character.

Nancy picked my brains, as a friend. For some years she underwent regular cervical smear screening. Her first abnormal smear presented with cervical intra-epithelial neoplasia (CIN) grade 1 in June 2018, treated in July. Despite that treatment, CIN grade 3 was present in the July biopsy; this was treated in September, but again the November biopsy continued to show CIN 3. Nancy was told this was almost certainly caused by human papilloma virus (HPV – known to be carcinogenic) and/or human herpes virus 1 (HHV 1 – probably carcinogenic). It was almost inevitable that her CIN 3 would progress to invasive cervical cancer and her gynaecologist recommended a full hysterectomy. This is how the surgeons think – you may not be able to control the warring parties, but you can at least remove the battle field! Nancy was booked for vaginal hysterectomy in the February. Could anything be done in the interim?

We were ploughing a new furrow here. But there was a clear two-pronged approach that we could put in place. First, cancer cells can only grow on sugar and are killed by vitamin C. Nancy immediately started a PK diet and took vitamin C to bowel tolerance. Second, we needed to kill the infectious driver of her CIN3. One of my most useful clinical tools is iodine since it contact-kills all microbes, but in the doses employed is not toxic to human cells. A little ingenuity was required to fashion a tool – we used iodine oil (100 ml of coconut fat mixed with 10 ml of Lugol's 15% iodine), warmed it to a runny state, soaked tampons in the mix and allowed them to cool. Nancy used these twice daily. To my surprise, panty-liners were not required.

*Footnote: Craig's father, Peter, was a Squadron Leader in the Royal Air Force Regiment, and he would love to tell of how he selected his 'volunteers'. One of his favourites was having the men on parade and marching up to one of them and presenting him with a toothbrush. Peter would ask, 'What is this, Gunner Smith?' and the answer sure enough was, 'Toothbrush, Sir!' Peter then proceeded with: 'You clearly have an aptitude for dentistry – detailed to the Sick Room.'

Nancy, being a tough character and well able to stand up to the demands of NHS consultants, insisted on a repeat cervical smear prior to surgery. The results were little short of astonishing and caused me to rush to my pantry for a bottle of champers. No CIN changes were visible, HPV gone, HHV gone, cervix normal, surgery cancelled. Wow – the potential of this treatment is little short of mind-boggling!

Chapter 76
Conception and after

Conception, pregnancy and paleo breast-feeding case histories
Infertility (occupational exposure to heavy metals)
The baby who slept (the benefits of a PK diet for mother and baby)

Infertility

When I first started getting interested in Ecological Medicine one of my mentors was Dr Honor Anthony. She often said that we see miracles every day. This is the case of a miracle baby – but by contrast with the Magic Circle* I am going to tell you how the trick was done.

Agnes and Jim consulted with me in December 2008. Numerous attempts to start a family had been tried and ended with difficulty conceiving, or early miscarriage. They had been offered in vitro fertilisation with implantation of the fertilised egg in the womb. Agnes and Jim had refused this. I had to agree with that decision – this approach to treatment lacked logic. Agnes and Jim had achieved fertilisation and implantation all on their own – the problem was *sustaining* a pregnancy.

The starting point for treating everything is to do a good paleo-ketogenic (PK) diet and take a basic package of nutritional supplements. I have never seen normal tests of micronutrients in someone eating a Western diet who is not taking supplements. These nutritional supplements include a good multivitamin, a multimineral, essential fatty acids and vitamins D and C.

However, the elephant in the room became apparent from Agnes's history – she worked as a restorer of stained glass windows and so she was occupationally exposed to toxic metals which were used to colour the glass. She was regularly exposed to cadmium yellow, cobalt blue, nickel violet, antimony white and other such toxic minerals.[†]

These minerals are readily absorbed by inhalation or ingestion. Their toxicity is made worse where there are micronutrient deficiencies. This is because, if the body becomes deficient in a micronutrient such as zinc, then it will use something that 'looks' like zinc in its place. This could be lead, cadmium, mercury or whatever.

---

*Footnote: By 'Magic Circle' I mean the grouping of magicians with the motto *indocilis privata loqui* ('not apt to disclose secrets') and not the top five law firms in London who share that nomenclature.

[†]Personal note from Craig: Reading this has triggered a thought for Craig. Craig's grandfather was a veteran of Ypres, and with hindsight probably suffered from PTSD. After the Great War, he took up a job with a tanning firm; he used cadmium (and other toxic elements, such as nickel, lead, mercury and arsenic) as a tanning agent. Some time after taking this job, Eddie began to suffer from (lifelong) joint and bone pain, and, on the one occasion that he mentioned it to the doctor, he was told that it was probably something to do with 'the War'. Thereafter Eddie just carried on. Perhaps he had something akin to Itai-Itai disease? Itai-itai disease ('it hurts-it hurts' disease) was the name given to the mass cadmium poisoning of Toyama Prefecture, Japan, starting around 1912, which results in joint and bone pain.

So these toxic minerals get incorporated into enzyme systems of the body, with the potential to wreak biochemical havoc. Clearly we had to look at her toxic load. A cheap and quick way to start would be hair analysis – but this is not a reliable test. One may be lucky and pick up a toxicity but so often there are false negatives. Nowadays I reckon the best test is to measure urine elements following the taking of a chelating agent – namely, DMSA (see page 15.4). This is an easy test to do – empty the bladder, take a dose of DMSA at the rate of 15 mg/kg body weight, collect all urine for the next six hours, measure the total volume and send a sample off to Biolab. This test can be accessed through Natural Health Worldwide:

www.naturalhealthworldwide.com.

DMSA can be purchased as captomer

www.supersmart.com/en--Detoxification-- DMSA-100-mg--0248

However, in 2008 I was using bloods tests. Results for toxic metals for Agnes were:

Agnes's results	Reference ranges
Lead 15 ug/l	(< 10.0 ug/l)
Antimony 2.5 ug/l	(< 2.0 ug/l)
Cadmium 7.5 ug/l	(< 2.0 ug/l)
Cobalt 6.0 ug/l	(<1.0 ug/l)
Nickel 9.5 ug/l	(<5.0 ug/l)

It must be remembered that the reference ranges are not normal; the normal range should be zero or very close to zero. This is because none of these toxic metals (barring cobalt which is the active principal of vitamin B12) has any known biological use in the body. Indeed lead, antimony, cadmium and nickel are all carcinogens. These 'normal ranges' simply reflect what is present in modern Western populations. This alone is an indication of what a toxic world we live in.

Further tests of DNA adducts were as follows:

Agnes's results	Reference ranges
Lead 4 ng/ml	(zero)
Nickel 16 mg/ml	(zero)
Cobalt 5 ng/ml	(zero)

And all of these were stuck on to her DNA. As I have said, DNA should be pristine – there should be nothing attached. Nickel was present in particularly high levels stuck on to the gene that codes for DNA ligase. This enzyme is vital for DNA repair and may impact directly on fertility and egg quality. We now had a biologically plausible explanation for Agnes's infertility.

The priority therefore was to get rid of these toxic metals. Firstly, she had to change her occupation to prevent further exposures. We then used four techniques to help her body eliminate the toxins:

1. Oral chelation therapy with DMSA – I use a weekly dose of 15 mg/kg of body weight. Because DMSA also chelates some of the friendly minerals, the other six days of the week one 'rescues' with a good multimineral.
2. Extra doses of zinc (30 mg), selenium (500 mcg) and magnesium (300 mg) to displace the toxic minerals from their binding sites. This was combined with glutathione (250 mg twice daily) – this 'grabs' the displaced toxic mineral so it can be peed out.
3. Extra vitamin C (5 g daily), which increases toxic metal excretion.
4. Iodine as iodoral (14.5 mg daily), which again increases toxic metal excretion.

Six months later we repeated the DNA adducts test and found the only toxic metal left was nickel, but the level had reduced substantially from 16 ng/ml to 7 ng/ml. Everything was moving nicely in the right direction. During this time, Agnes's partner Jim had joined in with the paleo-ketogenic diet and supplements. During this time his sperm count rose from 37 million per millilitre to 75 million per millilitre.

It was important for Nicky not to conceive during this time of detox – I did not want the baby to be exposed to these nasty toxins. I reckoned that another six months of detox and the green light could be given…

Two years later our miracle baby, Ben, was born fit and well, weighing 3.8 kg (8 lb 4 oz), following an uneventful pregnancy. Agnes[‡] was then 46. What a girl!

The baby who slept

Practising ecological medicine is exciting. It is also my hobby. I talk about it all the time and that means many of my friends and family have adopted the regimes. Michelle was one such. She became a neighbour in 2017, when she moved from Dorset so that her husband, Peter Wilson, could continue training locally at the top shooting ground, Griffin Lloyd. Peter won a gold medal at the 2012 London Olympics. He is also the current world record holder for the event, having scored 198 out of 200 at a World Cup event in Arizona during 2012.

Michelle and Peter became good friends. Baby Robyn was born August 2018. Throughout her pregnancy and breast-feeding Michelle did Groundhog Basic, to the letter, not even taking any of the liberties that I occasionally do. She ate the perfect PK diet, took supplements, kept fit and continued to use her brain. What happened?

Michelle had a trouble-free pregnancy and delivery. Eating PK meant her blood sugars were low and completely stable, so her insulin and adrenalin levels were not spiking. She did not gain excessive weight, her blood pressure was perfect, no stretch marks, no oedema and Bobs was born without complications.

Bobs was breast-fed and Michelle continued to eat PK. Since breast milk is simply a filtrate of blood, this meant that levels of sugar in the breast milk were low, there were no strong antigens from dairy, no toxic lectins from grains and no adrenalin surges from wobbly blood sugar levels. Of course, her breast milk was full of micronutrients, protective antibodies and vitamin C. How did this manifest in our Bobs (who, yes, I have adopted as a surrogate grand-daughter)? (I tend to do a lot of that these days. Now we want to open a 'school' at Upper Weston – a free venue for parents to home-educate their children with benign neglect. It will be called Warthog's PIE – 'politically incorrect education'. And yes, I love Harry Potter too!)

The most important outcome for Bobs and Michelle was sleep. Michelle's breast milk was high in fat and so Bobs was fuelling her body with fat. This is the most desirable fuel for the brain. In babies, 40% of all fuel used goes into brain development. Bobs's blood sugar would also be low and completely stable, so she was not spiking adrenalin. Adrenalin spikes are the most common cause of sleep disturbance in adults, and it is the same for babies. By 4 weeks of age Bobs was sleeping a regular 11 hours at night, and more in the day. Now at 9 months, she sleeps 13 hours at night together with a further four hours in the day. This means Michelle is well rested and has continued in her work as an artist. Locally she is known as Michelle Angelo – she is the most brilliant painter and drawer of horses and her works are in great demand – see www.mccullagh.co.uk/exhibitions/

[‡]**Footnote**: 'Agnes' is the Latinised form of the Greek name 'Αγνη' (Hagne), derived from 'αγνος' (hagnos) meaning chaste. Just like me (in Hebrew the meaning of the name Sarah is Princess), Agnes victoriously defied her name's meaning and did it anyway!

Because Michelle's breast milk was so low in sugar, Bobs did not develop a fermenting gut. This meant she never burped or posseted. She did vomit once when she was being weaned – an overdose of liver, avocado and coconut milk – all of which she loves! In the absence of sugar, microbes cannot survive and so Bobs never had oral thrush. At 4 months she picked up a bug which made her miserable and feverish for 24 hours – next day she was back to her normal, smiling, engaging self. At 8 months she had a few blisters on her side which I suspect was chicken-pox (I do hope so!); they went quickly with iodine oil ad lib, this time with no hint of systemic malaise.

Looking at this from an evolutionary perspective, all the above is highly desirable. A screaming, spewing baby dumping smelly gut contents in its wake, being carried by an exhausted Mother, is a beacon to all local predators to 'come and eat me'.

Midwives, health visitors, friends and families regularly congratulate Michelle on having such an easy baby. The main concern of the midwives was that Bobs was not gaining weight as fast as she should and recommended that Michelle wake her twice in the night for extra feeds! Our view was that if Bobs were hungry, she would tell us. Michelle let her sleep on. Shortly after, she was weaned onto coconut cream, avocado, liver, purple sprouting broccoli and linseed. Bobs is now a bonny little girl who continues to sleep 13 hours a night.

With the PK diet established and the first-aid kit stocked with vitamin C, iodine and coconut oil, the issue of vaccination fades into insignificance. More so, since we now know that acute febrile illnesses in childhood are protective against disease later on in life – diseases such as brain tumours. Indeed, it is biologically plausible that vaccination is driving our epidemics of autism, SEND (Special Educational Needs and Disabilities), allergy and autoimmunity (see Chapter 51). It is my view that the risk–benefit equation has now tilted firmly in the direction of not vaccinating. As I write I return from a conference where I again heard that viral vaccines contain 1.7 to 3.7 mcg of animal tissue per dose, of which 80% is human foetal cells and 20% chick cells – these may well be contaminated with other unidentified viruses. The only vaccination I would recommend is a single tetanus vaccination given intra-dermally (involves a much smaller dose but a better immune response), but this can be postponed until Bobs has got to the age when she is likely to plunge a dirty pitchfork into her foot.

Michelle has mastered the intellectual high ground and defended it. I confidently predict a bright future for our Bobs.

Chapter 77
Paediatrics/problems in childhood

Paediatrics – case histories
The baby who cried (milk allergy and Western diet)
The deaf child (milk allergy)
Down's syndrome

The baby who cried

One cannot help but be influenced by events which happen to self and family – just as well perhaps because this is how many doctors become interested in ecological medicine. My introduction came in the form of Ruth – a baby with severe colic and projectile vomiting which kept her awake day and night screaming and in pain. She was mine and nothing I did seemed to help. I thought I was going to be the perfect breast-feeding mother but here I was, falling at the first hurdle with weeks of pure misery. I can remember my then husband saying, 'You're the effing doctor – you sort it out!' I felt completely inadequate.

I cannot recall what it was that made me change my diet, but I cut out all dairy products. The result was, for me, a medical miracle. My daughter's gut settled at once, she became smiley and happy and slept contentedly through the night. On one occasion, when I inadvertently drank a drop of cow's milk, this resulted in a further miserable night of howling baby with me furious at my own stupidity. Ruth was clearly cow's milk allergic and has remained so.

What is so astonishing is that this relationship between dairy allergy, projectile vomiting and colic appears nowhere in the medical textbooks, either then or now. But this clinical gem has been of great use to me throughout my medical career.

Ten years later I had moved to the Welsh borders and was doing a GP locum role. 'Please could you visit Nina – she's ill again?' The diagnosis was easy – indeed I was able make it before even opening the front door. Those screams of misery were instantly recognisable, together with, as the door was opened, the white gob of snotty material on mother's lapel. However, the story that Ann told me was even more distressing than my own. Nina had suffered severe colic since birth some 10 weeks previous. She had been plied with all sorts of medications at the instigation of her GP and health visitor. These included a preparation of gripe water in which the main constituent was alcohol – out of interest I took a slurp of it and immediately felt heady – there was more alcohol in it than in a pre-dinner cocktail. In desperation, the family had agreed that Nina should be admitted to hospital for further investigation. The conclusion of that hospital trip was that

Nina was 'expressing symptoms of a stressful relationship between Mum and Dad'. The solution was for Mum and Dad to undergo counselling therapy. It is not often that I am convulsed by a combination of amusement and horror, but this was one such occasion.

So, I dived into my car, nipped down to the local supermarket and returned with a tin of Wysoy (soy infant formula). I had to do this because Ann was completely disbelieving of my diagnosis. 'Surely the hospital consultants would know about this?' I knew that if I did not take direct action, Ann would not either. I also recommended making up the Wysoy with bottled water... and left Ann in charge.

I revisited two days later. The house was silent. Ann had lost her Art Nouveau gobby badge. (En vogue experimental artist Inés Cámara Leret produces crystal artwork from spit; Ann and child were years ahead of their time!) Ann was smiling too. The parental counselling sessions had been cancelled and the reputation of the paediatricians trashed.

Dairy allergy is extremely common. What is so interesting is that if dairy products are continued, then the target organ changes. The baby may well grow out of the colic (typically at 13 weeks), but then another department is affected. What follows may be toddler diarrhoea, chronic catarrhal conditions with snotty nose or glue ears. Later we see eczema and asthma, then recurrent tonsillitis. The teenager develops migraine or irritable bowel syndrome. The adult presents with arthritis. The poor patient is referred from one hospital department to another with none making a proper diagnosis (for a proper diagnosis, one needs to discern causation) but instead dishing out nonsense 'diagnoses' like 'growing pains', 'abdominal migraine', 'sickly child' or 'moody mare'. Worse, potentially dangerous symptom-suppressing medication is prescribed.

Dairy allergy runs very strongly in families – often associated with the bright, blond(e) and blue eyed. Almost always in making a diagnosis of dairy allergy I can find a first-degree relative who also suffers. My special interest is chronic fatigue syndrome – I estimate a fifth of patients I see present with a history of dairy allergy, then pick up Epstein-Barr virus (glandular fever or 'mono') and switch into a post-viral chronic fatigue syndrome. I suspect many acquire moulds growing in their airways, especially sinuses. Such inoculation results from exposure to moulds in water-damaged buildings or, for us country folk, mouldy hay and straw. These further damage us through chronic mould infection, chronic poisoning by mycotoxins and chronic allergic reactions to moulds. Allergic reactions are such a wasteful expenditure of energy and my CFS patients can ill afford this. Actually, none of us can afford to waste energy. In fact, the word allergy derives from the Greek *allos* (other) and *ergia* (activity or energy), and so literally 'allergy' is expenditure of energy on *other* (things).

Indeed, dairy products are remarkably dangerous foods. Allergy aside, they are a risk factor for cancer, heart disease, osteoporosis and autoimmunity. Whilst they are essential for young mammals to grow rapidly, and so evade predation, they are a disaster for mature mammals. When challenged by the question, 'Are dairy products not natural foods?' a long-standing advocate of paleo diets (Dr Loran Cordain), replied, 'Have you ever tried milking a wild bison?'

As I get older, and perhaps wiser (although many would dispute this!) my medicine becomes simpler. The simple things, done really well, get you a long way. Dietary changes should be central to the treatment of all conditions – this means eating the evolutionarily correct paleo-ketogenic (PK) diet. The *Why* is detailed in our book *Diabetes – delicious diets, not dangerous drugs* and the *How* in our book *The PK Cookbook – go paleo-ketogenic and get the best of both worlds.*

The deaf child

It was an embarrassing and humbling feature of my early days in General Practice that I learned more from my patients than they from me. During the early 1980s the only tool that I knew to employ was the diet that cut out grains, dairy and yeast. So, when Ruth brought Colleen, aged 3, along to see me for advice about management of her eczema I knew before they even sat down what the treatment programme was going to be. Even today, I spend much more time on the *How* to put the difficult interventions in place than the *Why*, so much of the consultation time was spent on shopping and cooking tips. As we chatted, I became aware that Colleen was taking little interest... to learn that she had been diagnosed deaf, probably since birth, was registered disabled as such and had a place at deaf school reserved. I thought no more about this until the first follow-up consultation two months later.

On their return my immediate concern was that I had picked up the wrong set of clinical notes. Yes, the names were correct, but the subject of obvious excitement should have been Colleen's skin, but was actually about hearing. It was obvious that Colleen was now responding to noise and, as a result, was starting to talk. Indeed, with time her hearing became normal, she developed perfect speech and is now working as a lawyer earning considerably more than I ever did. Clever girl!

We pondered over the mechanism of this restoration of hearing. It had to be allergy. It is a feature of dairy products that they tend to be catarrh-forming. I do not yet know the mechanism of this. When I searched on the Internet on this this question, the main study that came up refuted such a link... but then it had been bank-rolled by the Dairy Council of California. Another case of follow the money. The bones of the ear – the hammer, anvil and stirrup – which allow the transmission of movement from a vibrating eardrum to the cochlear, where the nerve endings to transmit sound to the brain are, are the smallest in the body and easily impaired. A middle ear full of snot would do the trick nicely. The ENT consultants call this glue ear. This reminds me of my good friend and colleague and Reader in Allergy and Immunology, discussing the essential characteristics of that amazing material we call mucus:

> ...*You may know it as snot, but it is my bread and butter.*
> Dr David Freed 1945 – 2007

With this discovery suddenly, like Walter Mitty, I could see my name amongst the medical magnificents with appropriate paraphernalia: Dame Sarah Myhill, polished oak boards with my name emblazoned and numerous invitations for lectures and honorary degrees. All I had to do was write the case history paper and it would be published with a fanfare of glory. I wrote enthusiastically to the consultant who had made the diagnosis of congenital deafness inviting a joint paper. He wrote back. 'That is not possible – I must have got the diagnosis wrong in the first place.' Just as Colleen had deafness caused by her allergy to dairy, the consultant had intellectual deafness and blindness caused by his medical training. No, he did not want a joint paper. From this case I did not just learn that dairy products may cause deafness but also that, in the medical profession, you are not allowed to be enthusiastic, and certainly not to have new ideas or make outrageous diagnoses. This amounts to quackery and one risks Establishment opprobrium. I now do that in spades!

A case of Down's syndrome

We all know that Down's syndrome is a congenital abnormality caused by an extra chromosome. It is characterised by many features, but those that most interfere with a productive life include intellectual impairment and physical fatigue. Doctors offer no treatment for Down's because nothing can be done about the genes. However, we do know that all disease involves an interaction between genes and theenvironment. So, when I was consulted by Sonia about her daughter Sarah, who had Down's syndrome, we wondered what could be done to optimise Sarah's physical and mental functioning. At that time, I had stumbled across the work of Dr Henry Turkel. He was a physician who treated Down's as a clinician should – looking at the clinical picture and wondering about mechanisms. The picture that he saw was similar to that of hypothyroidism and allergies. Indeed, physical fatigue, mental retardation, macroglossia (large tongue) and oedema are common features. These children were treated with ecological medicine which included diet, micronutrient supplements, digestive enzymes and correction of hypothyroidism. Turkel described this as 'removal of the harmful expression of the excessive genes'. His work was completely rejected by the Establishment because it did not conform to the drug model. Indeed, his paper (Turkel, 1975) describing his attempt to gain official recognition for the effectiveness of his therapy opens with:

> In 1959, before the U.S. Food and Drug Administration lapsed into insanity...[1]

What Turkel was doing was not only biologically plausible but of demonstrable benefit. Risks and side effects were zero. He found that the earlier treatments were applied the better the result. Sonia put Turkel's techniques to her daughter, Sarah. Sarah was in her early teens when work was started. Essentially, she received Groundhog Basic (page A1.1) with the bolt-on extras for correction of thyroid and digestive function. In the 1980s, GPs were much less controlled and had many more clinical freedoms. Sarah's GP was supportive and prescribed the necessary thyroid hormones and pancreatic enzymes. Sarah blossomed. Her energy improved, she needed less sleep, she grew, her brain woke up. Age 18 she got herself a job at a garden centre and tea shop. With her loving personality, which is a particular feature of people with Down's, she became a favourite with the punters. She was able to work and to live independently with minimal supervision. Sonia was so proud. So was I.

Reference

1. Turkel H. Medical Amelioration of Down's Syndrome Incorporating the Orthomolecular Approach. *Orthomolecular Psychiatry* 1975; 4(2): 102-115. http://orthomolecular.org/library/jom/1975/pdf/1975-v04n02-p102.pdf

Chapter 78
Haematology/ blood problems

The pancytopenia of chronic disease – chronic Epstein-Barr virus

Lennie presented with the clinical picture of myalgic encephalitis (ME). What this means in terms of mechanisms is that not only did he have symptoms of poor energy delivery but also of inflammation. I reckon these days that we can correct poor energy delivery mechanisms reliably well (see Chapter 30). The greatest challenge now is the inflammation element. In Lennie's case, he had clear symptoms of inflammation – his immune system was activated because of either chronic infection, allergy or autoimmunity.

In Lennie's case, he had been previously bitten by a tick. But then so have many of us! A tick bite followed by ME is not sufficient to diagnose Lyme disease. We have the same problem with Epstein-Barr virus (EBV). We know from the work of Dr Martin Lerner that EBV is causally involved in 80% of PWME (people with myalgic encephalitis). But that is not sufficient to diagnosed chronic EBV. My clinical life has been revolutionised by Armin laboratories. This is for a number of reasons. Firstly, Dr Armin has developed an EliSpot test. This is a measure of gamma interferon produced by white blood cells when they are brought into contact with the putative microbe. What this tells us is not just what the body has been exposed to in the past but how white cells are responding to it now – the point being that a high EliSpot reading is the best indicator that the patient is currently infected with and busy fighting infection. This is a good predictor of response to treatment. Secondly, Armin laboratories give us a detailed haematology report. Almost invariably with a chronic infection we see low levels of white cells, often a low red cell count, and sometimes low platelets.

In Lennie's case, his EliSpot for Lyme was a low result suggesting Lyme was not the issue. By contrast, he had a very high EliSpot for EBV. Relevant haematology was as follows:

Table 78.1: Lennie's haematology results, implications and treatments

Significant result	What it means	Comments – action
Haemoglobin 131 g/l – low (Reference range 135-175 g/l)	The bone marrow is going slow for one of three reasons: (1) it does not have the raw materials and/or	Lennie had a high homocysteine level, suggesting poor B12 availability, so we started vitamin B12 by injection
	(2) it does not have the energy and/or	Due to poor mitochondrial and poor thyroid function (see Chapter 30)
	(3) there is excessive demand for red cells so supply cannot keep up with demand	He had no blood loss from the gut or haemolysis (ruptured red blood cells)
Red cell count 4.45 million cells/ mcl – low (Reference range 4.7-6.1 million cells/mcl)	Ditto all the above	PK diet and nutritional supplements (see Chapter 21)
White cell count 3.04 x 10⁹/l – low (Reference range 4-11 x 10⁹/l) Lymphocytes 0.7 x 10⁹/l – low (Reference range 1-4.8 10⁹/l)	Ditto all the above AND the white cell soldiers being used up in the battle against chronic infection	Provide the raw materials and energy Reduce the work of the immune system with Groundhog Chronic (page A3.1)
Platelets 116 x 10⁹/l – low (Reference range 150-400 10⁹/l)	Ditto all the above	Provide the raw materials and energy for the bone marrow to recover
CD8 + CD57 absolute 36* – very low (Reference range 100–700*)	There is a low level of activated T cells – ie, there are not enough soldiers to fight the battle	Ditto all the above

The battle against any chronic infection is not a battle but a war. I have seen a few patients who have a post EBV ME, tested positive with EliSpot, received antivirals but not responded. They had not put in place Groundhog Chronic, were not eating a PK diet, and were not taking vitamin C, nor doing regimes to improve energy delivery mechanisms. EBV is a swine of a virus that we have to fight with every available weapon.

Lennie had to first establish Groundhog Chronic before considering antivirals. He had been diagnosed with probable idiopathic thrombocytopenic purpura, an autoimmune condition (treatment: lifelong monitoring and steroids if the count goes dangerously low). What he

---

Footnote: These tests give an absolute cell count of CD8 and CD57 natural killer (NK) cells per litre of blood.

actually had was pancytopenia, with all cell lines (red, white and platelets) depressed. What is so interesting is that his haematology improved markedly, and within two months his platelets, white cell count and red cell count had all normalised.

His current counts are as follows:

Haemoglobin 149 g/l	(was 131 g/l)
Red cell count 4.71 million cells/mcl	(was 4.45 million cells/mcl)
White cell count 6.8 c 10^9/l	(was 3.04 x 10^9/l)
Lymphocytes 2.2 x 10^9/l	(was 0.7 x 10^9/l)
Platelets 194 x 10^9/l	(was 116 x 10^9/l)
CD57 + NK 65*	(was 36*)

We are about to start prescription antivirals, and now with an immune system working better we have a much better chance of success. Do it all, Lennie!

Chapter 79
Current cases – worked examples

The cases in this chapter all come from real patients who I am currently working with. You can see how rapidly eco-medicine is evolving as the management strategies below may be different from the case histories which have gone before. I am learning from my patients all the time and this book will need regular updating – already I need to expand the section on mycotoxins, as illustrated by the case history below.

The idea of the 'management frames' given here is to illustrate how you can do this yourself – the approach will be constantly changing. The following examples show how to put into practice the management frames of Chapter 10.

Well done, is better than well said.
Benjamin Franklin (January 17, 1706 – April 17, 1790; one of the Founding Fathers of the United States of America)

1. New patient – student, male, 18, with chronic fatigue syndrome

Table 79.1: Management framework – patient 1's history

Onset	Symptoms	Mechanism	See Chapter:
Child	Episodes of violent vomiting – knocked out for a few days – recurrent	Allergy	7 – Inflammation symptoms
2012	ME/CFS diagnosed when at 8-9 years old		5 – Fatigue

Onset	Symptoms	Mechanism	See Chapter:
	Epididymitis x 2. Used NSAIDs and antibiotics one time	Allergy to microbes from the fermenting gut	7 – Inflammation symptoms
	Paced ++ and home schooled – then back to school	Rest allowed energy for healing	
2014	Relapsed. Seen every six weeks at Paediatric CFS Department who advised graded exercise but became much worse as a result	Dear oh dear – a condition that is defined by exercise intolerance will be made worse by such!	

Table 79.2: Management framework – patient 1's test results

Test	Significant result	What it means	Action	See Chapter:
2011 CDSA	Elastase 242 ugE1/g – low normal	Possibly poor pancreatic function	May need pancreatic enzymes to digest foods	11 – Fuel in the tank, gut function
	Eosinophil x 4.5 x 10^9 /l – a bit high	Mild inflammation		16 – Inflammation mechanisms
	Beta glucuronidase 5,751 U/g Low n-butyrate 6.5 micromol/g	Upper fermenting gut caused by anaerobes	Starve the bugs out with PK diet Kill then with vitamin C to bowel tolerance	21 – The PK diet 31 – Vitamin C
	Aerobes x 1	Upper fermenting gut caused by aerobes		
	Pulse 60 bpm – too slow	Hypothyroid	Start thyroid glandulars (TG) as below	30 – Tools to improve energy delivery mechanisms
	'Lyme negative last year' (Sample sent to Porton Down, Wiltshire)	This lab seems to have a high incidence of false negative results for Lyme	Do not trust this test – do all else first and if not making progress then look for the infectious hole in the energy bucket	See our book *The Infection Game*

IgG food test	Egg, wheat, gluten, dairy	I do not trust these results	Use your own detective work – trial and error	7 – Inflammation symptoms
	Ferritin 31 ug/l	Suggest hypochlorhydria (low stomach acid) – you need an acid stomach to absorb minerals	Starve the bugs out with PK diet Kill then with vitamin C to bowel tolerance	21 – The PK diet 31 – Vitamin C
TFTs	TSH 2.54 mIU/l	Low or normal TSH never excludes the possibility of secondary hypothyroidism due to poor pituitary function; indeed, this is the commonest cause of hypothyroidism in CFS/ME	Start thyroid glandular (TG) as below	30 – Tools to improve energy delivery mechanisms
	T4 12.9 pmol/l (reference range 7.9-13.3 pmol/l)	This range is set ridiculously low; my lab's is 12-22. There is clear biochemical scope for a trial of thyroid hormones	We have to go very slowly here so suggest: Get PK-adapted first TG 15 mg on rising for one weeks If all well increase to TG 15 mg on rising + 15 mg at midday for one weeks. If all well, increase in 15 mg increments to 30 mg + 30 mg Re-check the bloods Monitor pulse and blood pressure – pulse should be less than 90 bpm, blood pressure 120/80 Hg mm or less Most people need 90-150 mg Too much thyroid hormone feels as if you have drunk 20 cups of coffee! Any problems, get in touch with me by email at once The commonest cause of problems is metabolic syndrome because this spikes adrenalin – you must be PK adapted	30 – Tools to improve energy delivery mechanisms
	D3 90 nmol/l	I like to see this between 100 and 200 nmol/l	Sunshine salt has 5,000 iu per 5 g dose	21 – PK diet

Table 79.3: Management framework – patient 1's symptoms

Symptoms	Mechanism	Action	See Chapter:
Fatigue not improved much by rest Pacing, rest	Poor energy delivery	Getting you right is like conducting an orchestra – we need to get all the players in place, playing at the same time to get a result See our book *Diagnosis and Treatment of Chronic Fatigue Syndrome and Myalgic Encephalitis* – *it's mitochondria not hypochondria*	11 – Fuel in the tank 12 – Mitochondrial engine 13 – Thyroid accelerator and adrenal gear box
15 minutes per day doing: 1-2 hours walking or gentle cycling 15 minutes stretching daily = 1-2 hours per week 30/100	Clinical score 30/100	Do not exercise too much yet as this will slow recovery. Wait until wild horses can't hold you back!	
Cannot tolerate oral minerals e.g. Biocare, so take organic minerals: Vitamin D 4000 iu + Vitamin K2 200 ug Phosphatidylserine 300 mg Vitamin C 1000 mg twice daily Eskimo3 oil 3 caps twice daily Topical multi-mineral spray B12 spray	Basic package of supplements Intolerance of supplements is often a fermenting gut issue You need the correct balance of omega-6 to omega-3 which should be 4:1 – you may have too much omega-3; suggest swap to hemp oil which has the correct ratio	Once you are PK-adapted you should tolerate oral supplements: Multivitamin Hemp oil 1 dessertspoon plus VegEPA 4 capsules for four months, then 2 daily long-term Sunshine salt – supplies all the minerals plus 5000 iu vitamin D3 and 5000 mcgm of B12 Vitamin C as ascorbic acid to bowel tolerance	21 – PK diet and essential micronutrients 31 – Vitamin C
Tried PK diet but no difference noted and, as cannot eat dairy and eggs, it became very limiting and he was losing weight so we returned to a paleo + pretty low-carb diet:*	Diet – great start! Suspect he has ketogenic hypoglycaemia possibly due to hypothyroidism – this is the elephant in the room: powering the body with sugar and carbs when the evolutionarily correct fuels are fat and fibre	We must get to full PK diet – do core temps as below and start thyroid glandulars then you will be able to manage PK Boosting the thyroid will help a lot – you burn fat with thyroid hormones instead of adrenal hormones Expect to get DDD reactions	28 – Diet, detox and die-off (DDD) reactions

There are carbs in this diet from fruit, potato, humus, seeds, crisps	Metabolic syndrome (which is defined by the contents of the supermarket trolley!)	PK diet, thyroid glandulars	
Sleep – drop off at around 11:00-11.30pm …wake around 8:00-8.30 am Quality: Varies with how feeling. Can be uninterrupted during a good spell or wake repeatedly and need to empty bladder or bowels until 1 am. Melatonin helpful	Sleep: With metabolic syndrome blood sugar levels fall at night and this spikes adrenalin levels, wakes you up 'Owl' (drop off to sleep late and wake late) You need three groups of hormone to correct your diurnal rhythm: – dark triggers melatonin production which – stimulates the pituitary so TSH spikes at midnight, then – T4 spikes at 4 am and T3 at 5 am, which stimulates the production of adrenal hormones, which wake you up.	PK diet See Chapter 22 (work in progress) – use a sleep dream We need to do a balancing act of melatonin, thyroid glandular (TG) and adrenal glandular (AG) to restore the diurnal rhythm but the dose very much depends on the individual's core temperatures – see 'Conducting the orchestra', Chapter 30 Example: start with melatonin 3 mg slow-release, 1 at night Adrenal glandular 125 mg in the morning Thyroid glandular 15 mg in the morning… and build all these three up in balance with each other. Most people end up needing melatonin 3-9 mg, TG 60-150 mg and AG 250-750 mg daily	14 – Sleep – why and how we sleep 22 – Sleep – why we sleep poorly and how to fix
Mother and grandmother have both had ME/CFS, migraines and food intolerances Acetyl L-carnitine 200 mg twice daily D-ribose in drinks when remember – no improvement noticed Ubiquinol 100 mg Niacinamide 1500 mg	Mitochondria come down the female line. Mitochondrial function improves reliably well with the regimes – I know! We published a scientific paper supporting this[1]	Carry on with these supplements – in order of importance: niacinamide 1500 mg ubiquinol 100mg magnesium 300 mg carnitine 500 mg D-ribose 5-15 g daily or as a rescue remedy if you really overdo things BUT this must be part of your carb count in the PK diet	12 – The mitochondrial engine

*Breakfast: Bacon, linseed bread with pate, sometimes fruit
Lunch: Veg soup, linseed bread or baked potato, mixed salad/raw veg
Supper: Meat (sometimes fish), raw veg and not much carbohydrate
Snacks: Nuts; humus with seed crackers (homemade) or crisps; dark chocolate (dairy-free); sometimes fruit; sometimes homemade snack bars made of nuts, seeds and a little dried fruit
Drinks: Water, tea – black, green and mint
Does not eat wheat, dairy (any kind) and currently no eggs.

Symptoms	Mechanism	Action	See Chapter:
Chronic constipation – Movicol one sachet daily Pulse rate 60 bpm 'Owl' T4 12.9 pmol/l Mum has thyroid cysts (hypothyroid)	Clinically hypothyroid with biochemical scope for a trial of TG	Start TG as above	
		Anyone who is hypothyroid will almost certainly be iodine deficient – take Lugol's iodine 15% 4 drops daily for four months to replete, then 2 drops daily for life	32 – Iodine
		THEN You need to fine tune the CFS orchestra – http://drmyhill.co.uk/ wiki/Conducting_the_CFS_ orchestra Measure your core temp regularly through the day and graph the results The average core temperature is a measure of thyroid function	30 – Tools to improve energy delivery mechanisms
Ashwagandha 100 mg twice daily	Adrenal	The fluctuations are a measure of adrenal function	30 – Tools to improve energy delivery mechanisms

Abdominal problems – IBS Migraines/cyclical vomiting syndrome every six weeks – when 7-8 years old – treated with Sumatriptan, Ondansetron and Ibuprofen lysine. Turned into more classical migraines and not very often now Grandmother and mother: migraines and food intolerances, Grandmother: problems with pollen and chemicals Pollen – fexofenadine Chemical sensitivity	Allergy to foods and/or to microbes BUT there is also an energy delivery aspect to migraine – sorting the thyroid may help greatly	PK diet Ascorbic acid helps a lot to switch off allergies We could try at any time: low dose naltrexone (1 mg at night, building up to 4 mg, or 50 mg in 50 ml i.e. 1 mg/ml) Pollen is sticky stuff and water soluble – washing the face with water or having a shower gets rid of pollen very well	36 – Tools to switch off inflammation
IBS with pain and nausea – restricted diet may have helped abdominal symptoms Movicol one sachet daily Buscopan = no benefit Cannot tolerate oral minerals	Fermenting gut	Starve the little wretches out with a PK diet Kill 'em with vitamin C to bowel tolerance	21 – PK diet 31 – Vitamin C
Appendectomy when nearly 8 years old	MAY make you more susceptible to gut dysbiosis issues	PK diet	21 – PK diet 31 – Vitamin C

Symptoms	Mechanism	Action	See Chapter:
Epididymitis Joint pain (often precedes ME flare) Sleep disturbed by peeing	Allergy to microbes from the fermenting gut Could be allergy to foods, or allergy to microbes from the fermenting gut – these easily spill over from the gut into the bloodstream (this is called bacterial translocation); these microbes then drive inflammatory reactions at distal sites	Starve the little wretches out with a PK diet Kill 'em with vitamin C to bowel tolerance	21 – PK diet 31 – Vitamin C
	Chronic infection	This is always possible, but all the above done well will help to deal with such . Wait and see – we may have to do tests for infection later if we are not making clinical progress	See our book *The Infection Game*
No dental work	Great!	The PK diet prevents dental decay	
L glutathione reduced 250 mg once daily 5-methyltetrahydrofolic acid once daily Trimethyl glycine 3 g Methylcobalbamin 1000 ug dissolvable once daily SAMe 400 mg once daily on empty stomach Ionic zinc Nascent iodine	Detox Reduces homocysteine	Carry on – all the above further helps detox Vitamin C to bowel tolerance Iodine as Lugol's 15% (8 mg iodine per drop) 4 drops daily	34 – Detoxing
	Connective tissue/bone		
Astaxanthin 12 mg once daily	Antioxidant	Fine to carry on Finally, remember all the above have the potential to make you worse in the short term – so be kind to yourself!	28 – Diet, detox and die-off reactions

2. Dental nurse, insurance-industry receptionist, bar maid 1986, now 32

Table 79.4: Patient 2's test results

Test	Significant result	What it means	Action	Chapter/page in *Diagnosis and Treatment of CFS and ME* 2nd edition(CFS), *Ecological Medicine* (EM) or *PK Cookbook*
CFS Panel:* ATP Profiles	Mitochondrial energy score (MES) 0.74 Page 75 in CFS book	Mitochondria functioning at 74% compared with the lowest limit of population reference range (1.00–3.00)	Needs correcting – it takes about four months of the regimes (and good absorption from the gut) for mitochondrial function to recover BUT this tells me there are other causes of fatigue since we cannot explain it in terms of pure mitochondrial dysfunction	CFS Chapter 4, pages 59-71, 369
	ATP levels 2.22 nmols/106 cells – low normal	Low ATP is a result of poor mitochondrial function but D-ribose is helpful to restore levels if one has overdone things	D-ribose 5-15 g daily or as a rescue remedy if you really overdo things BUT this must be part of your carb count in the PK diet	CFS Chapter 4, pages 76-77

*Footnote: Please note the 'CFS Panel' is not generally available. There is another laboratory currently working to provide this test. However, the regimes to improve mitochondrial function work reliably well so I think I am justified in tempting you all with these results.

Test	Significant result	What it means	Action	Chapter/page in *Diagnosis and Treatment of CFS and ME* 2nd edition(CFS), *Ecological Medicine* (EM) or *PK Cookbook*
	Ratio ATP/ ATPMg 0.54 (despite 100 mg Mg daily)	Very poor result – unusual to see such a low level. There may be a nutritional deficiency of Mg but low Mg is also a result of poor mitochondrial energy production – a typical vicious cycle With the EDS there must be leaky membranes and this compounds the problem	300 mg elemental magnesium by mouth (and vitamin D 5000 iu, essential for its absorption) Sunshine salt for life (5 g contains 5000 iu vitamin D) Mg by injection may be helpful. With this result I can supply – suggest ½ ml magnesium sulphate subcutaneously daily	CFS Chapter 4, pages 77-78
ADP to ATP conversion	ADP to ATP efficiency 60.7% – low normal	Slow conversion of ADP to ATP because of nutritional deficiencies…	B12 injections 0.5 mg daily See deficiencies below	CFS Page 80
Blocking 3.6%		Good		CFS Chapter 4, page 81 Chapter 20
	Excess ADP 28.8%	ATP cannot get from mitochondria into the cell where it is needed	My guess is blocking is from products of the fermenting gut… wait and see	CFS Chapter 20

	ADP blocked 74.7%	High normal – it is possible there is uncoupling of demand and supply so ATP is wasted	I suspect this is an adrenal/thyroid issue – i.e. a mismatch between energy demand and energy delivery. Sort the thyroid and adrenals	
CF DNA 7.8 ug DNA per dl plasma		Good		CFS Chapter 3, page 48 Chapter 4, pages 71-72
Nutritional deficiencies	indicated by...	Mitochondria do not have sufficient raw materials to function normally	Take supplements as per below...	
Niacin 15.8 ug/ml		Low normal	This is such an important intermediary that arguably you should be taking 1500mg slow release niacinamide for life	CFS Chapter 4, pages 73 and 78-79
Superoxide dismutase studies: Zinc/copper SODase 305 enzyme units Extracellular SODase 36 enzyme units	SODase 38% Manganese SODase 112 enzyme units	Rather poor result due to low Mn	Manganese 5 mg with lunch for four months Sunshine salt for life 1 tspn i.e. 5 g	CFS Chapter 4, page 72
	Glutathione peroxidase 70 U/g Hb	Just normal – possibly low selenium	Sunshine salt for life	CFS Chapter 4, page 73

Test	Significant result	What it means	Action	Chapter/page in *Diagnosis and Treatment of CFS and ME* 2nd edition(CFS), *Ecological Medicine* (EM) or *PK Cookbook*
	Glutathione 1.55 mmol/l	Glutathione deficient	Glutathione 250 mg for at least four months; arguably we should all be taking glutathione 250 mg for life because we live in such a toxic world	CFS Chapter 4, page 73
		You need an acid stomach to absorb minerals – possible hypochlorhydria? The commonest cause of this is upper fermenting gut	PK diet Vitamin C to bowel tolerance	EM Chapter 21 – PK diet Chapter 31 – Vitamin C
	Carnitine 29.4 umol/l	VERY poor – you need carnitine to transport the acetate 'fuel' into mitochondria – i.e. fuel delivery is impaired	Acetyl L carnitine 2 g daily for four months. Then 500 mg daily or eat lots of meat and tackle hypochlorhydria (you need an acid stomach to digest meat)	CFS Chapter 4, pages 73 and 79
	Co-Q10 0.61 umol/l	I like to see this >2.0	Ubiquinol 200 mg for four months then reduce to maintenance dose of 100 mg, possibly for life	
		A combination of blocking and deficiency is typical of the upper fermenting gut	PK diet	EM Chapter 28 – PK diet *PK Cookbook*

	Serum zinc 10.8 umol/l	Low	Sunshine salt for life	EM Chapter 28 – PK diet
	Coeliac IgA 1.31 mg/dl Tissue transglutaminase 0.2 U/ml	This suggests an allergic tendency; I think there should be no antibodies – i.e. a normal result should be zero	The risk factors for autoimmunity and allergy are: **Dairy** and **gluten** – PK diet Vaccination – avoid Vitamin D deficiency – take Sunshine salt ALSO think about toxic metal triggers (dental work, tattoos, vaccination, surgical implants)	EM Chapter 16 – Inflammation mechanisms
	HbA1c 37 mmol/mol (reference range 20-41)	A measure of sugar stuck on to haemoglobin – this reflects the average blood sugar over the past three months. This lab's range is set a bit high. My lab's is 22-38.	At the time of this test the carb intake was too high – PK diet	EM Chapter 28 – PK diet
Bone	Vitamin D 49 nmol/l (reference range 30-60nmol/l)	This lab's range is set very low. I like to see vitamin D between 100 and 200 Very poor result – this may partly explain the low Mg level – vitamin D needed to absorb it	Sunshine salt for life	
Liver function tests	Bilirubin 11 umol/l	Good – I like to see this below 12. Glutathione is doing a good job	Carry on with glutathione 250 mg for life	
	Alanine aminotransferase 25 U/l	I like to see this below 20 – mild enzyme induction, probably from products of the fermenting gut	PK diet Vitamin C to bowel tolerance	

Test	Significant result	What it means	Action	Chapter/page in *Diagnosis and Treatment of CFS and ME* 2nd edition(CFS), *Ecological Medicine* (EM) or *PK Cookbook*
	Gamma glutaryl transferase 15U/l	Good – I like to see this below 20		
Ferritin 55.1 ug/l				
B12 436 ng/ml		I like to see this high – ideally >2000 but certainly >1000	I think the B12 injections are a good idea – I call B12 the 'multitasker'	EM Chapter 33 – Vitamin B12
	Folate 4.8 ng/ml	Low normal. With large blood cells there may be a methylation problem	Possibly measure homocysteine – high homocysteine is a major risk factor for CFS and arterial disease If found to be high, first degree relatives should be screened (Definitely measure for reasons below)	EM Chapter 42 – Cardiology
Thyroid function tests (TFTs)	TSH (thyroid stimulating hormone) 0.93 mIU/l	Low or normal TSH never excludes the possibility of secondary hypothyroidism due to poor pituitary function; indeed this is the commonest cause of hypothyroidism in CFS/ME		EM Chapter 41 – Endocrinology

	T4 17 pmol/l	Again this does not tell us much. Some do not feel well until their T4 is at 30, OR there may be thyroid hormone receptor resistance	Fine tune the CFS orchestra – see Chapter 3 http://drmyhill.co.uk/wiki/Conducting_the_CFS_orchestra Measure your core temperature regularly through the day and graph the results The average core temperature is a measure of thyroid function The fluctuations are a measure of adrenal function	EM Chapter 30 – Tools to improve energy delivery mechanisms
Es	Urea 3.1 mmol/l	Low – suggests a low-protein diet	Protein is vital for our biological infrastructure	
Haem	White cell count (WCC) 9.6 x 10^9/l (ref 4-11 x 10^9/l)	The normal range is negatively skewed so I expect to see a result of 4-6. This result is a bit high suggesting chronic infection	The starting point to treat all chronic infection is to improve the immune defences with Groundhog Chronic	EM Appendix 3 – Groundhog Chronic
	Lymphocytes 3.7 (1.2-3.56 x 10^9/l)	High – due to virus?	Ditto above. If we are not making progress then consider specific antivirals for specific viruses (but we do not have antivirals for all known viruses)	The Infection Game
	Mean corpuscular volume 105.2 fl (reference range 80-96 fl)	The red cells are too big. Either you are hypothyroid...	See below... trial of thyroid glandulars	EM Chapter 30 – Improving energy delivery mechanisms

Test	Significant result	What it means	Action	Chapter/page in *Diagnosis and Treatment of CFS and ME* 2nd edition(CFS), *Ecological Medicine* (EM) or *PK Cookbook*
		OR a poor methylator	Measure homocysteine (it is possible your GP can do this test). High homocysteine is a risk factor for fatigue but also for arterial disease, cancer and dementia SO this is an important test not least of all because if positive then we must screen all first degree relatives as high homocysteine runs in families	EM Chapter 42 – Cardiology
Liver function tests (LFTs)	Globulin 19 g/l (reference range 19-35 g/l)	A bit low. This is the group of immunoproteins that fight infection. Immunity may not be good	Improve the defences with Groundhog Chronic	EM Appendix 3 – Groundhog Chronic
Bone marrow (ouch!)		This is 'non-diagnostic' BUT Dr Gilete, Barcelona report (https://drgilete.com), states 'presence of CMV (cyto-megalo virus) and EBV (Epstein-Barr virus) in bone marrow trephine	I think this is very significant. Suspect there is an immunological hole in the energy bucket	*The Infection Game*

Viral antibodies	CMV IgG positive EBV IgG positive	Very common triggers of post-viral CFS (PVCFS)	Groundhog Chronic. My guess is we will need valacyclovir; it works for EBV. It has some activity against CMV	*The Infection Game*
MRI of head and neck	Large range of movement	Ehlers-Danlos syndrome (EDS). I am no expert, and I cannot see the whole jaw, but it looks undershot... and may be narrowing the airway? But I am not sure	May result in obstructive sleep apnoea May be narrowed because of poor jaw alignment May be narrowed by the oedema of hypothyroidism or allergy	
Hydrogen breath test	Positive	Upper fermenting gut	Starve the little wretches out with a PK diet Kill 'em with vitamin C to bowel tolerance Sigh, yes, all roads lead to Rome!	EM Chapter 21 – PK diet Chapter 31 – Vitamin C
Tilt table test	Postural orthostatic tachycardia syndrome	The heart is not beating powerfully as a pump which means it cannot sustain your blood pressure when you are upright	Improve energy delivery mechanisms	EM Chapter 30 – Tools to improve energy
Mast cell activation test	Negative	This does not mean you are not allergic		

Table 79.5: Management framework – patient 2's history

Onset	Symptoms	Mechanism	See *Ecological Medicine* Chapter:
As a toddler aged 3-4 years	Disturbed sleep, until the age of 5, sent to a sleep therapist Possible asthmatic, sinus complications	Probably allergy Allergy to **dairy**, possibly yeast	7 – Inflammation symptoms
Aged 5 years	Alopecia	Autoimmunity – MUST avoid vaccination for life	13 – Inflammation mechanisms
Aged 2-3 years onwards	'Growing pains' (doctor's diagnosis), including head/neck aches, joints, muscles	This is allergy to **dairy**	7 – Inflammation symptoms
Aged 11 years	Suspected meningitis	Poor immunity?	7 – Inflammation symptoms
Aged 12 years	Pityriasis rosea	Probably viral – suggests poor immunity at that time	36 – Tools to switch off inflammation
Aged 13-17 years	Pill	Immunosuppressive – this would not have improved defences against EBV…	9 – Hormonal clinical pictures
		…and is major risk factor for cervical cancer. NEVER take the Pill or hormone replacement therapy (HRT)	54 – Women's health
Aged 17 years	Glandular fever resulted in a severe deterioration in her health from which she never recovered. Some symptoms (e.g. PEM/severe fatigue) appeared after these and the other illnesses/viruses listed separately	EBV is causally involved in 80% of PVCFS. Groundhog Chronic is the starting point to treat all chronic infections	Appendix 3 – Groundhog Chronic

Aged 19 years	Cervical intra-epithelial neoplasia grade 2/3 growths removed	Never take the Pill or HRT. See Chapter on iodine – I have had one patient get rid of HPV and genital herpes	75 – Women's health case history: pre-malignant cervix
Aged 20 years – birth of first child	Unable to work full time since	Obstetric bleed. I am thinking of Sheehan's syndrome, which may have knocked out the pituitary and so thyroid and adrenals	
Since 2008	Non-epileptic tonic clonic seizures	This is part of metabolic syndrome. The PK diet is a great treatment for seizures (see the film *Do no harm* with Meryl Streep). AND magnesium deficiency (see MAGPIE trial[2])	21 – PK diet
2008	Offered a gumshield	Hardly seems a proportionate response!	
2011	Polycystic ovarian syndrome (diagnosed on ultrasound scan)	This is part of metabolic syndrome	21 – PK diet
2017	Ehlers-Danlos syndrome (EDS) diagnosed Consultant recommends craniocervical fusion surgery	Cripes – I would be nervous of this See below	
Aged 26 years	Foetal loss at 20 weeks	Was the cause viral? Or high homocysteine? Or anti-phospholipid syndrome? Must measure homocysteine	42 – Cardiology and vascular medicine

Onset	Symptoms	Mechanism	See *Ecological Medicine* Chapter:
2018, age 32	Preliminary diagnosis of CFS although awaiting appointment at the Maudsley. NHS treatments tried, made symptoms worse	DO NOT do graded exercise!	
	Supplement regime and PK diet appear to have resulted in regular, morning bowel movements, timings of which were previously erratic	Great start	
	Sleep pattern, which was previously erratic, has stabilised	Ditto	
	Cannabis reduces pain levels somewhat, but has become less effective as time passes	It may be that CBD affords benefits because it is anti-retroviral Add in *Cistus incanus* tea 6 cups daily	See *The Infection Game* (revised reprint)

Table 79.6: Management framework – patient 2's symptoms

Symptoms and current strategies	Mechanism	Action	See Ecological Medicine (EM) chapter or other book:
Fatigue – excessive activity results in PEM (post exertional malaise) Muscle weakness, clumsy POTs	Poor energy delivery to the body	Getting you right is like conducting an orchestra – we need to get all the players in place, playing at the same time to get a result I suspect the big issues are: thyroid/adrenals and chronic infection with virus and possibly fungi	*Diagnosis and Management of Chronic Fatigue Syndrome and Myalgic Encephalitis – it's mitochondria not hypochondria*

Cognitive – poor memory and information processing	Poor energy delivery to the brain	Ditto above	
Sedentary, currently able to go out once a week for 10-20 minutes, occasionally 30/100	Clinical score on the Bell Disability Scale		
1 x BioCare Adult Multivitamin and Mineral 4 x VegEpa Omega-3 800 mg 1 x BioCare Essential Fatty Acids 3 x 1g Multimineral Mix 5 g Vitamin C as calcium ascorbate	Basic package of supplements	Well done – carry on But increase vitamin C to bowel tolerance (ascorbic acid is cheapest and best)	EM 21 – PK diet 31 – Vitamin C
1 x 100 mg food-state magnesium Blood pressure (BP) 112/56 mm Hg	Poor mitochondrial function – see above Rather low BP, ergo the heart is not beating powerfully	Carry on with PK diet Take the supplements as above	EM 21 – PK diet
Breakfast: Co-Yo yoghurt with nut selection Lunch: Chicken, courgette, pepper kebabs with coleslaw Supper: Tuna and olive salad Snacks: Pork scratchings Drinks: Coffee/organic tea, mineral water NB: On full PK Diet, intake of carbs limited to 15-20 g a day, 1400 kcal per day	Well done on the diet – the whole family should do this too	Carry on Make sure you are eating enough calories from fat The Grace coconut milk is ideal AND avocado	EM 21 – PK diet

Symptoms and current strategies	Mechanism	Action	See Ecological Medicine (EM) chapter or other book:
Non-epileptic tonic clonic seizures – for at least the past 10 years, around once a month, the majority of which happen between 28th of one month and 5th of the next	Metabolic syndrome	PK diet Correct magnesium I would be disappointed if this combination did not abolish the seizures	EM 21 – PK diet
Sleep Quantity: Drop off between 12:00 and 1:30 am, wake between 9:00 and 9:30 am Quality: Generally undisturbed but not refreshing	Sleep: With metabolic syndrome blood sugar levels fall at night and this spikes adrenalin, which wakes us up You may have ketogenic hypoglycaemia (a DDD reaction) 'Owl' You need three groups of hormone to correct your diurnal rhythm: (1) Melatonin – production triggered by dark (2) This stimulates the pituitary so TSH spikes at midnight (3) Then T4 spikes at 4 am, T3 at 5 am and this stimulates the production of adrenal hormones which wake you up The inflamed brain does not sleep	PK diet We need to do a balancing act of melatonin, thyroid glandular and adrenal glandular to restore your diurnal rhythm, but the dose very much depends on your core temperatures – see 'Conducting the orchestra' (Chapter 30) e.g. start with: melatonin 3 mg slow-release x 1 at night Adrenal glandular (AG) 125 mg in the morning Thyroid glandular (TG) 15 mg in the morning… and build all these three up in balance with each other. Most people end up needing melatonin 3-9 mg, TG 60-150 mg and AG 250-750 mg daily	EM 14 – Sleep: Why and how we sleep 22 – Sleep: Why we sleep poorly and how to fix it 28 – Diet, detox and die-off reactions 30 – Tools to improve energy delivery mechanisms

Slow digestive transit since birth of first child. Severe. Worsened by PEM/ fatigue, diet changes and stress. Constipation Puffy ankles Irregular periods Pulse 65 bpm OWL (drop off late and wake late)	Thyroid – I suspect hypothyroidism	We have to go very slowly here so suggest Get PK diet (adapted) first TG 15 mg on rising for one week. If all well go to TG 15 mg + 15 mg midday for one week If all goes well increase in 15 mg increments to 30 mg + 30 mg Recheck the bloods Monitor the pulse and BP – pulse should be less than 90 bpm, BP 120/80 mm Hg or less Most people need 90-150 mg Too much thyroid hormone feels as if you have drunk 20 cups of coffee! Any problems, get in touch with me by email at once. The commonest cause of problems is metabolic syndrome because this spikes adrenalin – you must be PK-adapted first	EM 30 – Tools to improve energy delivery mechanisms
		THEN you need to fine tune the CFS orchestra (Chapter 30) Measure your core temperature regularly through the day and graph the results The average core temp is a measure of thyroid function	Ditto
	Adrenal	The fluctuations are a measure of adrenal function	Ditto
Occipital/Parietal headaches, since childhood Pins and needles in limbs and muscle spasms, for at least a decade. Moderate to severe, with no apparent trigger Tinnitus IBS/gastro- oesophageal reflux (GORD) Hives, itching from unknown cause	Allergy – arthritis, muscle and joint pain are allergy	PK diet Vitamin C to bowel tolerance	EM 21 – PK diet 31 – Vitamin C

Symptoms and current strategies	Mechanism	Action	See Ecological Medicine (EM) chapter or other book:
Slow digestive transit/delayed gastric emptying results in carbs/ sugars causing SIBO Alcohol intolerant	Fermenting gut Poor detoxification in the liver	Starve the little wretches out with a PK diet Kill 'em with vitamin C to bowel tolerance	Ditto
Aching/weak joints, since childhood Poor skin quality – acne-prone Urinary urgency, incontinence	Allergy to microbes from the fermenting gut Could be allergy to foods, or allergy to microbes from the fermenting gut; these easily spill over from the gut into the bloodstream (this is called bacterial translocation). These microbes then drive inflammatory reactions at distal sites	Starve the little wretches out with a PK diet Kill 'em with vitamin C to bowel tolerance Ditto	
Test results: – chronically high WCC – high lymphocytes – positive antibodies to CMV and EBV – 'positive bone marrow' ME followed acute viral infection	Infection with virus	The starting point to treat all infection is Groundhog Chronic See how far that gets us – if you get stuck then consider tests	EM Appendix 3: Groundhog Chronic
		The four commonest infectious drivers of CFS are EBV, mycoplasma, Lyme and chronic fungal infection of the upper airways. The best test for the former three is EliSpot at Armin labs	*The Infection Game*

Black mould/damp spores in property Past medical history of sinusitis	Infection with yeast and/or fungus – see below	Measure urinary mycotoxins	
	Dental issues		
4 x 12.5 mg iodoral	Detox	Carry on with minerals Glutathione 250 mg daily Vitamin C to bowel tolerance. Iodine as Lugol's 15% (8 mg iodine per drop) x 4 drops daily (cheaper than iodoral)	EM 34 – Tools to detox
Asbestos exposure Smoker 5 per day	I am not worried about asbestos in the house – it is the fine dust that is the problem Not so happy about smoking!	Swap to vaping?	
EDS (mother and brother may have)	Connective tissue/bone will be leaky…	…and make all the above problems worse. There is no specific treatment. You have to do it all better than most. Bone broth provides all the raw materials for connective tissue	
28 – Diet, detox and diet reactions		Finally, remember all the above have the potential to make you worse in the short term, so be kind to yourself	EM

Table 79.7: Management framework – patient 2's results two months later to the Mycotox profile

Test	Significant result in ng/g creatinine	What it means – a normal result is ZERO – any amount is abnormal	The common range of positives is:	Notes – the principles of treating all these nasties are the same… see below
Mycotoxins in urine	Aflatoxin	3.5 – it is unusual to see this one; levels not too bad and will be contributing to the total load	3.5 to 20	From aspergillus – may come from fermented corn, peanuts and other nuts

Test	Significant result in ng/g creatinine	What it means – a normal result is ZERO – any amount is abnormal	The common range of positives is:	Notes – the principles of treating all these nasties are the same... see below
	Ochratoxin 13.44	Significantly high amount – this is the commonest mycotoxin I see in these tests	4 to 20	From the aspergillus and penicillium families Nephrotoxic, immune-toxic and carcinogenic Mainly from water-damaged buildings May drive Alzheimer's and Parkinson's
	Mycophenolic acid 9.54	Ditto – a significant exposure and these nasties will have an additional cocktail effect	5 to 50	From penicillium Immunosuppressant Associated with miscarriage and congenital malformations
	Citrinin <10	Detectable but low level, but again will add to the total load	10 to 50	From aspergillus, penicillium and monascus Immunosuppressant Can cause leaky mitochondrial membranes
		The above explains much – four different mycotoxins is unusual, especially the aflatoxin		Avoid – it is possible some of these come from the environment but I suspect many are in your airways and possibly gut

Table 79.8: Principles of treatment

Mechanism	Why	Action	*Ecological Medicine Chapter:*
Improve the immune defences	This is a war not a battle – without fighting the battle the fungi will simply recolonise for the same reasons they originally invaded	Groundhog Chronic PK diet Basic package of supplements Quality sleep Vitamin C to bowel tolerance and possibly other such... you will be doing much of this already	Appendix 3 – Groundhog Chronic
Water-damaged buildings will be mouldy	To prevent future inoculation with moulds and fungi	AVOID Any mould in your house? Exposure to water-damaged buildings?	
Damp environments e.g. cellars, Autumn, British/Irish weather... will be mouldy	To reduce the load of exogenous mycotoxins	AVOID Do your best – if the humidity is more than 40% moulds can grow Consider holiday in hot dry, cold dry, right on the coast (moulds cannot grow on salt water), above 1000 metres (air too thin to hold the moisture essential for moulds to grow) Indeed, this is a good test of mould allergy/toxicity – if one has much reduced symptoms when holidaying in a hot dry or cold dry, or right on the coast climate then one can infer mould allergy and/or toxicity because moulds cannot live in such environments or at least they live in much lower numbers[†]	

†Footnote: This is an example of that classic 'test' – the test of diagnostic hypothesis. If the patient feels better after applying an intervention (where that intervention is holidaying in said environments) or treatment based on a diagnostic hypothesis (here that hypothesis is mould allergy and/or toxicity) then one confirms the diagnostic hypothesis empirically.

Mechanism	Why	Action	Ecological Medicine Chapter:
Some foods are mouldy….	Aflatoxins are usually found in contaminated foods and they are less common nowadays so it is a bit odd to see this mycotoxin	Avoid	
Reduce the fungal load in the airways	To prevent endogenous production of mycotoxins	Use a salt pipe (cost about £15) – drizzle Lugol's iodine 15% 1-4 drops (whatever is tolerated) into the mouth-piece, sniff this up (to saturate upper and lower airways). Iodine is volatile. Use the valsalva manoeuvre to blow the iodine into the middle ear and sinuses (http://goflightmedicine.com/clearing-ears/) Keep going until the iodine smell goes (10-15 sniffs) – iodine gets everywhere and tiny amounts kill all microbes Do this at least three times daily but as often as convenient – indeed, any chronic infection, bacterial viral or fungal, would be killed with this	32 – Iodine The Infection Game
		If you can smell something then it is in the brain (the olfactory nerve is part of the brain). It may well be that iodine in the brain helps deal with toxicity and chronic infection there (dunno, but it seems a reasonable idea!)	
Reduce the fungal load in the gut	Ditto	PK diet Vitamin C to bowel tolerance Possibly add in nystatin powder (prescription only – I can supply)	Chapter 21 – PK diet Chapter 31 – Vitamin C
Get rid of any fungi on the skin	Ditto	Topical iodine – use iodine oil e.g. 100 ml coconut oil mixed with 10 ml of 15% Lugol's iodine. Apply ad lib	32 – Iodine

Get rid of any fungi in the perineum	Ditto	Make your own coconut oil/iodine mix as above and apply topically. A tampon soaked in this, inserted twice daily, works well	32 – Iodine
Treat possible infection elsewhere in body.....	ditto	Itraconazole 100 mg daily (prescription only) for some weeks (check LFTs at 1, 3 and 6 months). I think this would be a good idea considering your result	*The Infection Game*
Mop up mycotoxins in the gut (much of the load of mycotoxins will end up here)	...to reduce the mycotoxin load...	...with a clay such as Toxaprevent 3 grams at night, on an empty stomach away from food and supplements	
34 – Detoxing			
Sweat out mycotoxins with...	...to reduce the mycotoxin load...	...any heating regime e.g. FIR sauna, traditional sauna, hot bath with Epsom salts, sunbathing	
	34 – Detoxing		
		Expect die-off 'Herx' reactions that may last up to four weeks, possibly longer	28 – Diets, and die-off reactions
		Perhaps re-check urinary mycotoxins to make sure of progress – Brewer's experience is that one expects to reduce the load substantially, but perhaps not eliminate completely. Keep at it! As I have said, it is a war not a battle, and one that you must win	

References

1. Myhill S, Booth N, McLaren-Howard J. Targeting mitochondrial dysfunction in the treatment of Myalgic Encephalomyelitis/Chronic Fatigue Syndrome (ME/CFS) – a clinical audit. *Int J Clin Exp Med* 2013; 6(1): 1-15. www.ijcem.com / ISSN:1940-5901/IJCEM1207003

2. The Magpie Trial Collaborative Group. Do women with pre-eclampsia, and their babies, benefit from magnesium sulphate? The Magpie Trial: a randomised placebo-controlled trial. *Lancet* 2002; 359: 1877-1890. DOI: 10.1016/ s0140-6736(02)08778-0

PART VIII
Appendices

When to use Groundhog interventions

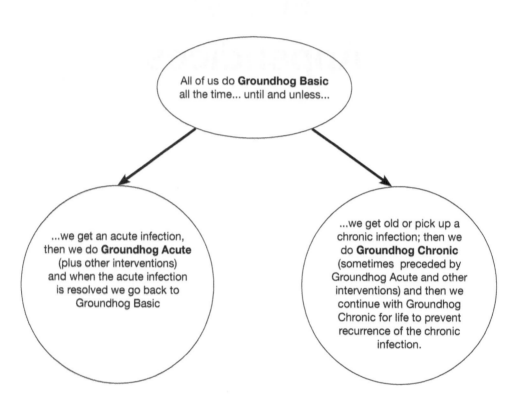

All of us do **Groundhog Basic** all the time... until and unless...

...we get an acute infection, then we do **Groundhog Acute** (plus other interventions) and when the acute infection is resolved we go back to Groundhog Basic

...we get old or pick up a chronic infection; then we do **Groundhog Chronic** (sometimes preceded by Groundhog Acute and other interventions) and then we continue with Groundhog Chronic for life to prevent recurrence of the chronic infection.

Appendix 1
Groundhog Basic

**– what we should all be doing all the time
– especially kids**

Because I constantly refer back to this basic approach, which is fundamental to the treatment of all infections, and by inference to the avoidance of the major killers [cancer, heart disease, dementia....] which are all driven by chronic infection, from here on I will call this Groundhog! In the film Groundhog Day, this refers to a time loop – this too is another sort of loop that bears constant repetition! The point here is that Groundhog done well will do much to prevent acute illness developing and chronic disease getting a foothold.

It is also the case that Groundhog will change through life as we are exposed to new infections and as our defences decline with age.

All should do the Groundhog Basic all (well most) of the time.

All should be prepared to upgrade to Groundhog Acute to deal with unexpected and sudden infectious challenges.

(Get that First Aid box stocked up now! See Appendix 2.)

All will need to move to Groundhog Chronic as we age and acquire an infectious load.

It is so important to have all the above in place and then at the first sign of any infection take vitamin C to bowel tolerance and use iodine for local infections because: You will feel much better very quickly!

- The immune system will not be so activated that it cannot turn off subsequently. So many patients I see with ME started their illness with an acute infection from which they never recovered – the immune system stayed switched on.

- The shorter and less severe the acute infection the less chance of switching on inappropriate immune reactions such as autoimmunity. Many viruses are associated with an arthritis, for example 'palindromic rheumatism.'* I think of this as viral allergy.

- The shorter and less severe the acute infection the less the chance that microbe has of making itself a permanent home in your body. Many diseases from Crohn's and cancer to polymyalgia and Parkinson's have an infectious driver.

Much of the graffiti (graffito is the singular of graffiti) found in Pompeii and Herculaneum

---

*Note: Palindromic rheumatism is rheumatism that comes and goes. The word 'palindrome' was coined by English playwright Ben Johnson in the 17th century from the Greek roots *palin* (πάλιν; 'again') and *dromos* (δρόμος; 'way', direction'). The first known palindrome, written as a graffito, and etched into the walls of a house in Herculaneum, reads thus: *'sator arepo tenet opera rotas* – 'The sower Arepo leads with his hand the plough' (idiomatic translation).

is somewhat bawdy, some of it focusing on what the local ladies of the fine houses would like to do with certain named gladiators or indeed vice-versa... the authors leave it to the readers to do their own research!

So, are you back with us yet?

On to the next Groundhog!

Table A1.1: Groundhog Basic

The Paleo-Ketogenic diet – high fat, high fibre, very low carb. Probiotic foods like kefir and sauerkraut No dairy or grains. 2 meals a day. No snacking.	See our books *Prevent and Cure Diabetes – delicious diets not dangerous drugs* for the WHY and *The PK cookbook – go paleo-ketogenic and get the best of both worlds* for the HOW
A basic package of nutritional supplements – multivitamins, multi-minerals and vitamin D	A good multivitamin and Sunshine salt 1 tsp daily with food. A dessert spoon of hemp oil
Vitamin C	Take vitamin C 5 grams last thing at night. This stays in the gut undiluted by food for best effect
Sleep 8-9 hours between 10pm and 7am	More in winter, less in summer
Exercise at least once a week when you push yourself to your limit	It is anaerobic exercise that produces lactic acid and stimulates new muscle fibres and new mitochondria
Herbs, spices and fungi in cooking	Use your favourite herbs, spices and fungi in cooking and food, and lots of them! Yum yum.
If fatigue is an issue – address energy delivery mechanisms as best you can	See our book *Diagnosing and treating Chronic fatigue syndrome and myalgic encephalitis: it's mitochondria not hypochondria*
Heat and light	Keep warm. Sunbathe at every opportunity.
Use your brain	Foresight: Avoid risky actions like kissing,[†] unprotected sex. Caution: Avoid vaccinations. Travel with care. Circumspection: Do not symptom suppress with drugs, treat breaches of the skin seriously.

[†]**Footnote:** Oscar Wilde knew this, perhaps for different reasons than the risk of infection, when he wrote that: 'A kiss may ruin a human life.'
Oscar Wilde, *A Woman of No Importance* (is there ever such a thing? Craig)
16 October 1854 – 30 November 1900

Appendix 2
Groundhog Acute

**– what we should all do at the first sign of any infection,
no matter what or where**

At the first sign of any infection you must immediately put in place Groundhog Acute. Do not forget what Dr Fred Klenner BS, MS, MD, FCCP, FAAFP (1907–1984) said: 'The patient should get large doses of vitamin C in all pathological conditions while the physician ponders the diagnosis.'

Strike soon and strike hard because time is of the essence. I repeat myself here – it is so important:

- You will feel much better very quickly
- Your immune system will not be so activated that it cannot turn off subsequently. So many patients I see with ME started their illness with an acute infection from which they never recovered – their immune system stayed switched on.
- The shorter and less severe the acute infection, the less the chance of switching on inappropriate immune reactions such as autoimmunity. Many viruses are associated with one type of arthritis or another – for example, 'palindromic rheumatism'. I think of this as 'viral allergy'.
- The shorter and less severe the acute infection, the less the chance a microbe has of making itself a permanent home in your body. Many diseases, from Crohn's and cancer to polymyalgia and Parkinson's, have an infectious driver.

Table A2.1: What to do at the first sign of the tingling, sore throat, runny nose, malaise, headache, cystitis, skin inflammation, insect bite or whatever

What to do...	...why and how
The paleo-ketogenic (PK) diet – high fat, high fibre, very low carb – for any infection Probiotic foods like kefir and sauerkraut No dairy or grains Just two meals a day with no snacking	See our books *Prevent and Cure Diabetes – delicious diets not dangerous drugs* for the WHY and *The PK Cookbook – go paleo-ketogenic and get the best of both worlds* for the HOW
You may consider fasting – this is essential for any acute gut infection	
Drink rehydrating fluids i.e. Sunshine salt 5 g in 1 litre of water ad lib	'Starve a cold, starve a fever' (No – not a typo – starve any short-lived infection)
Vitamin C to bowel tolerance: The need for vitamin C increases hugely with any infection. Interestingly, the bowel tolerance changes so one needs a much higher dose to get a loose bowel motion during an infection. If you do not have a very loose bowel motion within 1 hour of taking 10 g ascorbic acid, take another 10 g. Keep repeating until you get diarrhoea – that is what I mean by 'bowel tolerance'. Most people need 3-4 doses of 10 g to abolish symptoms	Vitamin C greatly reduces any viral, indeed any microbial, load in the gut. (Remember some of the infecting load of influenza virus will get stuck onto the sticky mucus which lines the lungs and is coughed up and swallowed) Vitamin C improves the acid bath of the stomach Vitamin C protects one from the inevitable free radical damage of an active immune system
A good multivitamin Sunshine salt 1 tsp daily in water Hemp oil 1 dsp	Sunshine salt in water for hydration because you should be fasting: 5 g (one tsp) in 1 litre of water provides a 0.5% solution
Take Lugol's iodine 12% 2 drops in a small glass of water every hour until symptoms resolve – swill it round your mouth, gargle, sniff and inhale the vapour	Just 30 seconds of direct contact with iodine kills all microbes
With respiratory symptoms, put 4 drops of Lugol's iodine 12% into a salt pipe and inhale for two minutes – do this at least four times a day. Apply a smear of iodine ointment inside the nostrils	30 seconds of direct contact with iodine kills all microbes. The salt pipe and ointment will contact-kill microbes on their way in or out, rendering you less infectious to others
Apply iodine ointment 10% (for example Betadine – Poridibe Iodine Ointment 10%w/w; this comes in handy 15 g tubes) to any bite, skin break or swelling	Contact-kills all microbes and is absorbed through the skin to kill invaders

Herbs, spices and fungi	If you are still struggling, then see our book *The Infection Game* to deal with complications of infections...
Rest – listen to your symptoms and abide by them. Sleep is even more important with illness than normally	I see so many people who push on through acute illness and risk a slow resolution of their disease with all the complications that accompany such. The immune system needs the energy to fight. I find vitamin C to bowel tolerance combined with a good night's sleep has kept me cold-free and flu-free for 35 years
Heat – keep warm	Fevers kill all microbes. Some people benefit from sauna-ing. Do not exercise!
Light – sunshine is best	Sunbathe if possible
Use your brain – do not suppress symptoms with drugs	Symptoms help the body fight infection. Anti-inflammatories inhibit healing and repair – they allow the microbes to make themselves permanently at home in the body
if you develop other acute symptoms... read on...	...turn to the relevant chapters... which all start with Groundhog Acute!

You may consider that doing all the above amounts to over-kill, but when that 'flu epidemic arrives, as it surely will, you will be very happy to have been prepared and to have these weapons to hand so that you, your family, friends and neighbours will survive. Stock up that first aid box now.

> *Be prepared.*
> Lord Baden-Powell in *Scouting for Boys*

and let us end with more wisdom from Benjamin Franklin (17 January 1706 – 17 April 1790)

> *By failing to prepare, you are preparing to fail.*

First-aid box contents

John Churchill, 1st Duke of Blenheim (26 May 1650 – 16 June 1722) was a successful general, partly because he made sure his armies were fully equipped for battle. The essence of success is to be prepared with the necessary to combat all enemies. Strike early and strike hard. Of John Churchill, Captain Robert Parker (who was at the Battle of Blenheim, 13 August 1704) wrote: '...it cannot be said that he ever slipped an opportunity of fighting...' We must be equally belligerent in our own individual battles, and part of this belligerence is preparedness, so keep the following in your own Battle First Aid Box. Use it at the first sign of attack.

Table A2.2: What to have in your Battle First Aid Box

For acute infections	Vitamin C as ascorbic acid – at least 500 gram (it is its own preservative so lasts for years) Lugol's iodine 15% – at least 50 ml (again, it is its own preservative so lasts for years)
Conjunctivitis, or indeed any eye infection	Iodine eye drops e.g. Minims povidine iodine 5% OR 2 drops of Lugol's iodine 15% in 5 ml of water. This does not sting the eyes and is the best killer of all microbes in the eye
Upper airways infections	Lugol's iodine – to use in a steam inhaler OR salt pipe into which drizzle 4 drops of Lugol's iodine 15% per dose
Skin breaches	Salt – 2 tsp (10 g) in 500 ml water (approx 1 pint) plus 20 ml Lugol's iodine 15%; use this ad lib to wash the wound. Once clean allow to dry Smother with iodine oil (coconut oil 100 ml with 10 ml of Lugol's iodine 15% mixed in) unless allergic to iodine Plaster or micropore to protect
Fractures	If the skin is broken – proceed as above. Immobilise If limb fracture, wrap in cotton wool to protect and bandage abundantly with vet wrap to splint it Next stop…casualty
Burns	As for skin breaches If a large burn, then use cling film to protect once cleaned (put the iodine ointment on the cling film first, then apply to the burn) Protect as per fracture above. Very large burn…next stop casualty
Sterile dressings	Melolin is a good all-rounder Large roll of cotton wool Crepe bandages (various sizes) and Micropore tape to protect any damaged area from further trauma Vet wrap bandage – wonderful stuff, especially if you are in the wilds, to hold it all together
Gastroenteritis	Sunshine salt – to make up a perfect rehydration drink mix 5 g (1 teaspoonful) in 1 litre of water, which gives a 0.5% solution
Urine infections	Multistix to test urine D mannose and potassium citrate
Consider acquiring antibiotics for intelligent use	These should not be necessary if you stick to Groundhog Basic and apply Groundhog Acute BUT I too live in the real world and am no paragon of virtue. So, if you slip off the band wagon:
	Amoxil 500 mg x 21 capsules for dental infection

	Cephalexin 500 mg three times daily for ENT and respiratory infections
	Doxycycline 100 mg twice daily for diverticulitis (DO NOT USE IN PREGNANCY OR FOR CHILDREN)
	Trimethoprim 200 g twice daily for urinary infection
	If you are susceptible to a particular infection then make sure you always hold the relevant antibiotic. The sooner you treat the less the damage... and always start with Groundhog Acute

Putting together such a Battle First Aid Box is as much an intellectual exercise as a practical one and this book, along with our books, *The Infection Game – life is an arms race* and *Prevent and Cure Diabetes – delicious diets, not dangerous drugs* give such intellectual imperative. As Shakespeare writes in Henry V: 'All things are ready, if our mind be so.' (Shakespeare, 1564 – 23 April 1616).

Appendix 3
Groundhog Chronic

– what we should all be doing increasingly as we age to live to our full potential

As we age, we acquire infections. My DNA is comprised 15% of retro virus. So is yours. I was inoculated with Salk polio vaccine between 1957 and 1966 so I will probably have simian virus 40, a known carcinogen. I am probably carrying the chickenpox, measles, mumps and rubella viruses because I suffered those as a child. I was also a bit spotty so *Proprionibacterium acnes* may be a potential problem. At least 90% of us have been infected with Epstein-Barr virus (EBV). I have been bitten by insects and ticks from all over the British Isles so I could also be carrying Lyme (*Borrelia burgdorferi*), bartonella, babesia and perhaps others. I have been a cat owner and could well test positive for bartonella on that account. I have suffered several fractures which have healed but I know within that scar issue will be lurking some microbes – feed them some sugar and they will multiply and give me arthritis. I have had dental abscesses in the past and have one root filling which undoubtedly will also harbour microbes. In the past, I have consumed a high-carb diet which inevitably results in fermenting gut. On the good side, my puritanical upbringing means I have been free from STDs (thank you, Mum!).

As you have read, we now know all these microbes have the potential to drive nasty diseases such as leukaemia, lymphoma, other cancers, dementia, Parkinson's, heart disease, autoimmunity and so on. I cannot eliminate them from my body; I have to live with them. I too am part of the Arms Race. Of course, this is a race I will (eventually) lose, but I will settle for losing it when I am 120. I am hoping that Groundhog Chronic will handicap my assailants and stack the odds in my favour.

So, as we age and/or acquire stealth infections, we all need Groundhog Chronic. It is an extension of Groundhog Basic. Most of us will end up doing something between the two according to their health and history. But as you get older, you have to work harder to stay well.

As Oscar Wilde (1854–1900) said, 'Youth is wasted on the young'.

Table A3.1: Groundhog Chronic

What to do	Why to do it	What I do (My patients always ask me what I do. I am no paragon of virtue, though I may have to become one eventually)
The Paleo-Ketogenic (PK) diet – high fat high fibre very low carb probiotic foods like kefir and sauerkraut no dairy or grains two meals a day and no snacking Source the best quality foods you can find and afford – organic is a great start	See our books *Prevent and Cure Diabetes – delicious diets not dangerous drugs* for the WHY and *The PK Cookbook – go paleo-ketogenic and get the best of both worlds* for the HOW	Yes, I do the PK diet 95% of the time. Glass of cider at weekends Other liberties if eating out or socialising... but my friends are all becoming PK-adapted too
Eat daily food within a 10-hour window of time...	...so there are 14 hours a day when your stomach is empty – this keeps it acid and so decreases the chances of microbes invading. It also maintains ketosis	Nearly there... breakfast at 8 am, supper at 6.30 pm
Consider episodic fasting one day a week	This gives the gut a lovely rest and a chance to heal and repair	I do this some weeks. The trouble is I am greedy and love food
A basic package of nutritional supplements – multivitamins, multi-minerals and vitamin D	A good multivitamin and Sunshine salt 1 tsp daily with food. Hemp oil 1 dsp	Yes
Glutathione 250 mg daily Iodine 25 mg weekly	We live in such a toxic world we are inevitably exposed. Glutathione and iodine are helpful detox molecules (but note, some people do not tolerate iodine in high doses)	Yes
Vitamin C to 90% of bowel tolerance, including 5 g last thing at night. Remember what your bowel can tolerate will change with age, diet and circumstance	With age, influenza becomes a major killer. With Groundhog interventions you need never even get it	Yes. I currently need 8 g in 24 hours BUT I never get colds or influenza that last more than 24 hours

What to do	Why to do it	What I do (My patients always ask me what I do. I am no paragon of virtue, though I may have to become one eventually)
Lugol's iodine 15% x 2 drops (or 12% x 3 drops) daily in water.	Swill around the mouth and swallow last thing at night	Yes
Make sure your First Aid box is stocked (see page A2.4)…	…so you have all your ammo to hand to hit new symptoms hard and fast	Yes, even when I go away, I take this – often to treat sickly others
Sleep 8-9 hours between 10 pm and 7 am Regular power nap in the day for 30 minutes to an hour	More in winter, less in summer Good sleep is as vital as a good diet	Yes
Exercise within limits. By this I mean you should feel fully recovered next day. If well enough, once a week push those limits, so you get your pulse up to 120 beats per min and all your muscles ache. It is never too late to start	No pain, no gain Muscle loss is part of ageing – exercise slows this right down Exercise helps to physically dislodge microbes from their hiding places; I suspect massage works similarly	Yes. Thankfully I am one of those who can and who enjoys exercise
Take supplements for the raw materials such as glucosamine for connective tissue. Bone broth is the best	With age we become less good at healing and repair	Yes
Herbs, spices and fungi in cooking	Use your favourite herbs, spices and fungi in food/cooking, and lots of them	Yes. Because I love food
Consider herbs and fungi to improve the defences – see our book *The Infection Game - life is an arms race*	Astragalus, cordyceps and rhodiola and the best	Sometimes when in stock and I remember
Address energy delivery mechanisms as below	See our book *Diagnosis and Treatment of Chronic Fatigue Syndrome and Myalgic Encephalitis: it's mitochondria not hypochondria*	Yes, Craig – I've got the book!

Take the mitochondrial package of supplements daily vis:
    CoQ10 100 g
    niacinamide slow-release 1500 mg
    acetyl L carnitine 500 mg
    D ribose 5-10 g at night if you have really overdone things
	With age, fatigue becomes an increasing issue because our mitochondrial engines start to slow down. The ageing process is determined by the health of our mitochondria. Look after them	Yes
		I don't take carnitine because I eat meat and my digestion is good

Mitochondria may be going slow because of toxins – consider tests of toxic load to see if you need to do any detox	A good all-rounder is Genova urine screen with DMSA 15 mg per kg of body weight. You can get this test through https://naturalhealthworldwide.com/	This is the only test I have ever done on myself – it showed background levels of toxic minerals
Check your living space for electromagnetic pollution	You can hire a detection meter from Healthy House www.healthy-house.co.uk/electro/meters-and-monitors	Yes, the cordless phone has gone. I never hold a mobile phone to my ear – I use the speaker I turn wi-fi off at night
Review any prescription medication – they are all potential toxins The need for drugs is likely to be symptomatic of failure to apply Groundhog	Ask yourself why you are taking drugs Once Groundhog is in place many drugs can be stopped. Taking prescription drugs is the fourth commonest cause of death in Westerners	I never take symptom-suppressing medication. This has allowed full and now pain-free recovery from three broken necks (horses again) and other fractures
Consider tests of adrenal and thyroid function since these glands fatigue with age and chronic infection	Thyroid blood tests and adrenal saliva tests are available through https://naturalhealthworldwide.com/ Core temperatures are helpful for fine-tuning adrenal and thyroid function with glandulars – see Chapter 30	I find natural glandulars (see page 30.5) very helpful and currently take thyroid glandular 60 mg in the morning and 30 mg at midday Adrenal glandular 500 mg once daily

What to do	Why to do it	What I do (My patients always ask me what I do. I am no paragon of virtue, though I may have to become one eventually)
Heat and light	Always keep warm. Sunbathe at every opportunity. Holidays in warm climates with sunbathing and swimming are excellent for killing infections and detoxing	I am a pyromaniac – my kitchen is lovely and warm with a wood-fired range I work in my conservatory with natural light I sunbathe as often as wet Wales permits Do not forget hyperthermia and light as a good treatment for chronic infections – see Chapter 24
Use your brain	Foresight: Avoid risky actions like kissing and unprotected sex Caution: Avoid vaccinations; choose travel destinations with care Circumspection: Do not suppress symptoms with drugs; treat breaches of the skin seriously	I have to say that with age this is much less of an issue! No vaccinations. No foreign travel except to the continent to see my daughter and to do lectures

If you are tiring from Groundhog, be inspired by these quotations:

We are what we repeatedly do. Excellence, then, is not an act, but a habit.
  Idiomatic translation by Will Durrant in *The Story of Philosophy* of the original,

Excellence is an art won by training and habituation.
  Aristotle, 384 BC – 322 BC

repetitio est mater studiorum – repetition is the mother of all learning.
  Old Latin proverb

consuetudinis magna vis est' – the force of habit is great.
  Cicero, 106 BC – 43 BC*

*Footnote: Assassinated for his opposition to Mark Antony, Cicero's last words were purportedly 'There is nothing proper about what you are doing, soldier, but do try to kill me properly.'

Appendix 4
Commonly used blood tests and what they mean

Poor interpretations have led to some serious mistakes throughout history. Even St Jerome, the patron saint of translators, fell victim: he translated the *Old Testamant* from Hebrew and made a simple error concerning the moment when Moses came down from Mount Sinai, with his head in 'radiance'. In Hebrew, *'karan'* is radiance, but because Hebrew is written without vowels, St. Jerome read *karan* as *keren*, which means 'horned'. Because of this mistake, there are many paintings and sculptures of Moses with horns. More recently, in 1980 Willie Ramírez was admitted to a Florida hospital in a comatose state. At the time of admission, an interpreter translated the Spanish term *'intoxicado'*, which means poisoned or having had an allergic reaction as 'intoxicated'. Willie, who was suffering from an intracerebral haemorrhage, was treated for an intentional drug overdose. As a result, he was left quadriplegic. This resulted in a $71million malpractice suit. Other examples of poor interpretation include those listed in Table A4.1.

Having said that, this Appendix really should not be necessary. However, I daily see medical tests that have been poorly interpreted so vital clues are missed. This is for several reasons:

- If a test result lies within the reference ranges, then the patient is told it is normal and that no action is required. However, reference ranges reflect population averages, while some individuals will function best at the top end of the range and others at the low end of the range.
- Population ranges may not reflect normal ranges. Ranges are arrived at by measuring the current population, which may not be 'normal'! The best example is levels of T4 in the blood: my lab's ref range is 12-22 pmol/l, but some NHS labs have ranges as low as 7-14. This will result in missing many cases of secondary hypothyroidism.
- A normal blood sugar level used to be 4-6.8 mmol/l, but now levels up to 11 may be considered acceptable because the population collectively has such poor control of blood sugar levels.

Table A4.1: Examples of significant errors in interpreting blood tests

Speaker	What they said/ intended	How it was interpreted
US President, Jimmy Carter, speaking to a Polish audience	'...I have come to learn your opinions and understand your desires for the future...'	'I desire the Poles carnally...'
HSBC marketing campaign	'Assume nothing'	'Do nothing...'
Japanese Prime Minister, Kantaro Suzuki, referring to the Potsdam conference in 1945 (The heads of government of the UK, US and USSR held this conference to consider post-war order, the formal peace treaty and countering the effects of the war... in so far as these three issues concerned the defeated Germany – the conference ended on 2 August 1945, well before V-J Day)	'No comment. We are still thinking about it'	'We are ignoring it in contempt.' On 6 August 1945 – four days after this comment was mis-translated – the American bomber 'Enola Gay' dropped a five-ton atomic bomb over the Japanese city of Hiroshima
During US President, Richard Nixon's, visit to China in 1972, Chinese premier Zhou Enlai famously said it was 'too early to tell' when evaluating the effects of the 'French Revolution'	Zhou Enlai was referring to the 1968 riots in Paris	The comments were interpreted as referring to the French Revolution in 1789 and the Western press inferred great wisdom in the Chinese Premier's words and compared how the East always takes the long view as opposed to the shabby short-term West!
Italian astronomer Giovanni Virginio Schiaparelli mapped Mars in 1877, calling dark and light areas on the planet's surface 'seas' and 'continents' and labelling what he thought were channels with the Italian word 'canali'.	Schiaparelli was trying to describe what he saw in everyday language	Canali was mistranslated as 'canals' and there followed a belief that 'life on Mars' had been established. Even respected figures such as US astronomer Percival Lowell mapped hundreds of these 'canals' between 1894 and 1895 and published three books on Mars with illustrations showing what he thought were artificial structures built to carry water by a brilliant race of engineers

- A range may be skewed.* A normal range for a white cell count is often 4-11 10⁹/l, but most run normally at 4-5. A white cell count running at 8-11 may point to chronic inflammation.

The key point is that tests are there to narrow the diagnosis, not to make it. All diagnosis is hypothesis which then depends on response to treatment. All diagnosis is therefore retrospective. The list below covers commonly done tests which I often see badly interpreted – it is not exhaustive!

Table A4.2: Commonly misinterpreted blood tests

Test	Significant result	What it means	Action
Full blood count	Haemoglobin should be: Men 140-160 g/l Women 130-145 g/l	Too low (anaemia) means either you are losing blood OR you are not making it fast enough because you are deficient in a raw material or lacking the energy for manufacture (see Chapter 57)	Do tests for faecal occult blood to check for gut losses, and faecal calprotectin both of which may indicate pathology Could the problem be heavy periods? Ferritin test to check for iron deficiency Measure vitamin B12 level
		If too high: Are you a smoker? (see Chapter 57) Polycythaemia rubra vera Carbon monoxide poisoning	Stop smoking and recheck See a doctor
	MCV (mean corpuscular volume – the size of red blood cells) should be 85–94 fL	If too high (above 94 fL) EITHER you are hypothyroid	Do thyroid function tests
		OR a poor methylator	Measure homocysteine level. It is possible your GP can do this test. High homocysteine is a risk factor for fatigue but also arterial disease, cancer and dementia, so this is an important test, not least because, if positive, then you must screen all first-degree relatives as high homocysteine runs in families (see Chapter 63)

*__Negative skew:__ A distribution is skewed if one of its tails is longer than the other. The distribution in Figure A4.1 has a negative skew since it has a long tail in the negative (left) direction:

Test	Significant result	What it means	Action
		Postal delay between blood taking and blood testing may cause a false macrocytosis (enlargement of red blood cells)	Check time between sample taking and testing
		If low, then there may be iron deficiency. Or this is an indicator of thalassaemia – a group of inherited conditions in which sufferers produce either no or too little haemoglobin	Check ferritin
	The WCC (white cell count) normal range is positively skewed, so I expect to see a result of 3.5-6 10⁹/l)	If too high, this may be a short-term response to acute infection so repeat in two weeks	If constantly high, then consult a doctor (cancers may present with high WCC). Look for causes of inflammation
		If too low, white cells are being used up fast to fight infection AND/OR There is a lack of raw materials AND/OR There is a lack of energy to make white cells	Improve energy delivery mechanisms Improve nutritional status Identify the infection (see our book *The Infection Game*) – the commonest offenders in ME are EBV (Epstein-Barr virus), Lyme disease (borreliosis) and mycoplasma
	The platelet count should be 200-350 10⁹/l	If too high, this may point to vitamin B12 deficiency	Measure active B12 levels and possibly homocysteine
		If too low, this may point to autoimmunity	See a doctor to consider Idiopathic thrombocytopenic purpura (ITP)? If below 100, see a doctor urgently
		It may mean poor bone marrow function	Check the quality and quantity of red cells and white cells – if all are low, then this is bone marrow suppression caused by possible exhaustion of chronic infection, poisoning, poor energy delivery mechanisms – investigate

	Healthy levels: ESR <5 mm/hour C reactive protein <1.0 nmol/l Plasma viscosity 1.5-1.65 mPA	These are all measures of inflammation. Reference ranges have all been increased because so many people are inflamed because of metabolic syndrome; an ESR of up to 20 is now considered acceptable!	If inflammatory markers are raised, always ask the question 'Why?' See Chapter 16
Cholesterol	Total cholesterol – be aware reference ranges are set too low; I like to see this at 4-7 mmol/l	If high, this may be due to hypothyroidism or vitamin D deficiency If too low, you will be starving the brain and immune system of this essential fat	Check thyroid function Measure vitamin D (I like to see this between 100 and 250 nmol/l) Eat a PK diet and get plenty of sunshine
	LDL cholesterol should be 2-4.4 mmol/l	Reference ranges for this important fat are set too low	
	HDL cholesterol should be 1.5-2.2 mmol/l	Again, reference ranges for this important fat are set too low	
	LDL:HDL ratio should be <2	If too high, this points to inflammation, but does not tell you why	Always ask the question 'Why?'
	HDL mmol/l % (this is calculated by dividing HDL cholesterol by total cholesterol)	If the percentage of the friendly HDL is low, then this is because HDL is being used up in the business of healing and repairing arteries – i.e. they are being damaged by something. This may be: metabolic syndrome and/or high homocysteine and/or chronic inflammation	Put in place interventions then repeat the test to check progress. The higher this result the better; on a good PK diet I expect this to be 40%

Test	Significant result	What it means	Action
	Triglycerides high Levels of <1.0 mmol/l are optimal	This MUST be an overnight fasting sample and should be below 1.0 mmol/l	Triglycerides may be raised if you have recently consumed medium chain fats (which is fine) OR because you have high insulin and high blood sugar, so insulin is changing sugar into triglycerides (not fine)
Electrolytes	Sodium – I like to see this at 139–142 mmol/l	If too low there is either a lack of salt in the diet or a salt-losing state e.g. diuretics or kidney failure	On a PK diet the need for salt increases – aim for 4 g daily (1 teaspoonful of Sunshine salt)
			If below 135 mmol/l you need to see a doctor as a matter of urgency
	Potassium (K**) – I like to see this at 4.0-4.4 mmol/l	If too high, there may have been a delay in transport – K easily leaks out of cells	Check time between sample taking and testing If above 4.9 mmol/l you need to see a doctor as a matter of urgency
		If low, too little in diet	The body cannot store potassium – you have to eat it daily; there is plenty in the PK diet Sunshine salt If below 3.5 mmol/l then see a doctor urgently
	Corrected calcium (mg/dl) = measured total Ca + 0.8 x (4.0 - serum albumin) where the measurement of total Ca is in units mg/dl and the serum albumin is in units g/dl	If low, this points to vitamin D deficiency	Measure vitamin D
		If high, then this must always be taken seriously	Consult a doctor urgently if above 2.8 mmol/l – you may have hyperparathyroidism

	Serum magnesium should be 0.8-0.95 mmol/l	Rarely done and not a reliable test of body stores. Most doctors do not understand the difference between a serum magnesium and a red cell magnesium. Serum levels must be kept within a tight range, or the heart stops. Therefore, serum levels are maintained at the expense of levels inside cells	Ignore if normal. If < 0.7 mmol/l then you are in serious trouble and need urgent medical attention
	Creatinine should be 80-115 umol/l	Too high suggests a high-protein diet and/ or high muscle mass OR Poor kidney function	Reduce protein intake and recheck Look for causes of kidney damage
		Too low points to a low-protein diet and/or low muscle mass Smaller people and women have less muscle mass so interpret this in that light	Eat more protein, take more exercise Smaller people and women may be perfectly fit but carry a smaller muscle mass
	Urea should be <7.0 mmol/l	Too high suggests dehydration	You need water AND fat AND salt to be properly hydrated
		High urea may accompany high creatinine	See creatinine above
	Uric acid is high if: >350 umol/l for men >300 umol/l for women	Uric acid is a mycotoxin	Look for a fungal issue (see Chapter 16)
		Too high may indicate poor antioxidant status	See Chapter 16

Test	Significant result	What it means	Action
	12-hour-fasting glucose should be 4.0-5.6 fl (ideally lower than 5.0)	If higher then you are on the way to diabetes If you are keto-adapted, then low blood sugar presents no problem at all	PK diet
	Glycosylated haemoglobin should be 22-38 mmol/mol 39-46 is prediabetes >46 is diabetes	A very useful test of average blood sugar over the previous three months. Ranges have changed recently because nearly all Westerners eat too much carb and are on the way to diabetes. How can the NHS deal with this? Move the goal posts!	PK diet See our book *Prevent and Cure Diabetes*
		The lower the better. On a good PK diet this may be less than 30. I would settle for less than 34.	
Liver function tests	Results should be: GGT (gamma-glutamyl transpeptidase) 6-20 IU/l ALT (alanine transaminase) 0-20 IU/l AST (aspartate aminotransferase) 0-20 IU/l	Standard reference ranges are all set higher than these here because so many people are poisoned Raised is due to enzyme induction to deal with toxins; this is not liver damage. However, if the alkaline phosphatase (see below) is also high then you are progressing to liver damage	The commonest toxins are: Alcohol, typically increases gamma GT Other drugs may also cause enzyme induction Consider toxins from the outside world – see Chapter 25 Consider products of the upper fermenting gut – see Chapter 15 Monitor alkaline phosphatase for liver damage
	Alkaline phosphatase should be <80 IU/l	Again reference ranges are often set higher for the above reasons If the alkaline phosphatase is high but GGT, ALT and AST are <20 then consider damage to bones	Find the cause!

	LDH (lactate dehydrogenase) should be 150-200 U/l	May indicate tissue damage in any part of the body; commonly liver, bones, heart, kidney	What is the cause of tissue damage? Consult a doctor.
		I suspect where there are poor energy delivery mechanisms with early switch into anaerobic metabolism, this enzyme is induced	Improve energy delivery mechanisms – see Chapter 30
	Bilirubin should be <12 umol/l	Too high means you are a slow detoxifier via glucuronidation and will be more susceptible to toxic stress Above 19 is called Gilbert's syndrome	Identify the cause of the toxic stress and mitigate – see Chapter 25. Take glutathione 250 mg for life to improve liver detox
Bone health		Normal 'bone markers' does not exclude osteoporosis	The best test for osteoporosis is a heel bone density scan which is accurate and involves no dangerous X-rays
	Phosphate should be 0.97-1.20 mmol/l	Too high...	Check for kidney disease (see doctor)
		Too low points to vitamin D deficiency	Measure vitamin D Check for kidney disease and parathormone levels (see doctor)
	Ferritin should be: Men 30-300 ng/ml Women 30-150 ng/ml	Too low points to iron deficiency	Either you are losing blood OR lacking iron. This may be due to lack of iron in the diet (meat) OR malabsorption. You need an acid stomach to absorb iron. One cause of this is upper fermenting gut due to too much carbohydrate in the diet
		Too high points to inflammation	Look for causes of inflammation – see Chapter 16

Test	Significant result	What it means	Action
Prostate markers	PSA <2.0 ng/ml	PSA reflects the amount of prostate tissue present. Western diets high in carbs and dairy stimulate prostate growth; this means reference ranges have been changed so older men have a higher range	Regardless of the result, do the PK diet
		If high, remember it is the rate of change that suggests malignancy, not the absolute amount	Keep rechecking monthly and arrange for an MRI scan of the prostate gland Go PK – this may shrink the prostate gland and reduce the PSA – see Chapter 46
	Total vitamin B12 200-900 ng/ml I like to see this over 2000	'Normal' ranges simply reflect enough to prevent pernicious anaemia but not what is needed for optimal biochemical function. Much of total blood B12 is inactive	A normal vitamin B12 level never predicts a response to B12 by injection – see Chapter 33 Neither does it accurately predict the level of active B12
	A better measure is active B12 (HoloTC) >50 pg/ml		To be sure, also measure homocysteine
Homo-cysteine	I like to see this below 10 umol/l (many lab reference ranges are <15)	High homocysteine means poor methylation. This is an essential biochemical tool to allow one to 'read' DNA (for protein synthesis), to detoxify, to synthesise enzymes and much more. Being a poor methylator is a MAJOR risk factor for arterial disease, dementia, cancer and degenerative disease	To normalise levels you need methylated B vitamins – see Chapter 42

Thyroid function	TSH (thyroid stimulating hormone) should be <1.5 mIU/l	Low or normal TSH never excludes the possibility of secondary hypothyroidism due to poor pituitary function	Also see Chapter 41. A TSH tells us little but it is relied upon far too heavily by many doctors to determine the dose of thyroid hormone.
	Free T4 (thyroxin) should be 12-22pmol/l	Check the reference range – some NHS ranges are as low as 7-14 pmol/l…	…but some people do not feel well until running at 30 pmol/l – see also Chapter 41
	Free T3 should be 3.1-6.8 pmol/l	Ditto above	Ditto
		If T3 is low compared with T4, this suggests poor conversion of inactive T4 to active T3	This is T3 hypothyroidism. You may need a T3 supplement
		If TSH is high despite good levels of T4 and T3, this points to thyroid hormone receptor resistance	…in which case consider measuring reverse T3. Look for a toxic cause – see Chapters 8, 15, 25 and 34
	High reverse T3 0.13 to 0.35 nmol/l (reference range: 0.13-0.35 nmol/l)	If high, this points to thyroid hormone receptor resistance – in this event the blood tests are not helpful	You must rely on the clinical picture to determine the dose of thyroid hormone

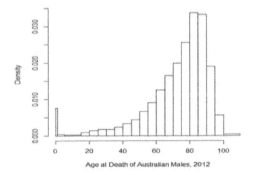

Figure A4.1: Histogram of age at death of Australian males in 2012

†**Linguistic note:** Why is the symbol for potassium 'K'? 'Potassium' is derived from the English word 'potash'. The chemical symbol K comes from '*kalium*', the Mediaeval Latin for potash, which may have derived from the arabic word '*qali*', meaning alkali. Interested readers should see https://en.wikipedia.org/wiki/ Symbol_(chemistry)

Appendix 5
Chronic inflammation

Stealth infections
– principles of diagnosis
– which tests to do

'Stealth' as a means of escape from being attacked occurs everywhere in Nature. Moths have developed 'stealth coating' so as to avoid being eaten by bats. The furry coating on the moths' thorax absorbs the sonar signals bats use to locate their prey. So, moths got there millions of years before the United States Air Force![1]

There may be clues from the clinical picture – the patient's symptoms and signs (see below) – but the definite diagnosis will require laboratory tests. These are expensive, but we can increase the chances of a positive diagnosis by first considering the symptoms and signs.

A vital and powerful symptom of a chronic stealth infection is failure to respond to Groundhog interventions. Regardless of whether you do or do not test positive for a chronic stealth infection, Groundhog must be in place for long-term good health, especially for old crones like me – so just do it and do it now. Indeed, I know that many of my patients must have been cured through Groundhog alone. I say that because these stealth infections are common, so many of my patients who recovered must, unknowingly, have suffered from them.

Symptoms and signs of chronic infection

History
This is perhaps the most important tool for diagnosis. Start when the symptoms began – which may be decades before. The list below is not comprehensive but is put in order of probability based on my clinical experience.

Table A5.1: Patient history indicative of chronic infection

Symptoms started...	Possible diagnosis	Useful tests to support diagnosis in order of priority
Sudden flu-like illness, fever, malaise. Feeling ghastly – unable to do anything, let alone work! Bedbound for some days. Perhaps swollen glands in neck, armpits, groin? Perhaps went a bit yellow? Perhaps pericarditis and chest pain? At the time blood tests may have been 'a bit wrong but nothing to worry about'?	HHV 4 glandular fever	Armin laboratory tests: Elispot, IgG antibody titre, IgM antibody titre, DNA by PCR. Tests available from www.naturalhealthworldwide.com A raised IgG is typically interpreted as evidence of past exposure ergo no treatment necessary but it does not exclude the possibility that a microbe is driving pathology
Ditto	HHV6 roseola	IgG/IgM antibodies DNA PCR
Ditto	Coxsackie virus	IgG/IgA antibodies.
Ditto	HHV 5 Cytomegalovirus (CMV)	Elispot
Above with localising signs e.g. shingles, chickenpox. Cold sores, genital herpes are also caused by herpes virus but rarely trigger CFS/ME	Other herpes viruses. All herpes viruses target the brain and immune system. Once in the body all herpes viruses persist for life	Elispot for varicella zoster (shingles/chicken pox) Elispot HSV 1 HSV2 IgG antibody titre
Vaccination – I estimate that one in 10 of my CFS/ME patients have had their disease triggered or worsened by vaccination	These are designed to switch on the immune system with the potential to trigger autoimmunity and allergy	There may be positive IgG titres to virus
	We know some retroviruses have been present in vaccination, such as SV 40. The jury is still out with respect to XMRV	It is almost impossible to get retroviral tests done

Symptoms started...	Possible diagnosis	Useful tests to support diagnosis in order of priority
Acute gastroenteritis (or indeed any gut symptom such as pain, bloating, reflux, diarrhoea, constipation, abnormally formed stools)	Fermenting gut Inflammatory bowel disease (MAP) Parasite or unfriendly gut microbes e.g. *Helicobacter pylori*, giardia, amoebiasis, blastocystis hominis	Comprehensive digestive stool analysis e.g. from Doctors Data or Genova. I know of no commercial test for MAP (*Mycobacterium avium paratuberculosis*) Other tests available from www.naturalhealthworldwide.com
Possibly a tick bite and bull's eye rash but probably none such. As with borrelia, babesia and bartonella, any insect bite could transmit many infections Possibly rash and arthritic condition Often no clear onset	Lyme disease – *Borrelia burgdorferi* *Borrelia myamotoi*	Armin labs: Elispot seraspot (often antibody tests are negative – this does not exclude the diagnosis). Tests available from www.naturalhealthworldwide.com
As with Borrelia, could be acquired through insect bites. Virtually all mammals harbour bartonella. Classically follows cat scratch, but absence of such does not exclude the diagnosis	Bartonella – may cause a PUO or FUO (pyrexia (or fever) of unknown origin)	Armin labs: Elispot IgG/IgM antibodies DNA PCR Tests available from www.naturalhealthworldwide.com
Insect bites	Babesia – may cause a PUO	Armin labs: Elispot IgG/IgM antibodies Babesia DNA PCR Tests available from www.naturalhealthworldwide.com
Insect bites	Rickettsia	Elispot Ehrlichia. Elispot Anaplasma
Insect bites	Yersinia	Elispot Yersinia

Chest infection or pneumonia (may be atypical 'walking pneumonia' i.e. the patient is not very ill). I seem to be seeing many new cases – at least 10 suspicious cases to date	*Mycoplasma pneumoniae*	IgG antibodies
Ditto	*Chlamydia pneumoniae*	Elispot IgG antibodies Tests available from www.naturalhealthworldwide.com
Sexually transmitted disease	*Chlamydia trachomatis* HIV, hepatitis C, syphilis, herpes, HPV, gonorrhoea, trichomonas, bacterial vaginosis	Get screening tests at a Special Clinic Elispot IgG antibodies
Recurrent chest, upper respiratory or sinus infections	Chronic septic focus e.g. bronchiectasis Fungal infection e.g. aspergillosis	Chest X ray, sputum sample (but often false negatives) Aspergillus precipitin test IgG IgM and IgA antibodies MycoTOX Profile (Mold Exposure) from Great Plains Laboratory
Joint pains and arthritis	Inflammation driven by allergy to microbes from the fermenting gut OR Allergy to a virus – so-called 'reactive arthritis'	No direct tests Auto-antibody studies may help Investigations for the fermenting gut: Comprehensive digestive stool analysis e.g. from Doctors Data or Genova Tests available from www.naturalhealthworldwide.com

Current symptoms and signs

Chronic infections often start with local symptoms of inflammation such as sore throat, head cold, chest infection, gastroenteritis, urinary tract infection or whatever, but as the microbe makes itself comfortably at home in your body then the symptoms become more general and, indeed, may start to trigger pathology. Many chronic so-called 'degenerative' conditions we know are driven by infection. This includes most cases of dementia (herpes viruses, Lyme), Parkinson's (Lyme), many cases of autoimmunity, cancer, arterial disease, arthritis and, of course, CFS/ME. Indeed, with any inflammatory pathology, always think and look for an infectious cause.

When I was at medical school I learned that syphilis was the 'great mimic' because it can cause almost any pathology. Syphilis had to be thought of in almost every differential diagnosis. Lyme too is caused by a spirochete (a spiral-shaped bacterium) with similar potential for damage and mimicry. This case report demonstrates the possibility: 'The initial electrodiagnostic test showed widespread active and chronic denervation findings. The initial physical and electrodiagnostic findings were suggestive of amyotrophic lateral sclerosis (ALS).* However, blood serology indicated possible Lyme disease. Thus, the patient was treated with doxycycline. The clinical and electrodiagnostic findings were resolved with the treatment.'[2]

Interpretation of tests

No test is perfect; all must be interpreted in the light of that patient's history... and all patients are unique. This is what makes medicine an art as much as a science. So much modern Western medicine has been condensed into simple algorithms based on a drug end-result so that real pathology is missed. Patients suffer and die needlessly. Nowhere is this a greater issue than with the interpretation of tests. Any result is taken as absolute. So often I see patients who have been told that all the test results are normal and so they are either not ill or hypochondriacs. Nowhere is this worse than in the field of CFS/ME.

There are several possible mechanisms that form the basis of tests to decide if chronic infection is present:

- A false negative result means: this does not exclude infection
- A false positive result means: there may be, or has been, microbe exposure but it is no longer a clinical problem.

You may need different tests for different microbes depending on where it is living in your body, and whether your immune system is fighting it with antibodies or with white cell foot soldiers.

Table A5.2: Tests for chronic infection

Test	Mechanism	Notes
Can that microbe be seen or grown in tissue culture?	Not all can be – e.g. viruses cannot be grown in culture	False negative results are common. A positive result makes it very likely you are harbouring that microbe.
PCR (polymerase chain reaction)	If positive, then that microbe is present...	...BUT false negatives abound. You will only get a positive result if the microbe you are looking for is present in the tissue sample that has been taken
Are there IgM antibodies to that microbe?	These are part of the acute immune response	If positive, then the immune system is fighting that microbe BUT false negatives abound with stealth infections

*Footnote: ALS is a form of motor neurone disease.

Are there IgG antibodies to that microbe?	These form part of immune memory	We commonly see a positive result which may well mean all is well – i.e. that microbe has been dealt with and kicked into touch by the immune system
		However, sometimes there are very high IgG responses which may suggest the immune system is still fighting a battle[†]
Are there IgA antibodies to that microbe?	Tests for IgA antibodies only apply to microbes living on mucous membranes, such as *Mycoplasma pneumoniae*	False negatives are possible
Elispot testing looks at how the white T cell soldiers are reacting with cytokines to a particular microbe (also known as 'lymphocyte transformation testing' because the normally quiet white cell soldiers transform into fighting lunatics)	This test is very sensitive, specific and clinically relevant	A positive result means the immune system is fighting that infection. This is a very good test for infection with: – a high level of sensitivity (i.e. false negatives are uncommon) and – a high level of specificity (i.e. it is the microbe you are looking at and not another)
White cell counts	May be high during acute infection	Help these with Groundhog Acute (page A2.1)
	May be low with chronic infection…	…as the immune system becomes exhausted because it is running out of raw materials or energy; treat this with Groundhog Chronic (page A3.1)

[†]**Footnote:** For example, finding a high IgG antibody titre is generally thought to be simply evidence of past infection. However, we know that all herpes viruses persist in the body for life – so if they have been there in the past they will be present today. Once comfortably installed in the body they have the potential to drive many other nasty diseases. Their targeting of the brain and immune system explains many symptoms. I suspect it is this group of viruses that are responsible for many cases of post-viral CFS/ME. Dr Martin Lerner showed that Epstein-Barr virus (also known as EBV, HHV4, mono and glandular fever) was causally involved in 81% of post-viral CFS. See our book *Diagnosis and Treatment of Chronic Fatigue Syndrome and Myalgic Encephalitis – it's mitochondria, not hypochondria* for much more detail on this. A general rule of thumb amongst clinicians is that if the antibody titre is five times higher than baseline, then an anti-viral strategy should be considered. What is so interesting is that Dr Lerner showed that the anti-viral titre (EBV nuclear antigen and EBV viral capsid antigen) fell with effective treatment and that this was paralleled by clinical improvement. This may allow an objective measure of progress. Armin laboratories now offer Elispot testing for EBV and this is a very useful tool. Again, as the immune system defeats the virus, the level of positivity comes down, making this is a very helpful clinical tool.

Summary

Diagnosis depends on:
- A high level of clinical suspicion – if you don't look you don't see
- Good tests and interpretation of such – in this respect diagnostic tests are essential
- Response to treatment – all diagnosis is hypothesis, which must then be put to the test. However, always remember this may not be the sole cause of symptoms.

At the same time, do not forget that once one infection is established, other microbes are more likely to get into the body, perhaps for the same reasons that the first microbes got in – that is, poor defences. So, the existence of one microbe may indicate that other, as yet unidentified, microbes may also be present. The point here is that it will never be sufficient just to target a particular microbe that has been identified. Improving the defences is as vital a part of attacking microbes, as is targeting particular microbes. Having had one debilitating infection, always return to Groundhog Chronic. You will find Craig and me there too!

Finally, I stress once again, that these chronic infections *do* exist and that tackling them can be the key to recovery for many patients. A famous European philosopher well sums up where we are at this moment in time:

> *There are two ways to be fooled. One is to believe what isn't true; the other is to refuse to believe what is true.*
> Søren Kierkegaard, Danish philosopher, 1813 – 1855

Do not be fooled either way.

References

1. Bristol University. Moths grow 'stealth' fur to thwart bats' sonar. *Daily Telegraph* 7 November 2018 – www.pressreader.com/uk/the-daily-telegraph/20181107/textview; Neil TR, Shen A, Drinkwater BW, Robert D, Holderied MW. Stealthy moths avoid bats with acoustic camouflage. Presented at the Acoustical Society of America's 176th meeting. (www.bristol.ac.uk/news/2018/november/moths.html)
2. Burakgazi AZ. Lyme disease-induced polyradiculopathy mimicking amyotrophic lateral sclerosis. *International Journal of Neuroscience* 2014; 124 (11): 859-862. www.tandfonline.com/doi/abs/10.3109/00207454.2013.879582

Appendix 6
Useful resources

Natural Health Worldwide
https://naturalhealthworldwide.com
You can see details of mobile phlebotomists
here:
https://naturalhealthworldwide.com/mobile-
phlebotomists/

Testing laboratories

All accessible via
https://naturalhealthworldwide.com

No practitioner referral is required for these
laboratories:

https://aonm.org

https://medichecks.com

https://www.mineralstate.co.uk

http://www.btsireland.com/joomla/

http://www.btsireland.com/joomla/

https://smartnutrition.co.uk/health-tests/

https://thriva.co

These laboratories require a practitioner
referral:

https://www.gdx.net/uk/

https://www.doctorsdata.com

https://www.greatplainslaboratory.com

https://www.biolab.co.uk

See here for MELISA test details: https://www.
biolab.co.uk/index.php/cmsid__biolab_tests_
referred_to_other_laboratories#melisa

https://regeneruslabs.com

Useful resources for allergies (including food), non-toxic and electrical sensitivity products

Detect & Protect
For the detection of electrosmog (invisible
electromagnetic radiation)
www.detect-protect.com/k/buzz/
whatiselectrosmog.htm

Earthing
For products that connect to earth's natural
energy
www.earthing.com/

Electric Forester
Do electromagnetic surveys and investigations
www.electricforester.co.uk/electricforester/
index.html

Electrosensitivity UK
This is a registered charity (reg number 1103018).
Address: BM BOX ES-UK, London WC1N 3XX
Tel: +44 (0)845 643 9748 – freely available UK
helpline staffed by volunteers.
www.es-uk.info

Friends of the Earth
www.foe.co.uk/

Garden Organic

Formerly known as Henry Doubleday Research Association, advice on how to garden organically whether your garden is large or small
www.gardenorganic.org.uk/

Gluten Free Society

For information about the effects of gluten on human health, tools to test for sensitivity and guidance on a gluten-free lifestyle.
Website: www.glutenfreesociety.org/gluten-and-the-autoimmune-disease-spectrum

The Healthy House Ltd

For an excellent range of products to help you detox your house including EMF detectors (just search for 'electrosmog detector' in their search box)
Tel: 0845 450 5950
Tel from a mobile phone: +44 (0)1453 752216
www.healthy-house.co.uk
See here for nontoxic cleaning products:
www.healthy-house.co.uk/cleaning

Powerwatch

A source of information about EMF issues
www.powerwatch.org.uk/
For products: www.emfields-solutions.com/

Soil Association

For information about what the standards are to be classed as 'organic'
www.soilassociation.org/

Tincture London nontoxic cleaning products
https://tincturelondon.com/collections/frontpage

Supplement resources

VegEpa

Concentrated EPA supplement in a fish-gel capsule from Igennus Ltd.
Tel: +44 (0) 845 13 00 424 or +44 (0) 845 13 00 424
sales@igennus.com
www.igennus.com

D-mannose

One typical product is:
https://uk.iherb.com/pr/Now-Foods-D-Mannose-500-mg-120-Veggie-Caps/525
– take 3 x 500 mg capsules one to three times a day

Potassium citrate

These are all example products with their respective doses:
- Effervescent tablets (brand Effercitrate) – take two tablets, up to three times a day, dissolved into a whole glassful of water.
- Liquid medicine (brand Cymaclear) – take two x 5 ml spoonfuls, stirred into a whole
- glassful of water. You can take up to three doses a day.
- Sachets (brand Cystopurin) – empty the contents of one sachet into a whole glassfulof water. Stir it well before drinking. Take one sachet, three times daily.

Iodine products

Iodoral can be obtained from
www.amazon.co.uk/Iodoral-12-5-mg-180-tablets/dp/B000X843VG
Lugol's iodine 12% can be obtained from
www.amazon.co.uk/Lugols-Iodine-12-Solution-30ml/dp/B00A25GCLO

Herbs
UK – www.indigo-herbs.co.uk
UK – www.hybridherbs.co.uk
USA – www.mountainroseherbs.com

Sunshine salt
One teaspoon (5 ml) contains all the minerals
and vitamin D needed for one day
sales@drmyhill.co.uk

Vitamins and non-herbal supplements
UK – www.salesatdrmyhill.co.uk
UK – www.biocare.co.uk
UK – www.naturesbest.co.uk
USA – www.swansonvitamins.com
USA – www.puritan.com

Other useful resources

Tempur Mattresses and Pillows
Tel: 0800 0111 083
customerservice@tempur.co.uk
http://uk.tempur.com/

Trace Element Services
www.traceelementservices.co.uk

For CFS/ME sufferers please see these two
webpages:
www.drmyhill.co.uk/wiki/Useful_aids_for_
CFS_and_ME_sufferers
www.drmyhill.co.uk/wiki/CFS/ME_support_
organisations

Index

By the same authors...

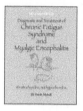

Diagnosis and Treatment of Chronic Fatigue Syndrome and Myalgic Encephalitis – it's mitochondria, not hypochondria explores the commonest symptom which people complain of – namely, fatigue – together with its pathological end result when this symptom is ignored. This is Dr Myhill's life's work. She has spent over 35 years in clinical practice, many months of academic research and the co-authoring of three scientific papers, all directed at solving this jigsaw puzzle of an illness. This book has application not just for the severely fatigued patient but also for the athlete looking for peak performance and for anyone wishing to increase their energy levels.

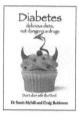

Prevent and Cure Diabetes – delicious diets not dangerous drugs All medical therapies should start with diet. Modern Western diets are driving our modern epidemics of diabetes, heart disease, cancer, and dementia; this process is called metabolic syndrome. *Prevent and Cure Diabetes* explains in detail why and how we have arrived at a situation where the real weapons of mass-destruction can be found in our kitchens. Importantly, it describes the vital steps every one of us can make to reverse this situation so that life can be lived to its full potential.

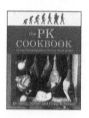

The PK Cookbook – go Paleo-Ketogenic and get the best of both worlds gives us the *how* of the PK diet while *Prevent and Cure Diabetes* gives us the *why*. This is the starting point for preventing and treating modern Western diseases, including diabetes, arterial disease, dementia, and cancer. Dietary changes are always the most difficult, but also the most important, intervention. This book is based on Dr Myhill's first-hand experience and research on developing a PK diet that is sustainable in the long term. Perhaps the most important feature of this diet is the PK bread – this has helped more people stick to this diet than all else.

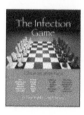

The Infection Game – life is an arms race tells us why modern life is an arms race, which infections are driving Western diseases and why we are currently losing this arms race, citing the clinical signs and symptoms that demonstrate this. Then comes the good news. There are chapters detailing the general approach to fighting infections followed by specific measures for specific infections, including EBV (glandular fever, 'mono'), Lyme disease, Bartonella and others. How to diagnose these infections is also covered and there are special sections on how to treat acute infections and also how to protect your microbiome. The vast majority of the approaches in this book are natural, including many herbal preparations, and can be done by the reader completely on their own, with no need to involve doctors.

Another important resource...

Natural Health Worldwide (NHW): Dr Myhill had the idea for, and funded, the development of, the website www.naturalhealthworldwide.com Once it had been set up, she divested herself of any pecuniary interest. NHW is a portal where any knowledgeable practitioner (medical doctor, qualified health professional or experienced patient) can register without any cost and offer their opinions to any patient. NHW practitioners offer consultations by telephone, email, Facetime, Skype or face-to-face, where appropriate. Some NHW-registered practitioners make no charge for their services, whereas others charge normal or reduced rates. Katie Twinn and Craig Robinson, who are the founders and administrators of Dr Myhill's Facebook groups (see https://drmyhill.co.uk/wiki/My_Social_Media_Presence) helped with the development of NHW and now deal with the everyday running of the site.